MyNursingLab for the
Practical/Vocational Nurse

Elaine U. Polan, RNC, MS, PhD
Supervisor
Practical Nursing Program
Vocational Education and Extension Board
Uniondale, New York

Daphne R. Taylor, RN, MS
Assistant Supervisor
Practical Nursing Program
Vocational Education and Extension Board
Uniondale, New York

Notice: Care has been taken to confirm the accuracy of the information presented in this book. The authors, editors, and the publisher, however, cannot accept any responsibility for errors or omissions or for consequences from application of the information in this book and make no warranty, express or implied, with respect to its contents.

The authors and the publisher have exerted every effort to ensure that drug selections and dosages set forth in this text are in accord with current recommendations and practice at time of publication. However, in view of ongoing research, changes in government regulations, and the constant flow of information relating to drug therapy and drug reactions, the reader is urged to check the package inserts of all drugs for any change in indications of dosage and for added warnings and precautions. This is particularly important when the recommended agent is a new and/or infrequently employed drug.

The authors and publisher disclaim all responsibility for any liability, loss, injury, or damage incurred as a consequence, directly or indirectly, of the use and application of any of the contents of this volume.

Publisher: Julie Levin Alexander
Editor in Chief: Maura Connor
Senior Acquisitions Editor: Kelly Trakalo
Development Editor: Rachel Bedard
Assistant Editor: Lauren Sweeney
Director of Marketing: David Gesell
Senior Marketing Manager: Harper Coles
Managing Editor, Production: Patrick Walsh
Production Liaison: Yagnesh Jani
Senior Operations Supervisor: Ilene Sanford
Senior Art Director: Maria Guglielmo-Walsh
Cover Designer: Kris Carney
Digital Media Product Manager: Travis Moses-Westphal
Printer/Binder: Edwards Brothers
Cover Images: Courtesy of Getty Images

A. SUKHDEO
VEEB STUDENT

10 9 8 7 6 5 4 3 2 1

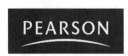
www.pearsonhighered.com

ISBN 10: 0-13-503458-2
ISBN 13: 978-0-13-503458-3

Preface

This *MyNursingLab* was specifically designed to help practical/vocational nursing students during their course of study and at the completion of their program. The entire practical/vocational nursing curriculum is presented in nine modules. Students can use any of the pre-tests to determine their level of competency at any point in their study. Based on their pre-test results, students then have the option to review course content found in the related modular outlines. Post-test questions help students to confirm mastery of the subject.

Pre-test and post-test questions are written using the latest NCLEX-PN® style. These include multiple-choice, fill-in-the blank, multiple-response, and ranking. Included in *MyNursingLab* are student remediation activities to foster understanding and individual learning styles. Additional questions, video clips, and animations are included to support the module's learning outcomes.

Faculty have the option of assigning portions of modules and tracking students' work and performance.

Table of Contents

My Nursing Lab/LPN and LVN

Module 1	**Math**		1
	1.1	Basic Arithmetic	4
	1.2	Working with Fractions	4
	1.3	Working with Decimals	11
	1.4	Working with Percents, Ratios, and Proportions	14
	1.5	Systems of Measurement	17
	1.6	Dosage Calculations for Medications	24
	1.7	Medication Administration	32
Module 2	**Fundamentals**		61
	2.1	Nursing Process	61
	2.2	The Health Team and Healthcare System	65
	2.3	Culture	68
	2.4	Legal and Ethical Issues	74
	2.5	Communication	79
	2.6	Vital Signs and Physical Assessment	83
	2.7	Admission/Transfer/Discharge/Documentation	89
	2.8	Comfort and Hygiene	92
	2.9	Safety and Infection Control	95
	2.10	Activity, Rest and Sleep	100
	2.11	Oxygenation	106
	2.12	Wound Care	110
	2.13	Nutrition, Fluids, Electrolytes, and Acid-Base Balance	117
	2.14	Elimination	129
	2.15	Sensory Perception and Pain	135
	2.16	Death and Dying	141
Module 3	**Medical-Surgical Nursing**		144
	3.1	Inflammation, Immunity, and Infection	144
	3.2	Caring for Surgical Clients	150
	3.3	Clients with Cancer	154

3.4	Disorders Affecting the Integumentary System	159
3.5	Musculoskeletal Disorders	170
3.6	Disorders Affecting the Nervous System	177
3.7	Disorders of the Eyes and Ears, the Sensory System	193
3.8	Endocrine System	201
3.9	Respiratory System	215
3.10	Diseases of the Circulatory System	226
3.11	Gastrointestinal Disorders	245
3.12	Reproductive Disorders	260
3.13	Genitourinary System	273

Module 4   **Growth and Development/Nursing Care of Children**   286

4.1	Growth and Development	286
4.2	Pediatric Disorders	300

Module 5.1   **Maternal-Newborn Nursing Care**   325

Module 6.1   **Older Adult Nursing Care**   357

Module 7.1   **Mental Health Nursing Care**   368

Module 8.1   **Disaster Nursing**   389

Module 9.1   **Leadership and Management**   399

PEARSON

MODULE 1

Math

Submodule 1.1 Basic Arithmetic

Learning Objectives

1.1.1 **Apply the principles of arithmetic to solve problems adding, subtracting, multiplying, and dividing whole numbers.**

1.1.2 **Identify the symbols used in Roman numerals and apply them to problem solving.**

I. **Adding, Subtracting, Multiplying, and Dividing Whole Numbers**

A. Addition

1. **Addition** is putting quantities together to obtain a total, called the *sum*.

2. Rules

   a. Numbers are lined up based on their value (units, tens, hundreds, etc.).

   b. Add upward.

   c. Check answer by adding downward.

      Example

      168 + 100 + 13 + 5 =

      Line up the numbers in columns.

$$
\begin{array}{r}
168 \\
100 \\
13 \\
+\ 5 \\
\hline
286 \ = \text{sum}
\end{array}
$$

B. Subtraction

1. **Subtraction** is taking a quantity away from a total and finding out what is left. The total before subtraction is the *subtrahend*. The number being subtracted is the *minuend*. The answer is the *remainder*.

2. Rules

   a. When the subtrahend (top digit) is smaller than the minuend (bottom digit) the minuend must go to its subtrahend neighbor (next number left) to ask for help or borrow ten.

   b. When the neighbor gives of himself he is now less in value by one.

    c.   Check your answer by adding the minuend to the answer.

       Example

       325 - 18 =

       Line up the numbers in columns.

```
  1
325 = subtrahend
-18 =  minuend
307 = remainder
```

C. Multiplication

    1. **Multiplication** is actually a shortcut to addition.

    2. Rules

       a.   Multiplicand is the digits to the left of the sign

       b.   Multiplier is the digits to the right of the sign.

       c.   Multiply from right to left skipping one unit of each digit.

       Example

       17 x 18 =

```
   17 = multiplicand
 x 18 = multiplier
  136
 + 17
  306 = product
```

D. Division

    1. **Division** is breaking down the whole into equal parts.

    2. Rules

       a.   Divisor is the number used to divide (right of division sign).

       b.   Dividend is the number being divided (left of division sign).

       c.   Quotient is the answer.

       Example

       2563 ÷ 22 =

```
116_____
22 |2563
   22++
   36
   22
   143
   132
    11
```

       Ans. = 116 remainder 11

II. Roman Numerals

A. Prescription and medical orders are often written in Roman numerals.

B. Addition is indicated when a numeral of lesser value follows one of greater value.

C. Subtraction is indicated when a numeral of lesser value precedes one of greater value as in IV (4), IX (9), XL (40), and XC (90).

D. Numerals of the same value are not repeated more than three times in a sequence.

E. Letters represent the number as follows:

1	I
5	V
10	X
50	L
100	C
500	D
1000	M
$\frac{1}{2}$	SS

Examples

8	=	VIII
9	=	IX
2009	=	MMIX

Additional Resources Found on MyNursingLab

MODULE 1

Math

Submodule 1.2 Working with Fractions

Learning Objectives

1.2.1 **Recognize the relative value of fractions and reduce them to their lowest terms.**

1.2.2 **Apply the principles of arithmetic to adding, subtracting, multiplying, and dividing fractions.**

    I.   **Adding, Subtracting, and Reducing Fractions**

        A. Essential Knowledge

            1.   A common fraction is part of a whole number.

            2.   In the fraction $\frac{2}{3}$, the 2 is the numerator and 3 is the denominator. The line separating the numerator from the denominator expresses division.

            3.   The **numerator** tells the number of parts or pieces that exist. (there are 2 in $\frac{2}{3}$).

            4.   The **denominator** tells how many parts the whole is divided into (in $\frac{2}{3}$ the whole is divided into 3 parts).

            5.   Types of fractions

                a. **Proper fraction** - the numerator is smaller than the denominator as in $\frac{2}{3}$. The fraction is less than 1.

                b. **Improper fraction** - the numerator is larger than the denominator, e.g., $\frac{8}{5}$. The fraction is greater than 1.

                c. **Mixed number** - contains a whole number and fraction, e.g., $1\frac{1}{3}$.

                d. **Complex fraction** – The number has a simple fraction in the numerator, the denominator, or both.

$$\frac{\frac{2}{3}}{\frac{1}{8}} \text{ or } \frac{\frac{1}{4}}{5}$$

B. Reducing fractions - A fraction is expressed in the lowest terms by two methods:

1. Reducing to lowest terms.

   a. Reducing fractions to their lowest terms is done by dividing the numerator (top) and the denominator (bottom) by the same number.

   e.g.: $\frac{25}{30} \div \frac{5}{5} = \frac{5}{6}$

2. Expressing as a mixed number.

C. Improper fractions as mixed numbers - Express improper fractions as mixed numbers by dividing the denominator into the numerator and placing the remainder over the denominator,

   e.g.: $\frac{8}{5} = 8 \div 5 = 1\frac{3}{5}$

D. Mixed numbers as improper fractions - Express mixed numbers as improper fractions by multiplying the whole number by the denominator and adding the numerator,

   e.g.: $3\frac{2}{3} = \frac{(3 \times 3) + 2}{3} = \frac{11}{3}$

E. Adding Common Fractions

1. Rule with **like denominators:** When the denominators are the same, add the numerators and reduce the fraction to its lowest terms.

   e.g.: $\frac{3}{5} + \frac{2}{5} = \frac{5}{5} = 1$

2. Rule with **unlike denominators:** Express the fraction as an equivalent fraction by finding the lowest common denominator (L.C.D.).

   Example:

   $\frac{2}{3} + \frac{4}{5}$

   Step I: Find the L.C.D. by multiplying both denominators = 15

   Step II: Divide one denominator into the LCD and multiply the answer by the numerator $= \frac{2}{3} \times \frac{5}{5} = \frac{10}{15}$

   Then do the same with the other fraction $\frac{4}{5} \times \frac{3}{3} = \frac{12}{15}$

   Step III: Add the fractions with like denominators and reduce to lowest terms
   $= \frac{10}{15} + \frac{12}{15} = \frac{22}{15} = 1\frac{7}{15}$

F.   Adding Mixed Numbers:

1.   Rule: Find the L.C.D. Add the fractions, then the whole numbers, and reduce.

Example

$$3\frac{3}{10} + 5\frac{3}{15} =$$

$$3\frac{3}{10} \times \frac{3}{3} = 3\frac{9}{30}$$

$$+ 5\frac{3}{15} \times \frac{2}{2} = 5\frac{6}{30}$$

$$8\frac{15}{30} \div \frac{15}{15} = 8\frac{1}{2}$$

Answer $= 8\frac{1}{2}$

G.   Subtracting Fractions

1.   Rule with **like denominators:** When denominators are the same, subtract the numerator and reduce the fraction.

Example

$$\frac{4}{5} - \frac{1}{5} = \frac{3}{5}$$

2.   Rule with **unlike denominators:**   Find the L.C.D. factor and subtract, then reduce the fraction to its lowest terms.

Example

$$\frac{5}{8} - \frac{1}{3} =$$

$$L.C.D. = 24$$

Factor:

$$\frac{5}{8} \times \frac{3}{3} = \frac{15}{24}$$

$$- \frac{1}{3} \times \frac{8}{8} = \frac{8}{24}$$

$$\frac{7}{24}$$

Answer $= \frac{7}{24}$

H. Subtracting Mixed Numbers

1. Find the L.C.D. and factor; subtract the fraction and then the whole number.

2. When the numerator of the fraction in the minuend is larger than the numerator in the subtrahend, it is necessary to borrow from the whole number in the subtrahend.

3. The borrowed number one is equal to the value of the L.C.D. Add that to the minuend and subtract.

Example

$$2\frac{2}{3} - 1\frac{3}{4}$$

L.C.D. = 12

borrow

1

$$2\frac{2}{3} \times \frac{4}{4} = 1\frac{8}{12} + \frac{12}{12} = 1\frac{20}{12}$$

$$-1\frac{3}{4} \times \frac{3}{3} = 1\frac{9}{12} = \qquad 1\frac{9}{12}$$

$$\frac{11}{12}$$

Answer $= \frac{11}{12}$

II. Multiplication and Division of Fractions

A. Multiplication of Fractions

1. Wherever possible, cancel the fraction first. Then multiply numerators and multiply denominators, and reduce (if possible) to the lowest terms.

2. Cancelling is choosing a number that will divide equally into both the numerator and the denominator. This can be performed as follows:

Example

$$\frac{\overset{1}{\cancel{2}}}{\underset{1}{\cancel{3}}} \times \frac{\overset{1}{\cancel{3}}}{\underset{2}{4}} = \frac{1}{2}$$

a. **You can cancel vertically or obliquely (diagonally),** dividing a number into a numerator and a denominator.

b. **You can never cancel horizontally** (numerator to numerator or denominator to denominator).

PEARSON

1. **Correct** cancellation (see the previous example):

2. **Incorrect** cancellation:

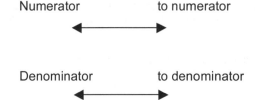

Numerator   to numerator

Denominator   to denominator

B. Multiplying mixed numbers

    1. Change the mixed number into an improper fraction, then cancel, multiply, reducing to the lowest terms.

       Example

$$5 \frac{1}{3} \times \frac{3}{5}$$

       Step I: Change $5 \frac{1}{3}$ to an improper fraction

       Step II: Cancel and then multiply $\frac{16}{3} \times \frac{3}{5} = \frac{16}{5}$

       Step III: Reduce the improper fraction to a mixed number and to lowest terms:

$$\frac{16}{5} = 3 \frac{1}{5}$$

    2. When multiplying a whole number and fraction, place whole number over 1.

C. Division of Fractions

    1. Rule: When dividing fractions, first invert the divisor (turn it upside down), then proceed as in multiplication.

    2. The divisor is the fraction to the right of the division sign.

       Example

$$\frac{1}{8} \div \frac{3}{4}$$

       Invert $\frac{3}{4}$ (the divisor) and change the division sign to a multiplication sign.

       Cancel and then multiply $= \frac{1}{8} \times \frac{4}{3} = \frac{1}{6}$

D. Dividing mixed numbers: Change the mixed number into an improper fraction. Invert the divisor, cancel, and then multiply.

Example:

$$5\frac{1}{2} \div 1\frac{2}{3}$$

Step I: Change the mixed numbers to improper fractions $\frac{11}{2} \div \frac{5}{3}$

Step II: Invert the divisor and change to a multiplication sign $\frac{11}{2} \times \frac{3}{5} = \frac{33}{10}$

Step III: Reduce the fraction to a mixed number and reduce to lowest terms.
$$\frac{33}{10} = \frac{3}{10}$$

III. Comparing Values of Fractions

A. When the denominators are the same, the fraction that has the largest numerator is largest and the fraction with the smallest numerator is smallest.

B. When the numerators are the same, the fraction with the smallest numerical denominator is the largest and the one with the largest numerical denominator is the smallest (9 halves is more than 9 hundredths).

C. Method One

1. When the denominators and numerators are different, find the least common denominator, raise each fraction to the same denominator, and then compare.

Example 1

Which is larger, $\frac{5}{8}$ or $\frac{7}{8}$?

Since the denominators are the same, the fraction with higher number in the numerator has the larger numerical value = $\frac{7}{8}$

Example 2

Which is smaller, $\frac{12}{7}$ or $\frac{12}{11}$?

Since the numerators are the same, the fraction with the smaller number in the denominator has the larger numerical value = $\frac{12}{7}$

Example 3

Which is larger, $\frac{7}{12}$ or $\frac{3}{5}$?

The numerator and denominator are different:

Step I: Find a common denominator = 60

Step II: Raise each fraction to that denominator:

$$\frac{7}{12} = \frac{35}{60}$$

$$\frac{3}{5} = \frac{36}{60}$$

Step III: Compare values: $\frac{35}{60}$ and $\frac{36}{60}$

$\frac{36}{60}$ or $\frac{3}{5}$ is the larger fraction

D. Method Two

   1. A simpler method used to compare fractions is cross-multiplication

      Step I: Cross-multiply each fraction.

      Step II: Place the product total over the numerator of each fraction you cross-multiplied.

      Step III: Compare the totals for both fractions.

   2. Rule

      a. The fraction with the larger total = the larger fraction

      b. The fraction with the smaller total = the smaller fraction

Example

Which is larger, $\frac{7}{12}$ or $\frac{3}{5}$?

  i.   12 x 3 = 36

  ii. 7 x 5 = 35

$$\overset{35}{\underset{}{\frac{7}{12}}} \ \text{or} \ \overset{36}{\underset{}{\frac{3}{5}}}$$

Since the number over the fraction $\frac{3}{5}$ (36) is the larger number, $\frac{3}{5}$ is the larger fraction.

Since the number over the fraction $\frac{7}{12}$ (35) is the smaller number, $\frac{7}{12}$ is the smaller fraction.

Additional Resources Found on MyNursingLab

MODULE 1

Math

Submodule 1.3 Working with Decimals

Learning Objectives

1.3.1   Identify the relative value of decimals.

1.3.2   Apply the principles of arithmetic to solve problems adding, subtracting, multiplying and dividing decimals.

I.   **Decimal Fractions**

A.   Decimals are fractions in which the denominators are expressed in powers of 10, 100, 1000 etc.

B.   The denominator is omitted and the decimal point used.

C.   Numbers that precede the decimal point are whole numbers, those that follow the decimal point are fractions.

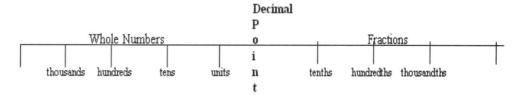

D.   Expressing common fractions as decimal fractions

1.   Divide the denominator of the fraction into the numerator.

2.   Place the decimal point after the numerator. Annex (add) as many zeros as decimal places needed.

   Example

   Change $\frac{1}{2}$ into a decimal (take 1 and divide it by 2)

$$\begin{array}{r} 0.5 \\ 2\overline{)1.0} \\ \underline{10} \end{array}$$

$$= 0.5$$

E.   Changing decimals to common fractions

1.   Give the decimal its denominator.

2.   Reduce to the lowest terms.

Example

Change 0.42 to a common fraction 0.42 ends at the 2nd decimal place. Determine the fraction by placing 1 below where the decimal point would be and annexing zeros in the denominator equal to the number of digits in the numerator (see below). Then reduce the fraction to its lowest terms.

decimal		
.	4	2
	tenth	hundredth
1	0	0

Reduce $\dfrac{42}{100} \div \dfrac{2}{2} = \dfrac{21}{50}$

Answer $0.42 = \dfrac{21}{50}$

II. Addition of Decimals

A. Place the decimal points under each other, keep the units together, and add.

Example

Add 1.25, 3.02, 0.12

```
   1.25
   3.02
 + 0.12
   4.39
```

III. Subtraction of Decimals

A. Place the decimal points under each other and subtract.

IV. Multiplication of Decimals

A. Multiply as for whole numbers.

B. Total the number of decimal places in the muliplicand and multiplier. You will use this number in the next step.

C. Beginning with the last digit to the right in the answer, count the number of places and place the decimal point.

Example

```
     7.5
 x   1.2
     150
     75
     900
```

There are two digits to the right of decimal points in the problem.

Answer = 9.00

V. Division of Decimals

A. Make the divisor a whole number by moving the decimal point the required number of places to the right.

B. The decimal point in the dividend must also be moved the same number of places to the right.

C. Place the decimal point in the quotient directly above the decimal point in the dividend. Divide as usual, annexing zeros as necessary.

Example

$5.25 \div 1.2$

```
        4.375
1.2 | 5.2500
      48 +++
      45
      36
       90
       84
      .60
       60
```

Answer = 4.375

$5.25 \div 1.2$

$= \dfrac{52.500}{12} = 4.375$

VI. Rounding Numbers

A. Decimals can be rounded off to the nearest tenth, hundredth, or thousandth.

B. If the digit to the right of the desired unit is less than 5, it is dropped.

C. If the digit to the right of the desired unit is 5 or more, add one to the preceding digit.

Example

Round off to the nearest tenth

$$\overset{+1}{2.55} = 2.6$$

VII. Valuing Decimals

A. Annex zeros to give both decimals the same denominator (the same number of decimal places).

B. Look at the numerical value of the two numbers.

C. The one with the larger numerical value is larger, and the one with the smaller numerical value is the smaller.

Example

Which of the following decimals has the greater value?

0.02 or 0.084

Annex one zero to give them both the same denominator making 0.020.
The value 0.020 or 0.084
84 is larger than 20

Answer = 0.084

Additional Resources Found on MyNursingLab

PEARSON

MODULE 1

Math

Submodule 1.4 Working with Percents, Ratios, and Proportions

Learning Objectives

1.4.1 **Identify the relative value of percents compared to other fractions, and solve problems using percentages.**

1.4.2 **Compare and contrast the value of ratio to other fractions and solve problems using ratios.**

1.4.3 **Given the properties, solve for the unknown in a proportion.**

    I. **Percentages**

        A. The percent sign represents a denominator of 100.

        B. To express a percent as a fraction, remove the sign and write the denominator, then reduce the fraction to its lowest terms.

            Example

            10% as a fraction

$$\frac{\cancel{10}}{\cancel{100}} = \frac{1}{10}$$

        C. To express a fraction as a percent, multiply by 100, reduce, and add the percent sign.

            Example

            $\frac{1}{5}$ as a percent

$$\frac{1}{\underset{1}{\cancel{5}}} \times \frac{\overset{20}{\cancel{100}}}{1} = 20\%$$

        D. To express a percent as a decimal, divide by 100 (move decimal point two places to the left).

            Example

            30% to decimal

            30 is a whole number, so the decimal point is to the right of the zero. Move it two places to the left and remove the percent sign.

                Answer = 0.3

PEARSON

E. To express a decimal as a percent, multiply by 100 (move the decimal point two places to the right) and add the percent sign.

Example

0.5 to percent 50 = 50%

II. Ratios

A. **Ratios** express the relationship between parts and the whole.

B. A common fraction can be expressed as a ratio.

C. The numerator is placed in front of the denominator.

D. The numbers are separated by a colon that means "is to."

Example

$\frac{1}{4}$ as a ratio is read "1 is to 4" or "1:4."

E. To express a percent as a ratio, drop the percent sign, place the number over 100, and reduce.

Example

50% as a ratio

$$\frac{\cancel{50}}{\cancel{100}}^{1}_{2} = \frac{1}{2} = 1:2$$

F. To express a decimal as a ratio, change it to a fraction by placing the decimal over its multiple of ten, remove the decimal point, and then reduce.

Example

$0.03 = \frac{.03}{100} = \frac{3}{100} = 3:100$

III. Proportions

A. A **proportion** consists of two equal ratios such as $\frac{1}{3} = \frac{4}{12}$

B. This statement can also be written using colons, as 1:3 :: 4:12.

1. The double colon stands for the symbol "=" and is read "as."

2. The single colon in ratios is read "is to."

3. The above proportion is read "one is to three as four is to twelve."

C. The terms in a proportion have names. The two middle terms are called the **means** the two outside terms are called the **extremes.**

```
     ┌ Extremes ┐
1 : 3   =   4:12
     └ Means ┘
```

D. In all proportions, the product of the means is equal to the product of the extremes.

Example

1 : 3 = 4 : 12

Means   3 x 4 = 12
Extremes   1 x 12 = 12

E. Most of the time when we are called to solve proportions, we only know three terms of the proportion (have values for three terms). The term that is not known is called the *unknown* and is represented by X. Use of ratio and proportion enables us to determine the fourth number.

Example

1:4 = 6:X

Step I: Multiply means; place to one side of an equal sign; 4 x 6 = 24

Step II: Multiply extremes; place to the other side of the equal sign; 1 x X = 1X

Step III: Divide each side of the equation by the number to the left of the X.

$$\frac{24}{1} = \frac{1X}{1}$$

X = 24 ÷ 1

Answer X = 24

F. Checking the answer to a proportion.

1. To proof the proportion, put 24 in place of X; 1:4 = 6:24

2. Multiply the means; 4 x 6 = 24

3. Multiply the extremes; 1 x 24 = 24

4. The answer is correct, since the product of the means is equal to the product of the extremes.

1:4 = 6:24

24 = 24

Additional Resources Found on MyNursingLab

MODULE 1

Math

Submodule 1.5 Systems of Measurement
(Metric, Apothecary, and Household)

Learning Objectives

1.5.1 List commonly used measures for metric weight, volume, and length and their abbreviations.

1.5.2 State the commonly used equivalents in the metric system.

1.5.3 Convert units of volume, weight, and length within the metric system.

1.5.4 Identify the commonly used measures in the apothecary and household systems, with their symbols or abbreviations.

1.5.5 List the commonly used equivalents within the apothecary and household systems.

1.5.6 Convert from one unit to another within the apothecary and household systems.

   I. **Metric System**

      A. The metric system has three units of measurement.

      B. The liter is the basic measurement for volume or capacity.

      C. The liter is approximately equal to one quart.

      D. The gram is the basic measurement for weight.

      E. The linear measure or unit of measure for length is the Meter.

      F. The meter is approximately equal to 39.4 inches.

      G. The metric system is based on the decimal system.

      H. Basic units of the metric system can be multiplied or divided by 10 or multiples of 10 such as 100 or 1,000.

      I. Quantities in the metric system are always expressed in Arabic numerals.

      J. Greek and Latin prefixes are added to the primary unit to indicate multiples and subdivisions of the basic unit.

         1. Prefixes for Larger Units

            a. Deka means 10

            b. Hecto means 100

            c. Kilo means 1,000

    2. Prefixes for Units Smaller than 1

       a. Deci means 0.1 or $\frac{1}{10}$

       b. Centi means 0.01 or $\frac{1}{100}$

       c. Milli means 0.001 or $\frac{1}{1,000}$

       d. Micro means 0.000001 or $\frac{1}{1,000,000}$

  K. Metric system incorporated in the decimal system

II. Common Metric Units Used in Nursing and Their Abbreviations

  A. Weight

    1. Kilogram   kg

    2. Gram   g

    3. Milligram   mg

    4. Micrograms   mcg

  B. Volume

    1. Liter   L

    2. Milliliter mL

       a. One cubic centimeter (cc) is often used in place of one milliliter.

       b. A milliliter of water occupies one cubic centimeter of space.

  C. Length

    1. Meter   m

    2. Centimeter cm

    3. Millimeter mm

III. Writing in the Metric System

  A. Write the amount first, followed by the abbreviation, e.g.: ten grams = 10 g

  B. Essential Learning (**memorize equivalents** in weight, volume, and length)

    1. Weight

       a. 1,000 micrograms (mcg)   =   1 milligram (mg)

       b. 1,000 milligrams   =   1 gram (g)

       c. 1,000 grams   =   1 kilogram (kg)

    2. Volume

       a. 1,000 milliliters (mL)   =   1 liter (L)

    3. Length

       a. 100 centimeters (cm)   =   1 meter (m)

       b. 1,000 millimeters (mm)   =   1 meter (m)

IV. Conversions Within the Metric System

A. When converting from a larger unit to a smaller unit of measure:

1. Multiply.

   Example

   Convert 2.5 g to mg

   Since gram is larger than milligram you would multiply.

   By what number? You know 1 g = 1,000 mg. Therefore you multiply by 1,000.

   2.5 g   = _____ mg

   2.5 x 1,000   = _____ 2,500 mg

   2.5 g   = _____ 2,500 mg

2. A simpler method is to move the decimal point three places to the <u>right</u> since there are three multiples of ten in one thousand (3 zeros in 1000).

   2500.   =_____ 2,500   mg

B. When converting from a **smaller unit** to a **larger unit** of measure

1. Divide.

   Example

   150 mg   =_____g

   Since milligrams are smaller than grams, you would divide.

   Since 1,000 mg = 1 g you would divide by 1000.

   150 mg   = _____ g

   150 ÷ 1000 = <u>0.15</u>

   150 mg   = _____ 0.15 g

2. A simpler method is to move the decimal point three places to the left because there are three multiples of ten in one thousand.

   .150 = 0.15 g

V. Apothecary System

A. The apothecary system is an old English system, the origin of which is not exactly known.

B. Roman numerals are used to express whole numbers.

C. Fractions are used to express less than one.

D. Numbers are placed **after** the unit of measure.

E. Abbreviations and symbols:

1. Solid Weights

   a. Grains   gr

2. Fluids

   a. Fluid ounce   no approved symbol

   b. Pint   pt

        c.   Quart   qt

        d.   Gallon   gal

3.   Fluid Measure

     a.   16 fluid ounces 1 pint

     b.   2 pints   1 quart

     c.   4 quarts   1 gallon

F. Conversions within the Apothecary System

    1. When converting a larger unit of measure to a smaller one, multiply.

    2. When converting a smaller unit of measure to a larger one, divide.

    3. Solve using ratio and proportion.

    4. Ratio expresses the relationship or comparison of one number to another.

    5. Ratio is a fraction written sideways. Ratio expresses the relationship or comparison of one number with another.

Example

$\dfrac{1}{3}$ written as a ratio is 1:3 and is read: "one is to three"

$\dfrac{1}{4}$ written as a ratio is 1:4 and is read: "one is to four"

    6. Proportion consists of two ratios (or fractions) which are equal in value

       Example: 1/3   =   2/6

                      or

             1/3   =   2: 6

     a. In a proportion the first and the last terms are called the extremes. The second and the third terms are called the means.

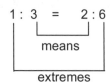

     b. In all proportions the product of the means equals the product of the extremes. If we multiply the means (3 x 2), the answer will be equal to that obtained by multiplying the extremes (1 x 6)

       Example: 3 x 2   =   1 x 6

                  6   =   6

     c. Use of ratio and proportion enables you to determine a fourth number (an unknown number) when you know the other 3 numbers.

7. Ratio and proportion in solving an apothecary conversion problem

   Example

   Convert 6 pints to quarts

   Step I: Start with a ratio of two known values. You should know 2 pints = 1 quart

   Step II: Set up a proportion that expresses the numerical relationship between pints and quarts to one side and the unknown quantity to the other side. This sets up the means and the extremes.

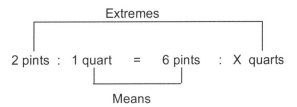

   Extremes

   2 pints : 1 quart = 6 pints : X quarts

   Means

   Step III: Multiply the means 1 x 6 = 6 and place 6 to the left side of the equal sign

   Step IV: Multiply the extremes = 2 x X = 2X and place 2X to the right of the equal sign

   Step V: Divide the number before X into both sides of the equation (meaning the number next to X must appear twice as the denominator and once as the numerator).

   $$\frac{6}{2} \quad = \quad \frac{2}{2}$$

   Step VI: Cancel.

   $$\frac{\cancel{6}^{\,3}}{\cancel{2}_{\,1}} \quad = \quad \frac{\cancel{2}^{\,1}X}{\cancel{2}_{\,1}}$$

   $$\frac{3}{1} \quad = \quad X \quad = \quad 3$$

   Step VII: Your answer will be expressed in the unit next to the X in the proportion.

   Answer = 3 quarts

8. To proof the proportion:

   a. Substitute your answer for X.

   b. Multiply the means.

   c. Multiply the extremes.

   d. The product of both the means and extremes must be equal.

      Example

      2 pints :   1 quart   = 6 pints : 3 quarts

      Means: 1 multiply by 6 = 6

      Extremes: 2 multiply by 3 = 6

      The answer is correct.

PEARSON

VI. Household Measures and Approximate Equivalents

A. Household System

1. Household measurements and equivalents are not scientifically accurate.

2. Used when proper equipment is not available, such as in community health nursing.

3. The household system is mainly used for liquid measure.

4. Household units and abbreviations.

   a. drops   gtt

   b. teaspoon   tsp

   c. tablespoon   tbsp

   d. ounces   oz

   e. cupfuls   c

   f. glassful   no abbreviation

5. Essential Learning (**memorize equivalents** within the household system)

   a. 60 gtt   =   1 tsp

   b. 3 tsp   =   1 tbsp

   c. 2 tbsp   =   1 oz

   d. 8 oz   =   1 measuring cupful

   e. 8 oz   =   1 glassful

VII. Conversion of Metric, Apothecary, and Household Units

A. Table of Equivalents

1. Essential Learning (**memorize equivalents** between each system)

   a. 2.2 lb   =   1 kg

   b. 1 gram   =   grain 15

   c. 60 milligrams   =   grain 1

   d. 1 milliliter   =   drops 15-16

   e. 5 milliliters   =   1 teaspoon = 60 gtt

   f. 30 milliliters   =   1 ounce = 2 tablespoons

   g. 1000 milliliters =   1 quart = 2 pints = 32 fluid ounces

2. Metric and apothecary equivalents

   a. 60 mg   =   1 grain

   b. 30 mg   = $\frac{1}{2}$ grain

   c. 15 mg   = $\frac{1}{4}$ grain

   d. 7.5 mg   = $\frac{1}{8}$ grain

PEARSON

3. Common apothecary equivalents that appear on labels with metric units:

   a. 0.6 mg   =   gr $\dfrac{1}{100}$

   b. 0.4 mg   =   gr $\dfrac{1}{150}$

   c. 0.3 mg   =   gr $\dfrac{1}{200}$

   d. 0.2 mg   =   gr $\dfrac{1}{300}$

   e. 0.1 mg   =   gr $\dfrac{1}{600}$

   Example

   Convert gr $\dfrac{1}{3}$ to mg.

   Step I: Write the known conversion as your first ratio; 1 gr : 60 mg.

   Step II: Write the second ratio starting with grains and let X represent the unknown;

   $$\dfrac{1}{3}\text{ gr}\ :\ X\ \text{mg}.$$

   Remember to place the equal sign between the ratios.

   $$1\text{ gr}\ :\ 60\text{ mg}\ =\ \dfrac{1}{3}\text{ gr}\ :\ X\text{ mg}$$

   Step III: Check to make sure the first and third terms express the same unit of measure and the second and fourth terms express the same unit of measure. Solve the proportion.

Additional Resources Found on MyNursingLab

MODULE 1

Math

Submodule 1.6 Dosage Calculations for Medications

Learning Objectives

1.6.1   **Read medication labels and use pertinent information to calculate the correct medication dosages.**

1.6.2   **Interpret the label of a powdered medication, reconstitute the powder, and determine the correct dosage to give.**

1.6.3   **Use the given formula to calculate intravenous fluid flow rate for gravity IV and electronic pump.**

1.6.4   **Interpret the order and label correctly, and calculate the heparin infusion rate.**

1.6.5   **Determine the safe dose by applying the appropriate formula for calculating pediatric dosages.**

1.6.6   **Given an insulin syringe, be able to read the syringe and draw up the correct dose.**

1.6.7   **Given a solution, be able to state the amount of solvent.**

   I.   Medication Calculations

   A.   A medication problem is made up mainly of two parts: the doctor's order and the ratio of the drug dispensed by the pharmacist.

   B.   Drugs can be ordered in the metric, apothecary, or household system.

   C.   The pharmacist can dispense drugs in the apothecary, metric, or household system.

   D.   All drugs dispensed by the pharmacist are given as a ratio.

   E.   The ratio can be the strength per volume (meaning a given amount of drug is diluted in a given amount of fluid) or a given strength of the drug per tablet or capsule.

   F.   Drug dispensed by the pharmacist is referred to in many terms:

   1.   "On hand"

   2.   "Supplied as"

   3.   "In stock"

   4.   "The label reads"

   G.   Reading Drug Labels

   1.   Total Volume per Vial

   2.   Problem without conversion of units: A physician has ordered Morphine sulfate 8 mg. Morphine sulfate is dispensed by the pharmacist in vials of 10 mg of morphine sulfate per one milliliter.

   How many milliliters would the client receive?

a. To solve a medication problem using ratio and proportion:

Step I: Rewrite the doctor's order.

Step II: Rewrite the supply on hand.

Doctor's order: 8 mg

On hand: 10 mg per mL

Step III: Check to make sure the doctor's order is in the same units of measure as the units on hand.

Step IV: If the units are different, then set up a proportion to convert the units on the doctor's orders to the units on hand.

Step V: If the doctor's order is in the same units as the units on hand, set up a proportion, writing (1) the ratio of the drug on hand, (2) equals, (3) the doctor's order to the unknown (X).

Ratio on hand   Doctor's Order   Unknown

10 mg : 1 mL =   8 mg   :   X mL

This kind of problem is always set up using the headings above.

Memorize:

Ratio of the drug on hand = Doctor's order: unknown

b. Solve the proportion.

10 mg : 1 mL = 8 mg : X mL

$$\frac{8}{10} = \frac{10X}{10}$$

$$X = 0.8 \text{ mL}$$

3. Problem with conversion of units

a. If the unit of measure of the drug you want to give is not the same as the unit of measure you have on hand, you must first convert to the same system.

Example:

The order says: Give morphine sulfate gr $\frac{1}{4}$ IM.

You have on hand morphine sulfate 30 mg in 2 mL.

Step I: Convert morphine sulfate gr $\frac{1}{4}$ to milligrams.

60 mg   : 1 gr = X mg : gr $\frac{1}{4}$

$$\frac{60}{1} \times \frac{1}{4} = \frac{60}{4} = \frac{15}{1}$$

$$\frac{1X}{1} = \frac{15}{1}$$

$$X = 15 \text{ mg}$$

Step II: You can now state the order: morphine 15 mg IM

Step III: You have on hand morphine 30 mg/2 mL. You must now determine the amount you would give.

Step IV: Set up the proportion.

$$30 \text{ mg} : 2 \text{ mL} = 15 \text{ mg} : X \text{ mL}$$

$$\frac{\cancel{30}}{\cancel{30}} \quad \frac{1}{1} = \frac{\cancel{30}X}{\cancel{30}X} = \frac{1}{1} = 1$$

$$X = 1 \text{ mL}$$

4. **Memorize:** When the units are different, the doctor's order must be converted to the units on hand!

II. Reconstitution of Medications

A. Reconstitution is necessary because certain drugs lose their potency in liquid form and so are packaged in powdered form.

B. These drugs must be reconstituted (have liquid added) prior to administration.

C. Although the pharmacist often reconstitutes powdered drugs for parenteral use, in some instances nurses perform this function.

D. The label or package insert contains specific information about the quantity of the drug, amount of diluent to add to the powder, the resulting strength per volume, and its shelf life.

E. The most frequently used diluent is sterile water for injection or sterile normal saline for injection.

F. When a diluent is added to a powder, the volume is often increased; this is called displacement.

G. For this reason the label may call for less diluent than the total volume of the prepared solution.

1. For example; add 2 mL of diluent to yield 2.5 mL prepared solution.

H. Once the powdered drug is reconstituted, the unused portion must be labeled, dated, refrigerated, and initialed.

Example:

Mefoxcin is supplied in a 1-g vial. The manufacturer's direction is to add 4 mL of diluent to the vial. This provides 0.5 g in 2.2 mL. The doctor's order is for 0.25 g. How much would you give?

$$0.5 \text{ g} : 2.2 \text{ mL} = 0.25 \text{ g} : X \text{ mL}$$

$$0.5 X = (2.2 \times 0.25) = 0.55$$

$$X = \frac{0.55}{0.5}$$

$$X = 1.1 \text{ mL}$$

III. Reading Drug Labels

    A. Use the label below to answer the following questions.

> **Pen G**
>
> IM or IV use
>
> **6 million units**
>
> | Amount of diluents | Units/mL |
> | --- | --- |
> | 15 mL | 100,000 units |
> | 20 mL | 400,000 units |
> | 25 mL | 800,000 units |
>
> Dilute with 0.9% NaCl.
> Use within 10 days.
> Refrigerate after mixing.

    B. The doctor ordered Pen G 750,000 units IM.

        1. Which strength will you use? _____ 800,000 units _____

        2. How many milliliters of diluent will be used to mix? ___ 25 mL _____

        3. What is the shelf life after reconstitution? _____ 10 days _____

        4. How many milliliters of medication will you give? __ Use a proportion to find 23.4. Round to 23 mL._____

IV. Intravenous Fluids

    A. When administering fluids intravenously, nurses must calculate and regulate the drops per minute in order to give a certain amount in the ordered period of time.

    B. The administration sets made by various manufacturers are constructed to yield varying numbers of drops per milliliter.

    C. This information may be found on the box containing the set.

        1. Examples are as follows:

            a. 10 drops/mL - Mead and Baxter

            b. 15 drops/mL - Abbott

            c. 20 drops/mL - Cutter

            d. 60 drops/mL - One example pediatric administration set made by various companies

    D. Steps involved in calculating flow rate when using an IV pump.

        1. $\dfrac{\text{Total mL fluid to be given}}{\text{Numbers of hours}}$ = desired mL/hr

        Example:

        Infuse 500 mL 0.9% NaCl over 6 hr by electronic pump.

$$\frac{500 \text{ mL}}{6} \quad = \quad 83 \text{ mL/hr}$$

2. A simplified formula for calculating drops per minute/flow rate is as follows:

   a. Formula I: If the fluid is ordered over several hours

$$\frac{\text{Amount of fluid in mL} \times \text{drop factor}}{\text{Time in hours} \quad \times \quad 60 \text{ min}}$$

   b. Formula II: If the fluid is ordered over several minutes

$$\frac{\text{Amount of fluid in mL} \times \text{drop factor}}{\text{Time in minutes}}$$

   c. Using Formula I, solve the following problem:

Example:

1000 mL 5% Dextrose in water in 2 hours using an IV

set calibrated at 15 gtt/mL

$$\frac{\overset{\displaystyle 125}{\cancel{\underset{\cancel{2}}{\cancel{1000}}}^{\cancel{250}}}}{\cancel{2}_{1}} \times \frac{\overset{1}{\cancel{15}}}{\cancel{60}_{\underset{1}{4}}}$$

Answer = Set up 125 gtt/min

   d. Calculated infusion flow rates are guidelines only.

   e. Maintaining the calculated rate of flow does not relieve nurses of their responsibility to observe for indications of too rapid or too slow infusion.

   f. Fulfilling one's obligation to speed up, slow down, or stop intravenous infusion at any time requires considerable nursing judgment based upon many factors.

V. Heparin Administration

   A. Heparin is weighed and measured in units.

   B. Heparin is given by subcutaneous or intravenous route.

   C. When given intravenously heparin can be IV push or by infusion.

   D. Intravenous infusion of heparin is usually delivered by electronic pump.

Example:

The physician orders heparin 30,000 units added to 1000 mL D5W to infuse at 1,200 units per hour. The IV is by electronic pump. What is the flow rate?

   Step I: Set up the first ratio of the proportion with the known ratio:

30,000 units : 1000 mL

   Step II: Set up the second ratio with the problem statement

1,200 units : X mL

Step III: Solve the proportion.

30,000 units : 1000 mL = 1,200 units : X mL

$$\frac{1200000}{30000} = \frac{30000X}{30000}$$

$$\frac{120}{3} = 40 \text{ mL/hr}$$

VI. Pediatric Dosages

A. Children's dosages are calculated according to weight or age.

B. You must know the average adult dosage.

C. It is also assumed that the average adult weight is 150 lb.

D. Clark's Rule (used when the **weight** of the child is available)

Formula I

$$\frac{\text{Child's weight in lb} \times \text{average adult dose}}{\text{Average adult weight} \quad (150 \text{ lb})} = \text{child dose}$$

E. Young's Rule (used when the **age** of the child is available)

Formula II

$$\frac{\text{Age of child in years} \times \text{average adult dose}}{\text{Age of child} + 12} = \text{child dose}$$

F. Fried's Rule (used for the child **under 2 years**)

Formula III

$$\frac{\text{Age in months} \times \text{average adult dose}}{\text{Average adult weight}} = \text{child dose}$$

G. The most accurate way to give medication to adults or children is by body Surface area.

H. This can be done in two ways. The simplest is the mg/kg method.

 1. Rules for mg/kg

   a. If the weight is in pounds, change to kilograms by dividing by 2.2.

   b. Then multiply by the recommended dose.

   c. Determine if the dose is safe.

   Example:

   The recommended dose for Meprobamate is 0.6 mg/kg/wt. What would a person weighing 88 lb receive?

   Step I: Change pounds to kilograms.

```
          040.
   22. ) 880.
          88
          0
```

   Step II: Multiply the weight by the dose.

$$40 \times 0.6 \quad = \quad \begin{array}{r} 40 \\ \times\, 0.6 \\ \hline 24.0 \end{array}$$

Answer: = Dose = 24 mg

VII. Insulin

A. Insulin is supplied and ordered in units.

B. The most commonly used strength of Insulin is units 100. Insulin is given using specially calibrated syringes.

C. 1 mL holds 100 units; 0.5 mL holds 50 units; 0.3 mL holds 30 units.

D. Types of Insulin

Rapid Acting	**Short Acting**	**Intermediate Acting**
Humalog	Regular	NPH
Novolog	Humulin R	Humulin N&L
Apidra	Novolin R	Novolin N&L

Long Acting
PZI
Ultralente
Humulin L
Lantus
Levimir

E. No calculation is needed if insulin syringes are available.

F. The nurse ensures the correct insulin and strength.

G. Draw up the ordered dose.

H. Sometimes an insulin syringe is not available and a tuberculin syringe must be used.

I. A tuberculin syringe is calibrated in milliliters and holds a volume of 1 milliliter.

J. Insulin is supplied in strength of U 100. This means 100 units of insulin per 1 mL.

Example:

Insulin 10 units of U 100 is to be given by tuberculin syringe. You would give _____ milliliter.

Set up the proportion:

100 units: 1 mL : : 10 units   : X mL

$$10 = 100\,X$$
$$X = 10 \div 100 \quad 100\,\overline{)\begin{array}{l} 00.1 \\ 10.0 \\ \underline{10.0} \end{array}} \quad = \; 0.1 \text{ mL}$$

K. A quicker solution to calculate the number of mL to be given is to take the order and divide it by 100 by moving the decimal two places to the left.

Example:

10 ÷ 100

10 = 0.1 mL by tuberculin syringe

L. Drawing up insulin in an insulin syringe

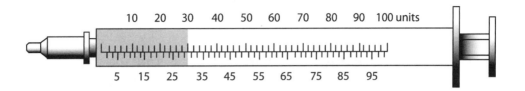

VIII. Solutions

A. As a nurse you may be asked to prepare a solution for a soak or irrigation.

B. The strength of the solution is expressed as a percent or a ratio; 1% means one part of every 100 pertaining to fluid.

1. Liquid drugs are measure in milliters

2. Solid drugs are measured in grams.

3. Therefore in a 1% solution there is 1 g to 100 mlL

Example:

Prepare 1,000 mL of a 10% solution of boric acid. How many grams of boric acid are needed?

Set up the proportion: 10 g : 100 mL =   X g : 1000 mL

$$100\, X = 10{,}000$$

$$X = 100\ g$$

Answer: You would add 100 g boric acid to 1000 mL of water.

Additional Resources Found on MyNursingLab

MODULE 1
Math
Submodule 1.7 Medication Administration

Learning Objectives

1.7.1 **Describe drug sources, uses, classification, legislation, and nursing responsibilities for medication administration.**

1.7.2 **Describe pharmacokinetics and pharmacodynamics.**

1.7.3 **Demonstrate proper drug administration for enteral, parenteral, and percutaneous routes.**

1.7.4 **Describe adverse drug reactions and interactions.**

1.7.5 **Describe proper medication administration using the nursing process.**

1.7.6 **Describe nursing care aimed at preventing medication errors.**

I. **Medication Administration** is one of the most important duties of the nurse and demands an intense level of concentration to be accurate.

   A. To ensure accuracy in medication administration, the nurse must have a good understanding of the basics of drug therapy.

   B. Drugs are chemical substances designed to create specific responses with living body tissues.

   C. Pharmacology is the science that studies drug action in the body.

   D. There are five branches of pharmacology:

      1. **Pharmaceutics:** the study of dissolution of drugs.

      2. **Pharmacodyamics:** the study of how drugs act in the body; the biochemical and physiological effect.

      3. **Pharmacokinetics:** the study of how drugs are metabolized.

      4. **Phamacotherapeutics**: the study of how drugs are used in the treatment of disease, most to least effective.

      5. **Toxicology:** the study of poisons, their causes, symptoms, diagnoses, and treatments.

II. **Drug Sources**

   A. Animal: Glandular secretions such as enzymes, serums, and vaccines are obtained from animals,. Drugs like insulin were originally obtained from the pancreases of cows, pigs, and sheep.

   B. Plants: All parts of the plant may be used: bark, roots, seeds, and other parts. Drugs like digitalis have their origin from a plant, in this case the purple foxglove.

C. Minerals: Organic or inorganic compounds and some synthetics are derived from a combination of man made and natural substances formulated in the laboratory. Most drugs are produced this way today to allow for greater volume at reduced costs.

D. Recombinant DNA Technology: Advances in the study of genetics have increased the production of drugs such as synthetic insulin and tissue plasminogen activators.

III. Drug Uses

A. Health maintenance: To keep the body functioning normally, for example, insulin

B. Prevention: To help to prevent diseases, for example, vaccines.

C. Diagnosis: To test or aid in diagnosis, for example, using barium or radio-opaque dyes disease.

D. Treatment: To reduce symptoms such as fever and vomiting.

E. Cure: To rid client of underlying health problem, for example, anticancer drugs to eradicate cancer or antibiotics to cure infection.

IV. Drug Names or Nomenclature

A. Chemical: Based on atomic and molecular structure of the drug. This drug name is in lowercase letters.

B. Generic or Nonproprietary: Names given to a drug when it is ready to be marketed. This name appears on label written in lowercase letters.

C. Trade/ Brand or proprietary: Given by manufacturer when a drug is ready to be distributed. On the label it is capitalized and carries the symbol R in upper right-hand corner. This means the drug is registered and use of the name is restricted to that manufacturer. A drug can have more than one brand name.

V. Drug Classification

A. Drugs are classified in five ways:

1. Site of action: where the drug is absorbed. Drugs that have a local action act at the site of administration. Drugs that have a systemic action are absorbed into the bloodstream.

2. Therapeutic use: the drug's action, for example, antifectives used to fight infections.

3. Chemical properties: the make-up of the drug, for example, beta blockers.

4. Body system: the system to be affected, for example, cardiovascular system drugs.

5. Legislation: the legal status of the drug, such as whether it is prescription/legend, nonprescription or over-the-counter (OTC), herbal, illicit/street drugs, and/or investigational.

VI. Prescription or Legend Drugs

A. Prescription or legend drugs carry the label, "Federal law prohibits use without a prescription," as they are considered to be harmful unless their use is supervised by a physician in a health care institution or at home.

VII. OTC or Nonprescription Drugs

A. OTC or nonprescription drugs are available for purchase without a prescription and are relatively safe.

B. Labeling for these drugs is carefully regulated to guide the consumer on when to seek medical supervision.

VIII. Controlled Substances

A. Controlled Substance: These drugs are regulated under the Controlled Substance Act of 1960 and are considered to be drugs that can lead to physical or psychological dependency.

B. The Controlled Substance Act designates drugs in five schedules based on their potential for abuse and their frequency of medical use.

C. This act is policed by the Drug Enforcement Agency (DEA) within the Department of Justice.

D. Schedule I: High potential for abuse and no current accepted medical use, e.g. heroin, marijuana, and LSD.

E. Schedule II: Abuse high, but with accepted medical use, e.g. morphine, Demerol, oxycodone, hydrocodone, amphetamines, and barbiturates.

F. Schedule III: Abuse decreased, with medical use increased, e.g., codeine mixtures, non-barbiturate sedatives and non-amphetamine stimulants.

G. Schedule IV: Abuse is low with medical use high, e.g., antianxiety drugs such as Valium and Librium.

H. Schedule V: Abuse potential low and medical use high. These are weak mixtures of codeine or morphine, e.g. antidiarrheal drugs such as Lomotil and cough mixtures such as Robitussin AC.

IX. Nursing Implications of Controlled Substance Act.

A. Controlled substances must be stored in a double-locked closet.

B. Wastage of controlled substance must be witnessed and cosigned.

C. Inventory is done on each shift and when receiving new stock.

D. Nurse must check to ensure seals are not broken on prefilled syringes.

E. Controlled substance drugs must be immediately logged out as they are removed.

X. Botanical /Herbal Drugs

A. Derived mainly from plants, many of these drugs have been used for thousands of years and in many cultures.

B. They are often used to complement traditional medicine or as alternative medicine.

C. About 80% of people worldwide and about 40% of people in the USA use some form of this medicine.

D. Herbal drugs, vitamins, and nutritional supplements are controlled substances.

E. In 1992, the National Institutes of Health established an Office of Alternative Medicine to study, document, and disseminate information on these drugs.

F. In 1994, the FDA established truth in labeling and advertising of herbal medicine.

G. The 1994, FDA regulations limited herbal drugs' claims to helping memory and regulating bowels.

XI. Investigational Drugs

A. These are new drugs in the initial stages of discovery and testing.

B. It takes 7 to 12 years to test new drugs.

C. This begins with *in vitro* testing in animal and human cells, then 1-2 years of animal testing. If the drug shows promise, the sponsor can apply to the FDA for Investigational New Drug status to begin testing in humans.

D. After approval, the FDA sets up a board made up of scientists, ethicists, and non-scientists to oversee the clinical research. The drug then enters three phases of clinical testing where all adverse reactions are monitored, recorded, and reported.

E. Phase 1: Uses a small sample of healthy individuals 4 to 6 weeks, to see side effects and to determine the dose that can be tolerated safely.

F. Phase 2: Uses a small sample of people with the disease for two years.

G. Phase 3: Uses a larger sample of people with the disease, using random double-blind studies for three years. If testing is successful, the drug is marketed with FDA approval and patented for 12 to 17 years.

H. Phase 4: This stage of testing involves post-market surveillance. This includes factory inspection for quality control and labeling.

I. MedWatch is an FDA monitoring system that encourages health care workers to report any adverse effects from drugs and any medical devices that cause harm to a client.

J. To report to MedWatch, suspicion is enough. Reporting can be anonymous: by telephone, in writing, or online.

XII. Standardization and Drug Reference

A. The *United States Pharmacopoeia* (USP), with the Food and Drug Administration (FDA), sets standard for drug purity and potency in this country and puts out a drug reference source for health care professionals.

B. The Physicians' Desk Reference (PDR) lists complete drug information, similar to that found in package inserts, and is a source for doctors and nurses.

C. There are several nurses' drug handbooks that use the nursing process approach.

XIII. Pregnancy Categories

A. Some drugs are recognized as teratogens. These are agents have the ability to induce birth defects if taken during pregnancy, especially in the first trimester.

B. Drugs are grouped into five pregnancy categories by the FDA based the effect on the developing fetus.

1. Category A: Sufficient human testing indicates no risk demonstrated.

2. Category B: Animal reproduction studies have not shown risk to the fetus and there are no adequate and well-controlled studies in pregnant women.

3. Category C: Risk cannot be ruled out--animal studies show risk. Human studies are lacking; however, potential benefits may outweigh the risk to the fetus.

4. Category D: ncreased risk shown in human fetuses. Benefit of drug may outweigh risk to fetus.

5. Category X; Contraindicated, meaning risks clearly outweigh benefits.

XIV. Drug Forms

    A. Tablets

        1. Tablets are the most popular dose form.

        2. **Tablets** are the drug in powdered form compressed in a mold.

        3. Tablets also contain inactive ingredients, such as cornstarch, to add bulk.

        4. When the cornstarch comes in contact with stomach fluids, it disintegrates easily and the drug is released.

        5. Tablets come in different forms which may be swallowed whole, chewed, placed under the tongue (sublingual), or between the cheek and gum (buccal).

        6. Sublingual tablets are placed under the tongue, dissolved by saliva and absorbed via the mucous membranes into the bloodstream.

        7. *Rule:* Sublingual tablets should not be swallowed with, or followed by, food or fluid or they will lose their effect.

        8. Some tablets are scored, meaning they are designed with markings or indentations to guide breaking into half or quarters.

        9. *Rule:* Never break a tablet that is not scored, as this can lead to dosage error.

      10. Some tablets have special coatings, such as wax matrix, or enteric coating. The purpose of these coatings is to prevent absorption in the stomach for two reasons:

           a. To protect the drug from being destroyed by gastric acids.

           b. To protect the stomach from irritation by the drug.

      11. Some tablets are called sustained-action or time-release; these medications are released over a specific period of time.

      12. *Rule:* Do not crush enteric-coated tablets and do not open time-released capsules, as this may decrease the efficacy of the drug.

    B. Capsules

        1. **Capsules** are the drug enclosed in a hard or soft outer gelatin coating.

        2. When the outer gelatin coating is hard, the drug is in powder or granule form. These granules may be time released.

        3. When the outer gelatin coating is soft, the drug is in oil or liquid form.

        4. Capsules are usually cylindrical in shape, but size varies.

        5. The purpose of having the drug in a capsule is to mask the smell and taste.

        6. *Rule:* These capsules should not be crushed or opened as they can lose their effect.

        7. Before opening a capsule, check with the pharmacy to ensure that the drug will not be toxic or lose its effect.

        8. Some soft capsules can be punctured with a needle and the contents removed for administration.

        9. Some time-released capsules can be opened and the pellets sprinkled on soft foods and swallowed (e.g., digestive enzymes).

      10. Capsules and tablets also carry abbreviations important to dosing, indicating onset of action and duration of effect:

           a. CR: Controlled Release

      b.   LA: Long Acting

      c.   DS: Double strength

      d.   SR: Sustained release

      e.   XL: Extra long acting

C. **Troches/Lozenges:** The drug comes in a flavored, candy-like base. As the candy dissolves, the medication is released, usually to relieve discomfort in the oral cavity or throat.

D. **Suppositories:**

   1.   The drug is combined in soap, oil, or gelatin with a cocoa butter base.

   2.   Suppositories are molded in a cone shape.

   3.   The cocoa butter is designed to melt when in contact with body heat.

   4.   Suppositories provide a local or systemic effect.

   5.   Suppositories can be administered in the rectum, vagina, or urethra.

E. **Liquid Suspensions**

   1.   The drug in the form of solid insoluble particles mixed in a liquid.

   2.   These must be shaken before pouring.

   3.   Small doses can be diluted in 5 mL of water.

   4.   Suspensions can be given orally or topically, but never intramuscularly or intravenously.

F. **Emulsions:**

   1.   The drug is in a milky suspension containing oil or fats in water with an emulsifying agent.

   2.   Emulsions can be used orally, topically, or intravenously.

   3.   They are shaken before use.

   4.   Client is seated upright when administration is oral to prevent aspiration.

G. **Elixir:** Drug dissolved in alcohol, water, and sugar. Used for drugs that cannot dissolve in water alone. Adding water will cause precipitation.

H. **Extract:** Usually a vegetable-based drug in concentrated form with an alcohol base.

I. **Spirits:** Volatile aromatic dissolved in alcohol.

J. **Tincture:** Drug extract in 10-20 % alcohol base. Adding water will cause precipitation.

K. **Syrups:** Drug dissolved in sugar and water.

L. **Significance:**

1. Drugs containing alcohol should not be given to clients with known allergy to alcohol.
2. Drugs containing alcohol must be tightly covered to prevent evaporation.
3. Drugs containing alcohol should not be given to clients on disulfiram (Antabuse).
4. Drugs containing sugar should not be given to diabetics.

XV. Principles of Drug Action

A. Pharmaceutics

1. Phase of dissolution. This phase studies how tablets or capsules disintegrate into smaller particles in the stomach.
2. Tablets that are enteric- or wax-matrix coated dissolve in an alkaline medium in the small intestines.
3. Only solid drugs go through the dissolution.

B. Pharmacokinetics is the study of how drugs act in the body. Drugs past through four distinct stages:

1. **Absorption.** This is the passage of the drugs from outside of the body to the blood stream.

   a. There are many ways in which drugs may enter the bloodstream depending on the route of administration. Examples:

      i. Oral – digestion processes bring drug to bloodstream through stomach or intestines

      ii. Inhalation – drug crosses into blood through the alveoli of the lungs during inspiration

      iii. IV – drug is placed directly into the bloodstream.

   b. Once the drug has reached the bloodstream, it is said to be free or unbound, meaning it is available for use by the body.

   c. The rate of absorption varies according to the drug route, solubility, and circulation.

   d. Route: Can place the drug near the site of absorption. For example, fluids given with oral drugs speed up absorption, and food given with oral drugs slows down absorption.

   e. Solubility: The speed by which the drug will dissolve to form a solution that can be readily absorbed into the cells.

   f. Drugs that are water- soluble or lipid- soluble drugs enter the systemic circulation more rapidly.

   g. Circulation: Decreased blood supply to an area, for reasons including edema, infection, congestion of the blood vessels, poor pumping ability of the heart, or low blood pressure slows the rate of absorption. If one of these factors applies to a client, the physician must be notified so a different route of administration can be used to overcome the problem.

2. **Distribution**

    a. The process by which the drug is carried from its site of absorption to the site of action.

    b. Drugs move from the blood stream via lymphatic tissue and capillaries across cell membranes to other tissues.

    c. The drug is carried rapidly to those organs with the greatest supply of blood, e.g., heart, liver, kidney, and brain.

    d. Once the drug reaches the blood stream, it must then progress to its particular site of action.

    e. In the bloodstream the drug actually divides into three forms:

        i. A portion that stays unbound or free

        ii. A portion of the drug binds with proteins, most commonly albumen. This remains pharmacologically inactive until released, and accounts for the largest portion of the drug in the body.

        iii. A portion of the drug binds with fat tissue.

    f. The body releases part of the protein-bound or lipid- bound drug to replace the portion of the free or unbound drug that has left the bloodstream.

    g. For a drug to reach its receptors, it must be circulated through the blood tream.

    h. An area or tissue of the body that has a good blood supply will have an increased supply of the drugs

    i. The drug will then have more opportunity to attach to receptors in that part of the body.

3. **Biotransformation**

    a. This is also called *metabolism*. It is the process by which the drug is detoxified and turned into harmless substances that are water–soluble.

    b. Biotransformation occurs in the liver through enzyme and chemical reactions.

    c. Therefore, it is important for a client receiving medication to have adequate liver function.

    d. Clients with liver disease need a smaller drug dose.

    e. Without biotransformation the drug continues to have its effect and accumulates in the body, eventually harming it.

    f. Under some conditions, the liver's ability to metabolize drugs is impaired, e.g. premature infants, neonates, the aged, and people with liver disease.

    g. Drug accumulation can lead to toxicity and damage to the body's cells.

4. **Excretion**

    a. Drugs are eliminated from the body through excretion.

    b. This may be through respiration, perspiration, or defecation.

    c. Most often excretion is through the kidneys, using the process of filtration.

    d. Other routes of elimination are via the feces, respiration, saliva, sweat, bile, and breast milk.

    e. Good kidney function is vital for the proper elimination of drugs.

    f.   If the drug or its transformed substances are not eliminated from the body, they build up and cause harm.

    g.   If a client has impaired kidney function, the dosage, the route, and even the drug itself may be changed because of the potential for accumulation.

5. **Drug Half-life**

    a.   Half-life. is the amount of time it takes for the body to inactivate half of the available drug.

    b.   This information is used in determining the proper dosage, dosage interval and route for specific drugs.

    c.   On average it takes a drug 5 - 6 half- life to leave the body.

    d.   Drugs with a short half- life of 2 to 4hours need to be administered frequently while drugs with a longer half- life of 12 to 24 hours need less frequent dosing.

    e.   Client with liver or kidney disease has altered half- life that can cause drug accumulation.

6. **Blood Plasma (Serum) Concentration**

    a.   Determine if an adequate amount of a drug is in the circulation.

    b.   The physician can order blood drawn to assess these levels.

    c.   Three commonly measured levels are therapeutic, peak and trough

    d.   Therapeutic: The level of drug in the blood stream that results in the desired or therapeutic effect.

    e.   Peak: Highest blood level of the drug.

    f.   Trough: Lowest blood level of the drug

7. **Pharmacodynamics**

    a.   Once drugs enter the bloodstream they have an affinity to certain cells these are called target cells.

    b.   Drugs exert their therapeutic effect at the target cells.

    c.   Drugs can affect cells in two ways by altering the cell's environment or cell action.

    d.   Drugs can alter cellular environment in two ways, chemically or physically.

        i.   Alteration in the chemical environment of a cell.

           (a) The cell environment can be altered chemically by the administration of drugs such as antacids that neutralize acidity of gastric fluids.

           (b) Antacids increase the pH of gastric content from 2 or 3 to 4 or 5.

        ii. Physical alteration in the cell's environment can be accomplished by a change in osmotic pressure, lubrication, absorption or surface tension on cell membrane.

           (a) Change in osmotic pressure: Occurs with the administration of drugs such as Milk of Magnesia. Cause the diffusion of fluid from plasma to distend the intestines and stimulate peristalsis.

           (b) Change in lubrication: Example is the administration of mineral oil to lubricate the bowel to ease the passage of the stool.

      (c) Change in absorption: Example is the administration of activated charcoal absorbing impurities or poison from stomach.

      (d) Change in surface tension on cell membrane: Example: administration of colace permits water and fats to enter the fecal mass to soften and allow easy passage.

e. Drugs alter cellular function: Drug cannot create new functions; however, when they form chemical bonds with specific receptor sites on cell membrane they can stimulate or depress the function of the cell.

  i. Depression

      (a) When a drug depresses cellular function, it lowers or lessens activity in a body organ or system.

      (b) The body system commonly affected systems are the respiratory, cardiac, and nervous system.

      (c) If a drug produces cardiac depression, there will be slowing of the pulse to extreme bradycardia or an irregular rhythm.

      (d) The physician must be notified immediately on noticing the decline in the pulse rate.

      (e) In general if a client's pulse is below 60 per minute, the physician may change the dosage or the drug.

  ii. Stimulation

      (a) Drugs that stimulate cellular function increase the function or the activity of a body organ.

      (b) The sites of action are the same as for depression; respiratory, cardiac, nervous, motor, mental and excretory.

      (c) The action would be the opposite of depression.

      (d) If a drug stimulates the heart this can result in a rapid heart rate, tachycardia, or irregular rhythm.

      (e) A heart rate of 100 beats /minutes or above calls for the drug to be held and the physician informed.

  iii. Receptor-mediated response

      (a) As the free drug is circulating in the bloodstream it comes in contact with chemicals on the cells to which it is attracted called receptors.

      (b) Receptors site is a place on the receptor where the drug becomes attached.

      (c) Once at the receptor site the drug's attachment can elicit two responses, agonist or antagonist.

        (1) Agonist drugs fit a receptor site exactly and have a strong attachment to it. Once the drug and the receptor site have attached, the drug elicits a response from the receptor. An example of a drug that uses this attachment is morphine.

        (2) Antagonist drugs also bind with receptors. They may attach strongly but not elicit a response. However, it does prevent other chemicals from reacting with the receptor simply because it is in the way. An example of a drug with that attachment is Narcan.

XVI. Drug Routes

A. **Enteral route** describes drugs given via the gastrointestinal tract such as oral or tubal.

   1. Oral drug form can be solids or liquid.

   2. Advantage easy, convenient, economical, and safe

   3. Disadvantage slow and unpredictable not suited for emergency and can cause irritation of the gastric mucosa.

   4. Gastric acids can destroy drugs; peristalsis can speed up or slow down absorption.

   5. Orally the drug passes into the digestive system and goes through all or part of the digestive processes.

   6. This means the drugs must survive these processes to be effective.

   7. The drug disintegrates and is dissolved in the stomach.

   8. Many drugs are absorbed into the bloodstream from the small intestines through the villi by a combination of osmosis, active transport, filtration and diffusion.

   9. Fluid moving from low to high concentration across a semi-permeable membrane.

   10. From the villi drugs travel via the mesenteric vessel.

   11. Tubal drugs are those given via a nasogastric, gastrostomy or jejunostomy tubes.

   12. Tubal medication is used to administer medication in a liquid form to clients unable to swallow such as unconscious or dysphagic clients.

B. **Parenteral route** describes drugs that pass the GI tract and goes from tissue the blood stream.

   1. Intravenous administration eliminates the need for the body to absorb the drugs because it is placed directly in the bloodstream.

   2. Therefore the IV route is the fastest acting

C. **Percutaneous route** describes drugs given via the skin or mucous membranes to include given topical, sublingual, buccal, inhalation drugs and drug instillation into the eyes, ears, nose, rectum, or vagina.

   1. They are not administered via the GI tract.

   2. Sublingual drugs are placed under the tongue and absorbed directly into the blood stream.

   3. Buccal drugs are placed between the cheek and gums and are absorbed directly into the blood stream through the mucous membrane.

   4. Topical drugs are applied externally and absorbed through the skin, such as lotions, ointments, and pastes.

   5. Transdermal drugs are released slowly into the skin via a patch or disk (certain contraceptives and nicotine, for example).

   6. Instillation drugs in a liquid form are instilled in a body cavity such as the eye, noses and ears.

      a. Insertion: Drug may be placed in a body cavity (such as the rectum or vagina) where the drug will dissolve at body temperature

   7. Inhaled: Drug given via the respiratory tract by nebulizer, or metered dose inhaler.

XVII. Adverse Drug Reaction

A. The primary effect of a drug is the desired or **therapeutic effect.**

B. **Secondary effects** are other effects of a drug, whether desirable or not.

C. **Adverse drug reactions,** side effects or untoward effects, are any unintended or undesired response to a drug.

D. Adverse reactions occur because of a lack of specific action exhibited by most drugs.

E. Adverse reactions have the potential to be serious either by leading to further illness, delayed recovery or even death.

F. Some adverse reactions are predictable, such as becoming drowsy after taking an antihistamine for a cold.

G. Some adverse reactions are unpredictable, such as allergic reactions.

    1. **Allergic reaction** or hypersensitivity is a response by the immune system to the presence of the drug in the body, even at very low levels.

        a. Allergic reactions are antigen - antibody reactions.

        b. The drug is considered an antigen or foreign protein.

        c. The mast cells reacting to the presence of the drug rupture and stimulate the production of proteins called antibodies.

        d. One of the substances produced is histamine that causes tissues to swell.

        e. This kind of reaction result in urticaria, which is rash, hives with itching.

        f. An allergic reaction can be mild or severe.

        g. A severe allergic reaction is called anaphylaxis.

            i. **Anaphylaxis,** because it can block the air passages, is a more serious allergic response that comes on suddenly and can lead to circulatory and respiratory collapse.

                (a) To have such a serious reaction there must be a previous exposure to the drug.

            ii. Another dangerous part of the allergic response is angioneurotic edema, which results in swelling of the eyelids, lips, mouth, and throat.

        h. Treatment of an allergic reaction

            i Administration of epinephrine 0.5 to 1 mg subcutaneous, intramuscular, or intravenous to dilate the bronchus and counteract respiratory depression and shock.

            ii Administration of the antihistamine Benadryl 25 to 50 mg orally or parenterally to decrease tissue swelling.

    2. **Idiosyncratic reaction** is an abnormal reaction to a drug at the first administration.

        a. The cause is not clear and could be the result of that person's genetics makeup.

        b. An example is giving an elderly person a sedative and instead of becoming drowsy which is normal reaction they become hyperactive.

3. Cumulative effect

   a. When the body is unable to break down or completely excrete the drug, the drugs build up to toxic levels in the body and can lead to toxicity.

   b. An example of a drug that can easily build up to toxic levels in the body is digoxin.

4. Toxic reaction

   a. Toxic reactions occur when the drug is given in high doses or a drug dose exceeds the therapeutic level.

   b. Commonly seen with decreased liver and kidney function

   c. Can be reversible or irreversible depending on the drug

   d. Some drugs have a high toxicity index or a narrow therapeutic margin, such as digoxin and lithium.

5. Tolerance

   a. **Tolerance** is decreased response to repeated doses of a drug that fails to produce the established effect.

   b. An example of tolerance is continued use of pain medication that results in a need for an increase in dose or frequency.

H. Drug Interactions

   1. Drugs are chemical substances that can react with other chemicals. As a result, the effect of one or both drug can be increased or decreased.

   2. This ability of chemicals to react to each other is called an interaction.

   3. The two common types of interaction are, drug-drug or drug-food.

   4. The nurse is responsible to check for these types of reaction before giving any drug.

   5. Drug to drug interactions:

      a. **Additive effect /summative interaction:** Two drugs taken together for an added effect because they have similar action, e.g., sedative + alcohol = sedation (1 + 1 = 2)

      b. **Potentiation/ synergism:** Two drugs with a different site or mechanism of action, when given together, have a greater effect than if either was given alone, e.g. Codeine + Tylenol (1 + 1 = 4).

      c. **Antagonism:** One drug negates the action of another drug, e.g., morphine + Narcan).

   6. Drug to food interactions:

      a. Incompatibility is seen when the chemicals in the drug cause the deterioration of another chemical structure in foods to either render the drug useless or more potent.

      b. For example, a monoamine oxidase inhibitor (MAOI) is prescribed for a client and the individual receives a protein, tryamine found in certain foods.

      c. This can lead to a hypertensive crisis.

XVIII. Factors Influencing Drug Action

A. Age

1. No two people respond to the same drug in exactly the same way. Older adults have increased reaction because body function decreases, so smaller doses are required.

2. Liver and kidney function decreases, causing a delay in all areas of drug metabolism.

3. Decreased gastric acidity and decreased gastric motility delay absorption.

4. Decrease saliva and dry mouth result in difficulty swallowing.

5. Increased body fat and decreased body water increase the accumulation of drugs and slow excretion.

6. Circulation slows and impairs the transport of drugs.

7. **Polypharmacy,** use of numerous drugs, leads to adverse drug reactions in the elderly.

8. Adverse effects on the older client are usually manifested as behavioral changes such as confusion, senility, fatigue, and weakness.

9. Prevention calls for frequent review of drug program, instructing family, and monitoring blood drug levels.

10. Children require a smaller dose because of decreased body fat and increased water content, immature liver and kidney function, along with decreased gastric acid, and increase transit time.

B. Weight

1. The average adult dose of a drug is based on a weight of 150 pounds.

2. Individuals who are overweight or under weight need to have their drug dosage determine.

3. Pediatric dosage is determined using the child weight and height to express dosage in body surface area.

C. Gender

1. Men tend to have more lean body mass than women. As a result, they need a larger drug dose. Women tend to have increased body fat and increased body water content, and as a result they need a decreased dosage.

D. Disease

1. Those that cause change in protein composition, kidney and liver disease, slowed circulation can lead to the accumulation of drugs with delayed distribution to tissues.

2. Diseases that increase the basal metabolic rate (BMR) such as in hyperthyroidism cause the rapid breakdown and excretion of drugs.

3. Hypothyroidism results in decreased BMR and breakdown and excretion of drugs in the body.

XIX. Medication Order

A. A medication order is needed for the administration of all drugs.

B. Physicians, physician assistants, nurse practitioners, midwives and dentists can write the medication orders.

C. Components of the medication order: date and time, client's name, drug name, drug dose, drug route, drug frequency, any special considerations, and signature.

D. Medication order can be computer-generated, manual, verbal, or telephone.

E. Computer-generated orders are more accurate because they can be scanned for safe dose, incompatibility allergy and high alert drugs.

F. The unit secretary can transcribe the medication order to the medication record.

G. The nurse is responsible for validation and interpretation of the medication order.

H. Types of orders:

1. Standing - until another order is written

2. Single - to be given once

3. Stat - to be given immediately

4. PRN – to be given when ever necessary

5. Verbal or telephone - taken in an emergency if the prescriber is not present or during a sterile procedure.

XX. Dispensing System

A. Computerized medication cart is an automated system that uses unit dose.

B. The cart contains medications that are frequently used in that unit.

C. It is the most cost -effective system and has the lowest error rate.

D. The nurse enters a code to access the cart and the medication is dispensed.

E. Unit dose: individual doses save time and reduce the need for dosage calculation and clients billed only for dosage used

F. The pharmacist refill medicine cart in a unit dose system daily

G. Floor stock multiple doses of frequently used medications are kept on the floor.

H. Readily available for use each time the client needs the drug.

I. It is cost effective but the error rate is high.

J. Individual prescription: used in home care 7 days to several week supply of medication, costly and error rate high.

XXI. Nursing Process and Drug Administration

A. This is the systematic gathering, organizing and interpretation of data to determine the clients nursing needs.

B. Assessment

1. Assessment begins with the gathering of subjective data and objective data.

2. Information needed on assessment, client's age, weight, height, diagnosis, allergies, lifestyle, habits, cognitive ability, sensory deficits, and support system.

3. Also need past medical history, surgical history, drug history including current drugs, over-the-counter drugs, herbal preparations, vitamins, contraceptive pills, and substances used for erectile dysfunction.

4. Question history of addiction to drugs or alcohol, and any drug reaction.

5. Complete physical assessment to gather baseline data, vital signs to include temperature, pulse, respiration, and blood pressure.

6. Assess lung sounds, bowel sounds, and circulation, and do a thorough examination of the skin.

7. Review pertinent laboratory tests.

C. Diagnosis

   1. Analyzing the collected data and making a statement covering the client problems.

   2. Any NANDA diagnosis can be used, but common ones are:

      a. Deficient Knowledge

      b. Noncompliance

      c. Ineffective Management of the Therapeutic Regimen

      d. Risk for Injury

D. Planning

   1. Stating the desired outcome and deciding what intervention will help including

   2. Setting goals and priorities

   3. Preparing client teaching materials

   4. Prepare for drug side effects by intervening e.g. stomach upset

   5. Making sure the drug is palatable

   6. Determining if there will be any drug incompatibility

   7. Determining if the route is safe

E. Implementation

   1. This step involves the administration of the drug, client teaching, or supervision.

   2. Implementation uses nursing judgment while observing the six rights.

   3. Implementation involves three types of nursing actions:

      a. Dependent, done based on the physician's orders

      b. Interdependent, done by consulting other members of the healthcare team to promote or restore health.

      c. Independent, done based on the nurse's education.

   4. Implementing the Five Rights

      a. Drug

         i. Use the 3 checks, check the label when the drug is remove, before dispense/pour, before return/discard.

         ii. Check carefully drugs with similar names or names that look alike or sounds alike.

         iii. Never use drugs from an unlabeled container; return to pharmacy for labeling and identification.

         iv. Never return drugs to a bottle once poured.

         v. Open unit dose package at the bedside.

         vi. Never administer a drug someone else has poured except multidose vials.

      vii. When opening multidose vial write, strength, date, and time prepared and signature.

      viii. Never leave medication at the bedside unless you have an order to self medicate

      ix. If there is uncertainty about the drug check the original doctor's order, doctor, charge, peer.

      x. Ask is the drug compatible with other drugs the client is taking?

  b. Dose

      i. Know the system of weight and measures.

      ii. Calculate accurately; always have someone else check.

      iii. Transcribe decimal with trailing zeros and zero before the decimal if no whole number.

      iv. Always determine if the dose is within safe limits, 10% variation allowed in the adult none in child.

      v. Have appropriate measuring devices when pouring liquid medicine and measure to the lowest point of the meniscus.

      vi. When drawing up from ampules or vials, or get rid of air bubbles to have the correct dose.

      vii. Check carefully if you have to give more than two tabs or more than 1 mL

  c. Client

      i. Need two forms of ID. Ask client to give name. Check ID bracelet.

      ii. Assess mental status; if impaired ask peer, family to identify client.

      iii. For children, can ask parents.

      iv. If the client questions anything, double-check from the beginning.

  d. Time

      i. Review symbols and abbreviations.

      ii. Make sure order specifies the time.

      iii. Some orders use meridian time, others use standard time.

      iv. Other drugs must be given at an exact time.

      v. Schedules are used to maintain a relatively constant blood drug level to achieve maximum effectiveness.

      vi. Give no more than ½ hour before or after drug is due.

      vii. Check if diagnostic test must be done prior to administering drug.

      viii. Some drugs given on an empty stomach e.g., ac; others are given after meals or p.c.

  e. Route

      i. Must know the route for each drug.

      ii. Route of administration affects the onset of action, side effects.

      iii. Always assess level of development to ensure route is safe.

    iv.   Gain the client's cooperation by explaining how the drug will be beneficial; do not force the client.

    v.   If several drugs must be given, give the most important first.

    vi.   Best vehicle to use with drugs is water.

    vii.   Always ask yourself if the route is compatible with the client's condition.

    viii.   If the client has nausea or vomits, withhold the drug and ask for the drug by rectal or parenteral route or give with food.

    ix.   If the client vomits within 20 minutes of receiving the drug, assess, measure vomitus, report, and await instructions; provide comfort measures; document.

f.   Chart

    i.   Document drug, dose, route, site, and date and time and client's response.

    ii.   Record and report adverse reaction to charge, doctor, pharmacist and complete drug reaction form.

    iii.   Record only after drug is given.

    iv.   If medication error occurs, inform charge nurse or doctor, and complete incidence report.

    v.   Chart fluid intake and health teaching.

g.   Evaluation

    i.   Assessing the effectiveness of the drugs. Questions to answer:

        (a) Did the medication alleviate the symptoms?

        (b) Were there any adverse reactions?

        (c) Does the client understand the purpose, precautions necessary when taking the drugs?

h.   Equipment

    i.   Gather cart, tray, cup, syringes, needles, alcohol prep, gloves, pill cutter and crusher, mortar and pestle, measuring cups, drinking cups, water, waste disposal, sharps, and stethoscope.

i.   Environment

    i.   Work away from traffic areas in an area that is quiet and free of distractions, with good lighting, a clean work surface, and clean hands.

    ii.   Most drugs are stored at room temperature; some are stored in refrigerator or frozen.

j.   Medication administration procedure

    i.   Check medication order against physician's order, medex, and/or medication administration record for completeness.

    ii.   Look up unfamiliar drugs. Be knowledgeable about drug actions, use, dosage, contraindications, precautions, interactions, adverse reactions, and nursing implications.

    iii.   Know the policy of the institution.

    iv.   In a manual system, check if the drug is on the unit, and reorder if necessary.

    v.   Assess, perform, or order any test or procedures to be done before the drug is given.

vi. Know and use only approved symbols and abbreviations.

vii. Give medications such as iron or diluted acids with a straw to prevent staining and weakening of the tooth enamel

viii. Never give a medication that is discolored , has precipitates, or has expired.

ix. If the client refuses the medication, don't force it, and find out why. Explain why the medication is being given. If the client still refuses, report to the charge nurse or doctor, record, and discard the medication unless it is a unit dose.

x. Stay with the client until the medication is swallowed.

xi. Check if client is NPO.

xii. Store internal and external medications separately.

xiii. Keep medications clean and, for sterile drugs, use aseptic technique.

xiv. Return in 20-30 minutes to assess client and medication effect.

xv. Ensure client safety at all times.

XXII. Medication Errors

A. Is a violation of one of the six rights.

B. Medication errors are reportable and are monitored by the United States Pharmacopoeia (U.S.P.) and Institute for Safe Medication Practices (I.S.M.P.), and by the Joint Commission (formerly called JCAHO).

C. These groups identify the number and type of medication errors reported and generate corrective measures to prevent repeated errors.

D. Medication errors cause 1 death per day and injure 1.3 million people annually.

E. USP, ISMP, and JCAHO national goal is the prevention of devastating medication error. They hope to accomplish this by education and teaching.

F. A medication error can occur anywhere in the distribution system, by nurse, doctor, or pharmacist.

G. Common causes of medication errors

1. Incorrect mathematical calculation, errors with decimal or zeros

2. Incorrectly reading the label

3. Poor packaging and labeling

4. Drugs that have names that look and sound alike

5. Inadequate knowledge of drugs

6. Improper use of abbreviations and illegible labeling

7. Failure to listen when a client questions a medication

8. Failure to educate clients about their medication

9. Failure to ID client

10. Failure to comply with policies and procedures

11. Increased workload

12. Poor reporting at shift change

13. Floating staff

14. Lack of critical thinking

H. How to overcome medication errors

1. Use of technology such as a computerized system and bar coding

2. Improvement in the nurse's knowledge of drug actions, uses side effects, expected dosage range, and contraindications.

3. Ability to think critically when applying the nursing process

4. Paying attention to details

5. Double-checking high-alert drugs (electrolytes, heparin, insulin, and morphine)

6. Therapeutic relationship and ability to listen

7. Clear written instructions

8. Use of appropriate measuring devices

9. Teaching for medications given in the home:

   a. Use reminders so they don't forget.

   b. Establish time to fit routine.

   c. Identify medication by name, not color.

   d. Use magnifying glass to help reading label.

   e. Use simply charts to emphasize time.

   f. Avoid medication in child-proof containers that make access difficult for the elderly.

   g. Prepour daily or weekly.

10. Critical thinking is applied in all phases of the nursing process. Critical thinking is needed for safe medication administration including:

    a. When calculating medication dosage.

    b. To challenge an order that is incorrect

    c. To distinguish between relevant and irrelevant information

    d. When reading a label and calculating dosages

    e. When selecting the correct type of syringe

    f. When clarifying that which is not understood.

XXIII. **Administration of Parenteral Medication and Fluids**

A. Parenteral administration

1. Parenteral medications are supplied as liquid or powder packaged in different ways.

   a. **Ampules:** single-use glass scored at the neck that holds liquid drug. To remove break and draw up without letting the needle tip touch the rim.

   b. **Vials:** plastic or glass containers, sealed, with metal cap and rubber diaphragm. Multi-dose or single doses; holds liquid or powder.

   c. **Mix O vial:** liquid separated from the powder by a rubber stopper; single use. Mix and use immediately.

    d. **Cartridges:** prefilled glass or plastic single dose containers. They need a special holder called a tubex or carpuject to release the medication.

    e. **Prepackaged syringes:** come in a single-dose syringe prepackaged with needle attached.

2. Parts of a syringe:

    a. Syringes are plastic and disposable; they are named based on their use or the quantity of fluids they hold (0.3 mL, to 50 or 60 mL).

    b. The barrel is the outer part with calibrations; this is not sterile.

    c. The plunger is the inner part that allows withdrawal and injection of fluid. This is always sterile.

    d. The tip holds the needle, styled in two ways -- plain or Luer-Lok.

3. Parts of a needle:

    a. Needles are stainless steel and disposable, named based on their diameter or gauge and length.

    b. The smaller the gauge the larger the diameter. The larger the gauge the smaller the diameter.

    c. Gauge goes from 14 to 30.

    d. The bevel is the tip and slanted area design to puncture the skin and cut with scalpel like precision.

    e. The shaft is sterile and is the part between the bevel and the hub and size is based on the length of the needle which could be 3/8 to 3 inches in length.

    f. The hub is the part that attaches to the needle and is also sterile.

4. Types of parenteral injections

    a. Intramuscular = Into a muscle

    b. Intravenous = Into a vein

    c. Subcutaneous = Into tissue beneath the skin

    d. Intradermal = Into the outer layer of the skin

    e. Intra- articular = Into the joint cavity

    f. Intrathecal = Into the spinal column

    g. Intracardiac = Into a chamber of the heart

    h. Intralesion = Into a lesion

5. Advantages of parenteral route

    a. Effective in an emergency or when client's LOC or mental status makes other routes difficult.

    b. Drugs not altered by gastric acids and cannot cause gastric irritation or be lost by vomiting.

    d. Precise dosage to targeted areas of the body.

6. Disadvantages of parenteral route

    a. Allergic reaction rapid

    b. Introduction of microbes leading to infection

   c. Injury to tissues such as blood vessels and nerves

   d. Breakage of the needle

   e. Injection in the wrong tissue could cause sterile abscess

   f. Could strike a bone

7. Assessment of site

   a. Inspect.

   b. Palpate to determine needle length and injection angle.

   c. Avoid lesions such as scars, moles, warts, or muscle wasting.

8. Intramuscular

   a. Used when the medication is irritating or painful.

   b. Absorption is fairly good as muscle has good blood supply.

   c. Syringe size 1-3 mL (cc).

   d. Needle length $\frac{1}{2}$ to $1\frac{1}{2}$ inches.

   e. Needle gauge 20-25

   f. Amount of fluid 1-3 mL, an average of 2 mL

   g. Angle of the injection 90 degrees.

9. Intramuscular sites

   a. Deltoid: site not fully developed until adolescence

      i. Used mainly for narcotics and sedative.

      ii. Cannot give more than 1 mL in this site.

      iii. Landmark: 2 to 3 fingers below the acromion process and for children 1 finger below.

   b. Dorsogluteal: injection into the gluteus maximus muscle

      i. Not used for children until they have been walking 1 full year or above age 3.

      ii. Landmark: Client in prone position toes pointed inwards to relax gluteal muscle and arms flexed towards the head.

      iii. Site can be landmark in two ways, one divide the buttocks into four equal parts and use the upper outer quadrant or quarter.

      iv. Draw an oblique line from the posterior superior iliac spine to the level of the great trochanter

   c. Ventrogluteal: injection into the gluteus medius and minimus muscle

      i. Landmark: Position clients to side with knees slightly bend and raised slightly towards the chest.

      ii. Use opposite hand. Place palm over the great trochanter of the femur and index finger on anterior superior iliac spine.

      iii. Spread fingers to form a V and give injection between the middle and index finger.

d.   Vastus lateralis: best site for children under 3

  i.   Landmark: One hand's breadth below the great and one hand's breadth above the knee.

  ii.   Lateralis to the side and the rectus femoris muscle to the anterior.

e.   Z track: A type of intramuscular injection recommended for drugs such as oil based meds, iron, or antibiotics.

  i.   Used a large muscle mass such as dorsogluteal or vastus lateralis.

  ii.   Prepare medication in the syringe expel air to get the exact dose.

  iii.   Draw up air into syringe 0.1 - 0. 2 ml air.

  iv.   Displace tissue to side.

  v.   Inject at a 90 degree angle.

  vi.   Aspirate to be sure you are not in a blood vessel.

  vii.   Inject slowly over 10 seconds.

  viii.   Release tissue, withdraw needle apply pressure do not massage.

10.   Subcutaneous/hypodermic:

a.   Used for drugs such as insulin and heparin.

b.   Syringe size 1-3 mL

c.   Needle length $\frac{3}{8}$ - $\frac{5}{8}$

d.   Needle gauge 25-27

e.   Amount fluid 1-2 mL (average 1 mL)

f.   Angle injection 45–90 degrees 90 for insulin and heparin.

g.   Sites: Over mid-deltoid muscle three fingers above elbow and below mid axilla line, lower abdomen 2 inches from umbilicus, upper anterior thigh, and subscapular region.

11.   Intradermal:

a.   Used for diagnostic purposes or allergic testing.

b.   Syringe size 1 cc

c.   Needle length $\frac{3}{8}$ - $\frac{5}{8}$

d.   Gauge 25 to 28

e.   Amount of fluid 0.01mL

f.   Angle of the injection 10 to 15 degrees

g.   Site: central forearm. Landmark, one hand's breadth above wrist using the anterior surface.

h.   Nursing judgment

  i.   Syringe selection based on amount of fluid

  ii.   Needle gauge selection based on viscosity of fluid

  iii.   Site selection based on drug route

      iv. Angle of needle based on type of injection and amount of tissue

      v. Site rotation for increased absorption, increased tissue integrity, decreased discomfort, and decreased lipodystrophy (fat atrophy) seen with insulin injection

B. Intravenous administration

  1. Advantage: large volumes of fluid can be delivered

  2. Uses

     a. Diagnostic therapeutic reasons.

     b. Maintain fluid electrolyte balance and provide nutrition.

     c. Doctor's order needed for type fluid, amount fluid, and infusion rate.

     d. Once on IV fluid, client must be on intake and output.

     e. Can be inserted peripherally or centrally.

  3. Peripheral line insertion

     a. IV solution comes in plastic bags that are sterile.

        i. Some are nonvented, meaning the atmospheric pressure pushes against the plastic to force fluid out.

        ii. Some are vented, meaning air must enter to allow flow; these are usually glass bottles.

        iii. IV solutions are in glass bottles because they are unstable in plastic.

        iv. Some are use-activated containers for piggyback administration, such as antibiotics.

        v. Use-activated containers have compartments with a permeable ingredient that forms an admixture when mixed.

        vi. Use-activated container are used for drugs with a short half-life.

     b. IV sets: are vented or nonvented, micro or macro, primary or secondary.

        i. Macro drip sets are calibrated 10 drops/milliliter, 15drops/milliliter, 20 drops/milliliter.

        ii. Micro drip sets are calibrated 60 drops/milliliter.

        iii. They are designed for use with gravity IV or for use with electronic infusion pump.

        iv. Primary sets are 66 to 100 inches long and contain a Y port with a resealable rubber.

        v. Primary IV sets have a back check valve to prevent solution from the secondary set from entering the primary line.

        vi. Secondary sets are 32 to 42 inches long, used for piggyback.

        vii. Metered volume chambers hold up to 150 mL and are used for children and critically ill adults to prevent overload.

     c. IV cannula

        i. Butterfly, inside-needle catheter and over-the-needle catheter

        ii. Sizes 16 to 24 gauge.

        iii. Dwell time on average 96 hours.

       iv. Gauge selection is based on the size of the vein and the length of therapy.

       v. 22 to 24 gauge for most fluids

  d. Add-on: stopcock used to control the direction of flow by manual manipulation

       i. J and U and T adapters and connections used at injection site help ease manipulation and access.

       ii. Filters are porous devices that prevent passage undesirable substances entering the blood stream.

       iii. Filters used for removal of particulate matter, dust, plastic and bacteria.

       iv. Most IV tubing has built-in filter, or filters can be added on

       v. There are three types of filter: membrane, depth, and screen.

       vi. The most common size filters are 0.22 to 220 microns.

  e. Pumps:

       i. Controller pumps count drops using gravity as a source of pressure; once kept 36 inches above the heart.

       ii. Volumetric pump use constant force to overcome pressures in lines and need special tubing.

       iii. Syringe pump use for giving analgesic; control rate by drives speed and syringe size.

       iv. Smart pumps used to aid the delivery of correct concentrations and dose of high alert drugs.

       v. Pump alarms warn of occlusion, air, but not for infiltration.

  f. Procedure for insertion

       i. Start with distal veins such as those in dorsum of hand and work upwards.

       ii. Select first veins in the non dominant hand.

       iii. Never use an arm with arteriovenous shunt, fistula, edema, areas with decreased sensation, or post mastectomy.

       iv. Avoid flex joints, such as those in legs.

       v. IVs placed in peripheral veins in the legs cause increased risk of thrombophlebitis.

       vi. Common veins selected are metacarpal, basilica, and cephalic.

       vii. Personnel who can start a peripheral IV: physicians, registered professional nurses, and practical nurses.

  g. Steps

       i. Check IV bag for leakage.

       ii. Check IV fluid; it must be crystal clear.

       iii. Do not use if cloudy, discolored, or beyond expiration date.

       iv. Fill drip chamber halfway; prime the tubing.

       v. Clean the skin with alcohol then iodine; some facilities use chlorohexidine.

       vi. Use universal precautions.

      vii. Check for latex allergy by asking if allergic to bananas, avocado, kiwi, or chestnuts.

      viii. Elevate solution 36 inches above the heart.

      ix. IV insertion causes some degree of pain; to decrease, use topical anesthesia.

      x. Topical anesthetic-use EMLA anesthetic; onset of action 5 to 6 minutes, peak in 1 to 2 hr

      xi. Reduce needlesticks by using visualization technology such as portable ultrasound.

      xii Must be trained to use technology and use must be documented.

      xiii. Clean skin with alcohol, then iodine or chlorohexidine.

      xiv. Catheter stabilization: use sterile tape, surgical strips, or manufacturer securement device.

      xv. Catheter stabilization decreases incidence of restarts, infection, infiltration, and extravasation.

      xvi. Always restart IV if complaint of pain, discomfort, or any complication.

4. Central lines

    a. The advantage of central lines is a decrease in complications.

    b. Common sites used: subclavian vein to superior vena cava to right atrium.

    c. Central lines can be short term (less than 30 days), intermediate (up to 42 days), or long term (more than 42 days).

    d. Long-term catheters are tunneled catheters.

    e. With tunneled catheters a portion of the catheter lies within the subcutaneous tissue before exiting the body.

    f. They are catheters such as Broviac, Hickman, and Groshong.

    g. Catheters can be single, double, or triple lumen.

    h. Some catheters are peripherally inserted, such as PICC lines.

        i. PICC lines are 20 to 24 inches in length and made from flexible soft material.

        ii. PICC lines can be advanced until the distal tip of the catheter rests in the superior vena cava.

        iii. Never take blood pressure on the arm with PICC insertion.

    i. Midline catheters are about 6 inches in length and are usually inserted in a large vein.

        i. Midline catheters are used when a peripheral line is needed with increase blood flow.

    j. X-ray confirmation is needed to check correct placement of PICC and subclavian lines.

    k. They are dressed using semi-permeable dressings.

    l. Can never be wet during shower or bath.

    m. Injection port must be cleaned with alcohol before each access.

    n. Infusion ports are catheters surgically placed into a blood vessel attached to a reservoir implanted under the skin for long-term chemotherapy.

PEARSON

5. Other types of IV

    a. IV bolus direct injection in the vein performed RN or MD

        i. Heparin lock catheter *in situ* in a vein serves as access to infuse fluids or drugs intermittently or continuously.

        ii. Hep lock allows the client free ambulating without IV pole or pump.

        iii. The line is flushed using 2 to 3 ml of normal saline or heparinized solution.

        iv. Flush using the acronym S.A.S.H:

            S   saline to determine potency

            A   administer medication

            S   saline to advance medication

            H   heparinized solution prevents blood clot in catheter

    b. IV Piggyback IV: added to another IV at the Y port

        i. Piggyback delivers drugs such as antibiotic by intermittent infusion (tandem).

        ii. When using piggyback, the primary line remains open.

        iii. Piggyback is positioned higher than the primary line to run by gravity.

        iv. At completion of piggyback, primary line will continue at a slow rate.

6. Possible complications

    a. Nonvesicant infiltration is the most common complication.

        i. Needle becomes dislodged, piercing the vein and allowing fluid to collect in surrounding tissue.

        ii. Infiltration can be placed on a scale according to severity from 0 (no symptoms) to 5 (severe pain and impairment).

        iii. Presenting signs and symptoms: area cold, shiny, swollen and painful.

        iv. Actions: inform charge nurse, doctor, stop the IV, remove, apply cold pack, elevate limb, and prepare new IV.

    b. Extravasation

        i. Infiltration of vesicant solution results in tissue breakdown or sloughing and necrosis.

        ii. Caused by infiltration of substances such as antineoplastic drugs and levophed.

        iii. Actions: report, stop infusion; the RN or MD can use a 3 cc syringe to withdraw as much medication as possible.

        iv. Catheter must be removed, apply ice pack x 30 minutes, and elevate extremity.

        v. Drugs like corticosteroids may be prescribed and administered.

    c. Thrombophlebitis

        i. *Thrombo* means clot, occurs on the walls of the vein.

        ii. *Phlebitis* is inflammation of the vein.

        iii. Clot and inflammation of the vein occur separately or together.

iv. Phlebitis can be mechanical, pertaining to problems with catheter ,or chemical, pertaining to problems with solution and from bacterial infection.

v. Signs and symptoms: redness, tenderness, streaking along vein, heat; vein feels cord-like.

vi. Severity can be placed on a scale of 0 (no pain) to 4+ pain.

vii. If infection, culture and sensitivity order for bacteriostatic ointment or course of antibiotics is given.

d. Pulmonary edema

i. Pulmonary edema is caused by overload of circulation due to rapid infusion of IV fluids.

ii. Most commonly seen in children, elderly, or cardiac clients.

iii. Sign and symptoms: increased pulse, increased blood pressure, dyspnea, frothy sputum, and crackles in lung.

iv. Actions: slow IV, keep vein open, and call for help.

v. Doctor will prescribe diuretics like lasix to get rid of fluid.

e. Pyrogenic reaction

i. Pyrogenic reaction results from bacterial contamination of IV fluid.

ii. Signs and symptoms: headaches, nausea and vomiting, fever and chills.

iii. Immediately stop and remove the IV; send fluid to pharmacy for analysis.

f. Catheter embolus

i. Catheter embolus results when a piece of catheter breaks off and travels in the bloodstream and obstructs blood flow.

ii. Signs and symptoms: pain along vein and shock.

iii. Immediate actions: notify charge nurse, remove IV, inspect catheter, save catheter.

iv. If broken, place a tourniquet on the limb high above insertion point to prevent catheter migration.

v. X-ray will be ordered by the doctor to locate the catheter.

vi. The client is prepared for surgery.

g. Air embolus

i. Air embolus occurs when a bolus of air from the IV line enters the bloodstream.

ii. This can occur while changing IV bag or if air in a central line enters the blood stream.

iii. Air embolus may enter the lung or heart and cause obstruction of blood flow.

iv. Signs and symptoms, are sudden onset anxiety, lightheadedness, confusion, shortness of breath, tachycardia, cyanosis and shock.

v. Immediate action, call for help, stay with client, place the client on left side with head lower to stop embolus from entering the heart.

vi. Stop infusion and inspect for empty bag, disconnection of IV line or a leak in system.

7. Assessment care of an intravenous infusion

    a. New order for IV fluid daily.

    b. Change IV solution q 24 hr.

    c. Change IV tubing q 48 - 72 hr.

    d. Change IV dressing q 24 - 48 hr.

    e. Change transparent dressings only as necessary.

    f. Watch for symptoms of complication, infiltration, phlebitis etc.

    g. No blood pressure in arm with PICC or midline catheter.

    h. Check placement in vein.

    i. Maintain the correct flow rate; check q 15-min to 1 hr.

    j. Use arm board to stabilize if needed.

Additional Resources Found on MyNursingLab

- Drug Metabolization animation
- Injections animation
- Pharmacology and the Elderly video

PEARSON

MODULE 2

Fundamentals

Submodule 2.1 Nursing Process

Learning Objectives

2.1.1   Describe the nursing process as it is used in nursing practice.

2.1.2   Describe the steps in the nursing process.

I.   **The Nursing Process**

    A   The nursing process is organized on the principles of scientific reasoning and is the base from which the nurse promotes and maintains the health of his or her clients.

    B.   It incorporates critical thinking to promote reasonable, sound nursing decisions and actions.

    C.   The nursing process is dynamic because it allows for changes and modification based on the client's needs and changing health status.

    D.   It is a continuous and overlapping process that allows individual care of the client in any care setting from hospital to community.

    E.   The nursing process consists of the following five parts: assessment, diagnosis, planning, implementation, and evaluation:

II.   **Steps of the Nursing Process**

    A.   Assessment

        1.   This is the phase in which data is collected and analyzed, and inferences are drawn from the information about the client. Data is collected from several sources.

            a.   Primary data is collected from the client.

            b.   Secondary data is collected from the client's family or medical records.

        2.   Initial nursing assessment is obtained by interview at the client's admission.

        3   The interview is set up and conducted using basic communication skills.

        4.   An assessment is called a focused assessment when it targets a specific nursing problem.

        5.   In a comprehensive assessment of the client the nurse collects both subjective and objective data.

        6.   Subjective data tells how clients view their health concerns and is the sharing of thoughts or feelings with the nurse.

        7.   Symptoms such as anxiety, stress, or pain are examples of subjective data.

        8.   Objective data is what the nurse observes and is measurable, descriptive,   and concise.

9. Examples of objective data are measurements of blood pressure and observation of a lesion on the skin.

10. Collection of data aids in the diagnosing, planning, implementing, and evaluation of client care. Data collected consists of:

    a. Biographical information.

    b. Past medical history.

    c. Family health history.

    d. Cultural practices.

    e. Spiritual practices.

    f. Present illness.

    g. Reason for seeking health care.

    h. Psychological coping.

    i. Observation of the client and the client's environment.

    j. Determination of functional status.

    k. Performance of physical exam from head to toe.

    l. Gathering of baseline vital signs, weight, height, and level of pain.

    m. Review of any diagnostic tests and laboratory tests.

    n. Collection of all laboratory specimens ordered.

11. Once accurate data is collected, it is analyzed, validated, and interpreted using critical thinking.

12. To validate data, consider the source and communicate with the client to check its accuracy.

13. Organize the collected data into patterns or clusters that reflect the client's needs for assistance or support

14. The pattern or clusters are then documented using Maslow's hierarchy of basic needs

B. Diagnosis

    1. The nursing diagnosis is a statement of the client's health problems.

    2. Nursing diagnosis differs from medical diagnosis.

    3. Medical diagnoses are based on disease pathology, signs, symptoms, diagnostic tests, and procedures.

    4. Nursing diagnoses are based on actual data about the human responses of the client to illness or to physical or psychological threats.

    5. These threats can be actual or potential.

    6. Actual threats are based on reported or observed symptoms.

    7. Potential threats are based on things for which the client is vulnerable and the nurse can intervene.

    8. The first part of the nursing diagnosis uses common language and standard statements endorsed by NANDA International. An example is Acute Pain.

9. The next part of the diagnosis describes the etiology, which is the set of social, environmental, situational, or physical factors that contribute to the client's problem.

10. These contributing factors serve to direct the nursing interventions.

11. The cause of the problem must be verified by the client to ensure its accuracy.

12. Prioritizing of the nursing diagnosis uses the nurse's judgment to determine which problem must be addressed first.

13. Maslow's theory of basic needs is the theory used to set priorities. This theory uses a ladder or hierarchy from basic need for survival to higher level needs.

14. Physiological needs are basic to survival and are the needs for food, air, water, shelter, rest, sleep, and elimination. These needs must be satisfied before the client can be concerned about other needs.

15. Safety and security are the client's need for physical and psychological wellbeing.

16. Love and belonging needs are those related to satisfying relationships and the giving and receiving of affection.

18. Self-esteem is feeling good about one's self.

19. Self-actualization relates to reaching one's full potential.

C. Planning

1. This step in the nursing process begins with the development of goals and nursing interventions to decrease or eliminate the client's identified problems.

2. The nurse develops goals and outcomes and nursing interventions in a written plan

3. Outcomes must be based on the client's assessed needs. They must be reasonable and within the client's ability to accomplish.

4. Outcomes must be measurable by observation of some specific criteria and by time frame.

5. Client goals can be short term, meaning the client can accomplish these in a few hours or a few days.

6. Long-term goals are those that can be accomplished in weeks or months and are those the client must ultimately reach.

7. Nursing interventions, actions, or nursing orders are written activities most likely to cause a positive outcome, either in the short term or long term. Client responses to interventions are part of client outcomes.

8. Nursing interventions are based on scientific rationales, reasoning, or evidence-based practice.

9. Care plans are written documents that guide the nurse in providing client care.

10. Care plans are developed after admission and change frequently to reflect the client's health status.

D. Implementation

1. The fourth step of the nursing process is providing actual care to the client based on clinical judgment and involves the delegating of care to licensed and unlicensed personnel.

2. The implementation of nursing care is designed to meet established goals and includes both physical and psychological care of clients and their environment.

3. In the implementation of care, the nurse takes actions (called interventions) that are dependent, interdependent, or independent.

4. Dependent actions are those that are carried out based on the doctor's order for medication or treatments.

5. Interdependent actions are those that the nurse that makes in collaboration with others while using nursing judgment. Example: giving PRN medication for a specific set of symptoms.

6. Independent actions are those made by the nurse based on the client's needs. No doctor's order is necessary; an example is a decision about ADL.

7. After implementation, documentation of all pertinent data related to the care given and the client's response to care it is very important.

E. Evaluation

1. This final step of the nursing process is client focused and measures the effectiveness of the care plan.

2. The client's response to care is analyzed, and factors that contribute to the success or failure of the plan are reviewed.

3. The goals that are achieved are labeled as such and those not achieved will trigger further assessment.

4. Evaluation should always lead to the revision of the plan of care and new goals and interventions designed to address unmet needs.

Additional Resources Found on MyNursingLab

- Thinking Critically, Making Decisions, Solving Problems video

MODULE 2

Fundamentals

Submodule 2.2 The Health Team and Healthcare System

Learning Objectives

2.2.1   List and describe the role of members of the health team.

2.2.2   Describe and explain three levels of health care.

I. Healthcare Team

   A.   The Licensed Practical Nurse (LPN) or Licensed Vocational Nurse (LVN)

     1.   Functions under direction of the registered nurse, licensed physician, or dentist in:

       a.   Disease prevention/Health promotion

       b.   Health teaching

       c.   Health counseling

       d.   Provision of supportive and restorative care

       e.   Administration of medication and therapeutic treatments

     2.   Makes pertinent observations, reports, and records

     3.   Assists in meeting client's physical, emotional, and psychological needs

     4.   May, under direction of RN, supervise nursing assistants/UAP, CNAs, etc.

     5.   Collaborates with other healthcare staff

     6.   Nurse Practice Acts varies from State to State – LPN/LVN should be familiar with laws that govern nursing in State where he/she practices; duties will vary with policies of different agencies and with conditions of employment.

   B.   The Registered Nurse

     1.   Diagnoses and treats human responses to actual or potential health problems through:

       a.   Disease prevention/Health promotion g

       b.   Health teaching

       c.   Health counseling

       d.   Provision of care supportive to or restorative of life and well-being

     2.   Executes medical regiments prescribed by licensed physician or dentist

     3.   Assesses total client care needs

     4.   Develops nursing care plan based upon client's diagnosis and psychological, emotional, and physical needs

     5.   Implements nursing intervention based upon medical regimen and nursing care plan

6. Evaluates client care plan

7. Revises and modifies nursing care plan to meet client's changing needs

8. Supervises and evaluates members of nursing team who assist implementing nursing care plan

9. Collaborates with other members of health care team

10. Audits and maintains nursing records

C. The Physician

1. Diagnoses client's illness by taking a complete history

2. Performs a thorough physical examination

3. Orders necessary diagnostic tests

4. Requests necessary consultants

5. Establishes a medical care plan for client which includes orders for medications, orders for specific therapeutic diets, orders for physiotherapy when necessary

6. Writes orders for client's degree of activity

7. Records daily progress notes describing client's reaction to therapeutic regimen

8. Records statement of medical goals for client

D. The Medical Social Worker

1. Aids client in dealing with social service agencies and community; helps client with third-party financial aid for Medicaid, etc

2. Aids client in making plans for future care

3. Studies client's home situation and counsels clients and family about client's illness

4. Provides referrals as needed

E. The Nutritionist

1. Supervises preparation of client's therapeutic diet

2. Consults with client about diet

F. The Physiotherapist

1. Aids in socialization of client

2. Uses group therapy techniques in working with handicapped clients

3. Aids clients who have limited motion in hands and fingers

4. Assists clients in achieving the activities of daily living

G. Occupational Therapist

1. Initiate the use of assistive devices to aid in activities of daily living

2. Identify problems with fine motor movement

3. Retrain muscles to improve activities of daily living

H. Speech Therapist

1. Provide rehabilitation for clients with speech or swallowing disorders

  I. Nursing Assistants

    1. Gives direct care to clients under supervision of the RN and LPN/LVN

    2. Helps other members of the nursing staff in giving client care

    3. Helps to maintain the proper client environment

  J. The Spiritual Advisor

    1. Helps clients to identify any emotional and physiological problems

    2. Helps clients to resolve these problems

    3. Gives spiritual comfort to clients

II. Levels of Health Care

  A. Primary-aimed at the promotion of health and disease prevention

  B. Secondary-aimed at early diagnosis and treatment

  C. Tertiary-aimed at rehabilitation to the individual's highest level of functioning

Additional Resources Found on MyNursingLab

MODULE 2

Fundamentals

Submodule 2.3 Culture

Learning Objectives

2.3.1   Define how culture and ethnicity affect values, beliefs, and behaviors.

2.3.2   Identify how cultural concepts affect healthcare delivery.

2.3.3   Describe different family structures and roles.

2.3.4   Describe the purpose of religion and its relevance to client care.

I. Theories of Culture

A. Nurses work with families, groups, individuals, and the community, and as a result they interact with many different cultures.

    1. Nursing theorist, Madeline Leininger, developed the theory of transcultural nursing as a framework within which the nurse views the client.

    2. Transcultural nursing proposed that the nurse make professional decisions by recognizing that clients belong to one world with many cultures.

    3. Transcultural nursing allows the nurse to care for clients anywhere in the world with respect and dignity.

B. The first step in providing transcultural nursing is to understand the different cultures in the world.

    1. Culture is a unique dynamic social pattern of behavior practiced by a group and passed down from one generation to another.

    2. Culture incorporates customs, values, beliefs, and ways of functioning typical to people who belong to that group.

    3. Learned interactions with other members determine how individuals interact within the wider population.

    4. Culture explains one pattern of thoughts and actions.

    5. Culture is dynamic. It changes over time through socialization with other communities. This adaptation allows the culture to survive.

    6. Culture can determine male/female roles, language use, styles of communication, health practices, child rearing practices, food preferences, and religious practices.

    7. Subcultures exist within dominant cultures, and a person can belong to more than one subculture. In subcultures the person interacts but retains the fundamental beliefs and even language of the primary culture.

    8. Subcultures include groups in a society to which individuals belong, such as community organizations, professions, and religious or other groups with their own rules and code of conduct.

II. Cultural Concepts

A. Terms and definitions

1. **Beliefs** determine socialization patterns, rituals, and problem solving within cultures.

2. **Values** provide the framework from which members of a culture determine what actions are considered good or bad.

3. **Norms** assign roles and ranking to each member within the culture, and also determine code of dress, manners, and basic rules on how members interact.

4. **Sanctions** are the punishment for violation of cultural laws, rules, and morals.

5. **Symbols** are the nonverbal communication patterns within a culture.

6. **Race** identifies people by biological differences such as skin color, hair texture, and eye color.

7. **Ethnicity** refers to values, ideals, attitudes, and behavior of people with a shared culture, race, or geographic area. Cultural diversity is evidenced by the many different cultural groups the nurse interacts with daily.

8. **Prejudice** is an unfair belief or bias (often unconscious and irrational) which is directed to a certain group of people.

9. **Ethnocentrism** is the belief that one's culture is better than another.

10. **Ethnocentrism** can lead to stereotyping (assigning common attributes to all members of a group) and prejudice).

11. **Racism** is a belief in the inferiority of people belonging to a different culture or having different physical characteristics.

12. **Discrimination** occurs when a group or individual is denied equality in treatment because of characteristic such as race, ethnicity, gender, or disability.

13. **Cultural sensitivity** is understanding, respecting, and being compassionate to people from different cultures.

B. Cultural awareness and tolerance by the nurse are essential to be sensitive and to show respect for clients from different cultures.

1. Components of cultural awareness:

   a. Knowing one's own culture

   b. Recognizing our own personal feelings

   c. Recognizing what makes us vulnerable

   d. Understanding our own personal values

   e. Knowing how the behavior of others affects us

C. The major cultural groups:

1. African Americans, Arab Americans, Asian Americans, European Americans, Hispanic Americans, and Native American.

   a. Many cultural groups have overlapping or similarities in beliefs and practices.

   b. Most cultural groups have a primary language and speak English plus their local or regional dialects.

   c. Families that are organized as matriarchal are African American and Native American.

d. Patriarchal family organization is seen among Arab Americans, Asian Americans, and Hispanic Americans.

e. European American families may be patriarchal or matriarchal.

2. African Americans

   a. Origins: the continent of Africa and the Caribbean.

   b. The primary language is English plus local regional dialects.

   c. Families are largely matriarchal with many single parent and extended families.

   d. Pregnancy and childbirth considered a natural process.

   e. Health and illness can be an act of God or due to exposure to cold temperatures or evil.

   f. Traditional medicines used along with herbal medicines

   g. Distrust of healthcare system

   h. Death is not seen as the end but chance of life in a better place.

3. Arab Americans

   a. Origins: the Middle East

   b. Most speak English but the primary language is Arabic.

   c. Many wear western clothing; others wear traditional clothes.

   d. Women may have to cover their head, face, wrists, and ankles.

   e. Families are patriarchal and include extended families with clearly defined roles by age and sex.

   f. Western medicine is practiced.

   g. During pregnancy or birthing, women are cared for by female healthcare professionals.

   h. Diet includes periods of fasting and periods of religious prayer scheduled during the day.

   i. Illness and death are seen as God's will and as punishment for sins.

4. Asian Americans

   a. Origins: regions of the Pacific.

   b. Most speak English, and primary language is country specific.

   c. Families are patriarchal and include extended families.

   d. Health is a balance of Yin and Yang which means positive/negative, hot/cold, opposing yet complementary phenomena.

   e. Western medicine is used along with traditional interventions of meditation, herbal medicine, and acupuncture.

   f. Pregnancy and childbirth is a period of contentment. Avoiding milk in the diet relieves many discomforts and promotes an active child.

   g. Death is seen as God's decision. Only women grieve openly.

5. European Americans:

    a. Families may be either patriarchal or matriarchal.

    b. Individuals are responsible for their own health.

    c. Western medicine used, incorporating any other treatment modality that has been researched and proven.

    d. View of death based on religion.

6. Hispanic Americans

    a. Origins: many countries in South America, and that makes this a very diverse culture.

    b. Spanish is the predominant language but many speak English.

    c. Family patterns are large extended families.

    d. Illness is caused by internal and external forces, imbalances in hot and cold, or supernatural forces.

    e. Western medicine is combined with the use of healers, and birthing is by lay midwives.

    f. Pregnancy is a happy natural process.

7. Native Americans

    a. Indigenous to the Americas

    b. Belong to different tribes

    c. Families are matriarchal and include extended families.

    d. Good health means that one is in harmony with the universe.

    e. Illness is due to imbalance in the universe.

    f. Western medicine is used along with the medicine man and herbal medicine.

    g. Pregnancy is natural, and birthing is attending by several close family members.

III. **Family**

A. Family is the basic organizing unit to which an individual belongs.

B. Families consist of two or more people who coexist based on shared values.

    1. The family functions include:

        a. Protecting its members from forces within or from the outside environment to allow for the survival of its members.

        b. Nurturing and providing love, affection, acceptance, and support of its members throughout their life cycle.

        c. Physical maintenance of its members in an environment where their basic needs for food, water, and shelter can be met.

        d. Socialization, the education of family members to enable them to function in the larger communities of school and work.

        e. Reproduction and recreation, which ensures the survival of the family.

    2. Types of families

        a. Nuclear family: Husband, wife, and children

b. Extended family: Husband, wife, children, and grandparents or other family

c. Single parent family: One parent and children

d. Blended or reconstituted family: Remarriage with children from both parents living together

e. Cohabiting family: Two people, man and woman, living together without legal marriage. This may also include children from other relationships or marriage.

f. Communal family: Groups living together with children, because they share similar values. All adults share in the discipline and nurturing of the children.

g. Foster or adoptive family: Family that raises children that are not their own; some arrangements are for temporary care, while others end with legal adoption.

h. Gay/Lesbian family: same-sex couples living together with their biological , foster, or adopted children.

3. Family Stages

a. Couple: Two people enter a relationship and move in together with the hope of marriage and a future together.

b. Childbearing: The first child arrives and calls for an adjustment in roles and routines.

c Grown children

d. Older family stage

4. Family Health

a. Family health is the means by which the family as a group integrates health practices as a part of their daily routines to promote the mental and physical health of each of its members.

b. A holistic approach to client care holds the nurse responsible for incorporating family health at the center of practice.

c. Family health is contingent on family rituals and family routines that help to promote adherence to established medical treatments.

d. These routines and rituals distinguish one family from another and set the foundation for families' ability to cope with issues of health promotion, disease prevention, or illness.

e. To help prevent family stress, family routines and rituals must include family members who live far away.

f. When family members become ill or disabled they usually are cared for by an older female relative, who often has her own medical problems.

g. Nurses must continually determine the impact of illness, disability, and recovery on a family.

h. How a family changes as a result of illness or disability depends on family resources and the coping strategies they have previously established.

i. Knowing who will be the caregiver for a sick or disabled family member

j. Setting respite, meaning who will relieve that member to prevent exhaustion and stress.

k. Communication links with the healthcare professional, pharmacy, or health insurance agents.

    l.   Transportation arrangements to and from appointments and activities.

    m. Handling economic issues and providing economic support

    n.   Shopping and preparation of healthy foods.

    o.   Patterns of sleeping of its member and who is the nighttime caregiver.

IV. Religion

A. Religion is part of spirituality.

B. Spirituality helps the individual to find a purpose for life.

C. Religion can be interwoven in culture and ethnicity.

D. Clients should be given every opportunity to have their spiritual needs satisfied.

E. Religious beliefs are critical in helping a client cope with illness as well as a means of promoting health and reducing stress.

F. Some of the common Christian religions practiced are Catholic and Protestant (including Baptist, Episcopalian, Presbyterian, Adventist, Lutheran, Seventh Day Adventist, Jehovah Witness, Christian Scientist, and Mormon). Nonchristian religions include Judaism, Buddhism, and Islam.

Additional Resources Found on MyNursingLab

MODULE 2

Fundamentals

Submodule 2.4 Legal and Ethical Issues

Learning Objectives

2.4.1   Describe legal and ethical aspects of nursing.

2.4.2   Discuss the importance of advance directives.

    I. **Legal Aspects of Nursing**

        A. Nurse Practice Act

            1. Laws pertaining to the practice of nursing vary from state to state.

            2. Other laws establish curriculum requirements for the approval of nursing schools (accreditation).

            3. State Boards of Nursing monitor nursing schools and approve new programs.

            4. State Boards of Nursing grant and renew licenses for qualified individuals.

            5. State Boards of Nursing investigate allegations of unsafe practice.

        B. Legal aspects of nursing

            1. The laws of the state control the practice of nursing in the state.

            2. The LPN/LVN is accountable for providing quality nursing care.

            3. Providing quality care will protect the LPN/LVN from criminal prosecution.

        C. The Patient's Bill of Rights

            1. The patient has a right to considerate and respectful care.

            2. The patient has the right to be treated with dignity.

            3. The patient has the right to obtain information concerning treatment.

            4. The patient has the right to receive information to make an informed consent.

            5. The patient has the right to refuse treatment.

            6. The patient has the right to privacy concerning medical care and records.

            7. The patient rightly can expect all records to be treated as confidential.

            8. The patient has a right to get a reasonable response from a hospital.

            9. The patient has a right to know the relationship of his or her hospital to other care agencies.

          10. The patient has a right to know if the hospital is involved in any experimentation.

          11. The patient has a right to expect reasonable continuity of care.

          12. The patient has a right to examine information regarding his or her bill.

          13. The patient has a right to know hospital regulations

D. Types of legal action

1. Civil: relates to the individual's right.

2. Criminal: involves the person and society.

E. Negligence or malpractice

1. Malpractice is misconduct by a professional person (e.g., LPN/LVN).

2. Negligence is conduct that falls below an acceptable established standard.

F. Elements required to prove negligence

1. Duty – The nurse did not provide care based on standards.

2. Breach of duty – the nurse did not adhere to an acceptable standard.

3. Proximate – the nurse left out an action or performed a questionable action (omission or commission)

4. Damages – the action resulted in injury in some way.

G. Torts

1. A wrong or injury done that involves violation of one's rights.

2. Unintentional tort: Act that results in unintended injury, or negligence

3. Intentional tort: Deliberate and willful act that results in injury or violation of one's rights.

4. Assault: Unjustified attempt or threat to touch someone

5. Battery: Actual physical harm to or touching someone

6. False imprisonment: Detaining someone against their will

7. Libel: Defamation through written communication

8. Slander: Defamation through oral communication

9. Abandonment: legal term that implies the healthcare worker has prematurely stopped care of the client.

H. Risk management

1. Process of identifying and reducing cost of anticipated losses.

2. Evaluation and review of all problems in the workplace.

3. Identifying common elements when error or injuries occur OK?

4. Develops methods to reduce their risk of occurrence.

I. Incident report

1. A primary tool of risk management

2. Completed by healthcare worker who makes discovery of an error

3. Is not punitive, but collects and reports factual data

4. Should include who, what, where, when, and actions taken at the time

5. Does not become part of the client's record.

J. Good Samaritan law

1. In some states, these provide legal immunity for rescuers who provide first aid in emergency.

2. These emergencies or accidents must be outside of the hospital.

3. Healthcare providers are held to a higher standard based on training.

K. Consent

1. Informed consent:

a. Must be signed by all clients before any kind of special or invasive procedure.

b. The client must be fully informed by the physician of all benefits and risks of procedures.

c. Consent is obtained by the physician and can be witnessed by the nurse.

II. Ethical Issues in Nursing

A. Nursing ethics

1. Ethics is a branch of philosophy that examines what is right and what is wrong

2. Nursing ethics provides the foundation and principles by which nurses practice.

3. Ethics has several branches

a. **Meta-ethics,** which explores is the nature of morality and is the basis for analyzing the nature of an ethical problem. Meta-ethics tells us what acts are considered good and what acts are considered bad.

b. **Normative ethics** is the study of how people should act and what should be done in a given situation.

c. **Bioethics** is concerned with questions of euthanasia, the allocation of health resources, and use of embryonic cells.

B. Nursing ethics is applied ethics involving the human rights of all people.

1. The code of nursing practice serves as a guide for each individual's obligation to practice nursing. These codes set standards of practice that are not negotiable. The standards provide nursing with a commitment to society and to patients seeking health care. They set a standard for responding to illness in all practice roles and all care settings.

2. Nursing ethics promotes autonomy, nonmaleficence, beneficence, justice, veracity, and fidelity.

3. Autonomy

a. Is respect for human dignity and rights regardless of the client's health problems, functional status, disease, disability, or proximity to death. It includes respecting human needs and values without prejudice for lifestyle, religion, or culture and honoring the person's choices.

b. A part of autonomy calls for collaboration, which is working towards a shared goal within the scope of practice. Collaboration calls for mutual recognition and respect for shared decision making among healthcare workers.

4. Nonmaleficence

   a. This is the obligation to do or cause no harm to another. In nonmaleficence the nurse cannot act to end a person's life but must advocate for the client. This role of advocate helps to minimize unwanted treatment such as interventions that cause the patient suffering.

   b. The withholding of lifesaving choices such as nutrition and hydration and maintenance of advance directive is included.

   c. Confidentiality protects participants in research, which needs legal authorization and an explanation of how data will be used and protected.

5. Beneficence

   a. This is the duty to treat clients well and maintain a balance between benefits and harm; this includes the right to self-determination.

   b. Clients have a moral and legal right to determine what will be done to them and to receive accurate, complete, dependable information

   c. Weighing the benefit of a treatment and available options and choice is the decision the client makes. Consideration must be given to the client to accept or not accept treatment, and to refuse or terminate treatment without undue influence or duress. Nurses must be supportive of their clients while they are making these decisions.

   d. Clients who cannot make decisions for themselves must have a designated surrogate

   e. In absence of a power of attorney or surrogate, the decision made for the client must consider past instructions given by the client and take into consideration the client's values.

   f. In some cultures the client may defer decision making to a family member or community, and this must be respected.

6. Justice

   a. This includes the equal distribution of health care resources regardless of the client's economic or cultural background.

   b. Justice means equal treatment for all clients and a commitment to integrity.

7. Fidelity

   a. Fidelity is the duty to do what was promised or be faithful.

   b. The nurse must think carefully before making a promise to a client and ensure it is reasonable and can be kept.

   c. Above all else, the nurse must honor commitments in a timely manner.

8. Veracity

   a. Veracity is the obligation to tell the truth to the client; this is the most difficult to keep.

   b. If the family or doctor wants to protect a dying client from the truth, the nurse may find himself or herself in a difficult situation.

9. Ethics committee

   a. A group of healthcare professionals (nurses, doctors, social workers, a lay person, ethicist, and the chaplain) who make ethical decision within a hospital.

   b. The ethics committee is appointed by the hospital executive board.

   c. The purpose is to review moral and ethical issues that arise during client care. These issues can be presented by medical or nursing staff, clients, or family members.

   d. The ethics committee also develops policies and guidelines to guide ethical and moral conduct and decision making in their institution.

III. Advance Directives

A. Act 1990 mandates all clients have right to have advance directives.

B. Provides clients with a chance to determine in advance their wishes regarding end of life decisions.

C. The Living Will states clients' wishes for end-of-life care if they are no longer competent.

D. Do Not Resuscitate (DNR) is a written medical order for end-of-life interventions. Each institution has a clear policy on DNR orders.

Additional Resources Found on MyNursingLab

- Collective Bargaining video

MODULE 2

Fundamentals

Submodule 2.5 Communication

Learning Objectives

2.5.1   Describe the communication process.

2.5.2   Distinguish between therapeutic and nontherapeutic communication.

    I.   Communication Process

      A. Communication is a vital link between clients, their families, nurses, and other healthcare workers.

      B. It is the exchange of information, feelings, or emotions.

      C. Communication begins at birth and continues throughout the life span.

        1. The communication process

          a. *Message:* what you want to say verbally or nonverbally.

          b. *Sender:* one who initiates the conversation and delivers the message.

          c. *Method:* means of sending communication; can be verbal, nonverbal, or both.

          d. *Receiver:* person to whom the message is sent.

          e. *Feedback:* the response (verbal or nonverbal) to the message.

        2. Types of communication

          a. *Verbal:* spoken or written word.

          b. *Nonverbal:* without expression through language (called body language).

        3. Mode of nonverbal communication

          a. Physical appearance and dress

          b. Body movement and posture

          c. Facial expression

          d. Gestures

          e. Eye contact

          f. Tone and volume of voice

          g. Touch

          h. Silence

        4. Personality types

          a. Passive or unassertive

          b. Aggressive

          c. Assertive

II. Therapeutic Communication

A. Styles of communication

1. *Social:* light and superficial between friends and family.

2. *Therapeutic communication:* promotes trust and good feelings; this is the style of communication between nurse and client.

B. Components of therapeutic communication

1. *Listening:* observation of nonverbal message as well as the interpretation of the spoken word.

2. *Warmth:* feeling of affection towards the client.

3. *Genuineness:* being honest, open, and truthful.

4. *Attentiveness:* concentrating completely on the client

5. *Empathy:* viewing from the client's perspective rather than adopting the client's beliefs and feelings

6. *Positive regard:* being nonjudgmental and respecting the client's beliefs and feelings

7. *Self-awareness:* knowing one's own thoughts and beliefs enough to be conscious of when they are different from the client's

C. Function of therapeutic communication

1. Decreasing anxiety by allowing the client to talk

2. Obtaining information to begin the nursing process

3. Giving the client information about the disease and treatment

4. Promoting trust and a good rapport with the client

D. Phases of therapeutic communication

1. *Orientation phase*: the nurse learns about the client and the client learns about the nurse; sometimes called opening phase. The goal is to build trust.

2. *Working phase*: the nurse helps the client explore his or her thoughts.

3. *Termination phase*: the nurse reviews and evaluates what was achieved and prepares for separation.

E. Factors affecting communication

1. *Congruence:* agreement between the verbal and nonverbal messages

2. *Time and setting:* what happens before the interaction, and the environment

3. *Proxemics:* the amount of space used for communication that allows both parties to feel comfortable. This comfortable distance varies with age, sex, and culture.

4. *Territoriality:* area and issues the individual considers his or her own.

5. *Space:* measure of distance

   a. Intimate space: from actual body contact to 18 inches away

   b. Personal space: 18 inches to 4 ft away

   c. Social space: 4 to 12 feet away

6. *Bias:* a prejudice or a negative belief about a particular group

7. *Physical impairment:* a deficit in some physical ability, such as hearing or vision

PEARSON

F. Blocks in communication

1. *Belittling:* making light of client's fears or beliefs, telling client what he or she thinks and feels is crazy, stupid, or not important.
   Example: "That's ridiculous."

2. *Disagreeing:* telling the client what he or she thinks or feels is wrong.
   Example: "That's not true."

3. *Agreeing:* telling the client what he or she is thinking and feeling is right.

4. *Defending:* telling the client he or she has no right to complain.
   Example: "You are not the only sick client here."

5. *Stereotyping:* generalizing that the client's feelings are like other people's in the client's group, and not allowing for any individual differences.
   Example: "You feel that way because you're young."

6. *False reassurance (reassuring):* telling the client everything will be all right even though the exact outcome cannot be determined.
   Example: "Don't worry. Everything will work out."

7. *Giving advice:* telling the client what he or she should do.
   Example: "I think you should."

8. *Changing the subject:* introducing a new subject to decrease the nurse's own anxiety

9. *Closed ended questions:* requires one word as an answer, yes or no, thus leaving the client no room for real expression.

10. *Why questions:* demanding an answer when the client may not be ready.
    Example: "Why didn't you call me right away?"

11. *Probing (or testing):* asking for more information than the client is comfortable sharing.

12. *Interpreting:* deciding what the client means without verifying it.
    Example: "You clearly have decided against chemotherapy."

G. Techniques to Improve Communication

1. *Give information:* provide facts about disease and treatments.

2. *Validation:* determine outcome: "Has the pain decreased?"

3. *Clarification:* try to make the message clear: "I am not sure I understand."

4. *Reflecting:* repeat the client's words as a way of inviting the client to say more about what he or she is feeling.

5. *Paraphrasing:* restate client's words slightly; often done in form of a question: "You think you may be nauseous?"

6. *Broad questions:* ask open-ended questions to encourage clients to elaborate on their feelings: "Tell me more about it."

7. *General leads:* let the client know you are listening: "And then…"

8. *Stating or making an observation:* verbalize observations: "You are trembling."

9. *Offering self (or silence):* sit for a while and be comfortable whether the client feels like talking or not: "I'll stay awhile if you'd like."

10. *Humor:* provide a light-hearted way of viewing the situation; aids in the healing process by boosting the immune system and reducing stress. Avoid cultural, ethnic, or religious humor.

11. *Summarizing: briefly state the key steps that have happened or the key points that have been ma*de.

H. Guidelines for the Interview

1. Assume a seated position; accept the client as a valued human being.

2. Provide privacy and watch your body language.

3. When seated, do not invade the client's personal space.

4. Respect differences in age, ethnicity, and culture.

5. Show interest in what the client is saying and be open minded.

6. Keep the language simple and clear; use words the client understands.

7. Start the conversation with open-ended questions.

8. Listen attentively; focus on what the client is saying.

9. Be consistent; do what you promise; be honest and be congruent.

10. Do not stare, because this increases anxiety.

11. Recognize symptoms of anxiety such as decreased concentration or communication.

12. If the client cries, don't focus on the crying.

13. Verbally identify the client's needs and ask for feedback.

14. If the client talks, then be sure to listen. Verbal and nonverbal responses must encourage further sharing of feelings.

Additional Resources Found on MyNursingLab
- Communication video
- Nonverbal Communication video

MODULE 2

Fundamentals

Submodule 2.6 Vital Signs and Physical Assessment

Learning Objectives

2.6.1 Describe the nursing responsibility in performing a physical assessment.

2.6.2 Describe methods used for taking, recording, and interpreting vital signs.

I. **Physical Assessment**

A. Usually taken by the physician or registered nurse; the LPN/LVN can contribute in the collection of data.

B. History and physical are important in helping with diagnosis and in planning total client care.

C. Physical examination

1. To obtain a determination of client's physical status.

2. For diagnosis of illness.

3. As a means of maintaining, gaining, and preserving health through early detection of disease.

4. For focused examination of the presenting problem.

5. Methods

a. *Inspection* – use of senses to observe the client and obtain normal and abnormal data

b. *Percussion* – tapping the body to detect changes in sound in chest and abdomen.

c. *Palpation* – feeling parts of the body with the hands to discover evidence of abnormalities in various organs.

d. *Auscultation* – using stethoscope to listen to sounds within the body; done before palpation and percussion, which can affect results.

6. Bowel sounds

a. Auscultate for bowel sounds in all quadrants.

b. Sounds are active/inactive.

7. Other routine tests – laboratory tests done as a part of a physical examination.

a. Many of these tests are done based on the client's disease state.

b. Routine tests include: urinalysis, complete blood chemistry profile, chest x-ray, and electrocardiogram.

C. Responsibilities of the LPN/LVN

1. Assist client onto examination table and drape client to avoid unnecessary exposure.

2. Prepare client physically and mentally for each step of examination. During the examination, help the client to relax by reassuring him or her.

3. Ensure privacy.

4. Maintain adequate lighting and ventilation.

5. Properly position client.

6 Arrange necessary equipment for examination.

II. Vital Signs

A. Temperature

1. Average body temperature range is from 36.1° -38°C (97-100.4°F).

2. Body temperature is lowest in the morning and highest in late afternoon or evening.

3. Body heat is produced by burning of calories which are generated in the muscles and secreting glands; heat is distributed to other parts of the body by the blood and blood vessels.

4. Body heat is eliminated through lungs by the breath, through the skin by perspiration, and with urine, feces, and saliva.

5. Body temperature is taken with a clinical thermometer or IVAC. A sudden fall in temperature may indicate shock, collapse, hemorrhage, or approach of death.

6. A sudden rise in temperature may indicate onset of disease, fatigue, worry, fear, or excitement.

7. Routes

a. Mouth (*oral*) – normal temperature is 97°F – 99°F; (37°C); clinical thermometer 2-4 minute electronic until reading indicated

i. Electronic thermometer

(a) Fast accurate and easy to use.

(b) Probe is placed in the client's mouth the same as clinical thermometer.

(c) Electronic thermometer must be kept clean and sterilized.

(d) Usually not used for client on isolation

b. Axilla (*axillary*) normal temperature is 97.6°F – 98°F (37.4° – 36.7°C) (axillary); temperature should not be taken if the client is so thin that there is a hollow under the arm or when client is perspiring so profusely that axillae cannot be kept dry for allotted time. The thermometer is placed in the armpit and left in place for ten minutes.

c. Rectum (*rectal*) – normal temperature is 98°F – 100 °F; (37.5°C); thermometer is inserted in rectum approximately one inch and left in place for 3-4 minutes; usually used for infants and children (although routine in some hospitals); rectal temperature is taken on unconscious clients.

i. Rectal temperature is most accurate of all methods used.

ii. Rectal thermometer should be held in place in children and the elderly.

iii. The thermometer should be lubricated.

iv. Thermometer should not be inserted too far, only 1 to 1½ inches (less in small children).

v. Rectal thermometers must be cleansed and disinfected according to hospital routine.

      d.   *Tympanic* (ear) – normal temperature 97°F – 99°F; placed in ear for 1-2 seconds

           i.   Client should not have anything hot or cold in the mouth.

           ii.   Thermometer should be held with lips but not teeth closed.

           iii.   If client is unconscious, delirious, disoriented, or has oral lesions, do not use oral method for taking temperature.

           iv.   Do not use for clients receiving oxygen after recent oral surgery or mouth trauma or with suicidal persons.

      e.   *Topical* strip -- placed on the skin or mucous membrane.

B. Pulse

    1. Taking the pulse

      a.   The pulse is a shock wave that travels along the fibers of the arteries with each contraction of the heart.

      b.   The pulse is taken by pressing an artery against a bone with the fingers and counting the pulsations for one minute.

      c.   The arteries most commonly used for taking the pulse are the radial, temporal, carotid, and femoral arteries.

      d.   Use a watch with a second hand and a pencil and pad.

      e.   Pulse is taken whenever the temperature is taken.

      f.   Pulse rate, rhythm, and volume are noted.

    2. Pulse rate

      a.   Normal pulse rate varies according to sex, age, size, position of client, and many other factors. Pulse sites include central (apical) and peripheral (temporal, carotid, brachial, radial, femoral, popliteal, and pedal

      b.   Average pulse rates:

           i.   Women: 70-80 beats per minute

           ii.   Men: 60-70 beats per minute

           iii.   Children: (over 7 years) 80-90 beats per minute

           iv.   Children: (one to seven years) 80-120 beats per minute

           v.   Infants: 110-160 beats per minute

      c.   Increase in pulse rate may be caused by excitement, emotional disturbance, use of certain drugs, elevated temperature, shock, some forms of heart disease, or exercise.

      d.   Decrease in pulse rate may be caused by certain drugs, disease, mental depression, or trauma. The pulse is slower when one is sleep.

    3. Rhythm

      a.   Spacing of beats is referred to as rhythm

      b.   May be regular or intermittent

      c.   Irregularity must be reported to the charge nurse.

4. Volume

   a. Refers to force of the pulse

   b. Varies with strength of the contraction and elasticity of blood vessels

   c. Descriptors include: strong, full, bounding, weak, or thready.

5. Variation in pulse rate:

   a. *Bradycardia:* slow heart rate, below 60 beats per minute.

   b. *Tachycardia:* rapid heart rate, above 100 beats per minute.

   c. *Irregular:* interval between beats is uneven.

   d. *Thready:* weak pulse, easily obliterated.

   e. *Bounding:* very strong pulse, hard to obliterate.

C. Respiration

1. Definition and techniques of taking respiration

   a. Respiration may be defined as the inhaling of oxygen and the exhaling of carbon dioxide.

   b. Normally, respiration is counted immediately following taking of the pulse, while the hand is still placed on the artery.

   c. Count the respiratory rate by watching the chest or abdomen rise and fall.

   d. The respirations are described by rate, depth, and regularity.

2. Respiratory rate

   a. Women: 18-20 respirations per minute

   b. Men: 14-18 respirations per minute

   c. Children: 20-30 respirations per minute

   d. Infants: 30-50 respirations per minute

   e. Variations in normal respiration may be due to nervousness, excitement, exercise, drugs, sleep, injuries, disease, certain drugs, shock, pain, gas poisoning, elevated body temperature, obstruction of the air passages, or high altitude.

3. Abnormal breathing patterns:

   a. *Bradypnea:* rate below 10 breaths per minute

   b. *Tachypnea:* rate above 20 breaths per minute

   c. *Biot's:* short irregular breaths followed by long irregular periods of apnea

   d. *Cheyne-Stokes:* pattern of very deep to very shallow breathing with periods of apnea

   e. *Kussmaul's:* increased rate and depth; above 20 breaths per minute

   f. *Dyspnea:* difficulty breathing

   g. *Orthopnea:* client can only breathe comfortably in upright position

   h. Abnormal lung sounds:

      i. *Crackles*: fine sounds as air moves through wet secretions

      ii. *Wheezing*: high-pitched musical sounds through narrowed passages

        iii. *Rhonchi*: low-pitched sounds on inspiration

        iv. *Stridor*: crowing sounds through partial obstruction

4. Pulse oximetry

  a. Noninvasive measurement of blood oxygen saturation.

  b. Normal reading in the adult: 95/100%.

  c. Hypoxia results in readings below 90%.

  d. Pulse oximetry 70% or below is life threatening.

  e. Clip probe to finger, toe, earlobe, or bridge of nose.

  f. Ensure area being used is clean and dry; remove nail polish.

  g. Rotate site every 4 hours for tissue integrity.

D. Blood pressure

1. Definition:

  a. Pressure exerted by the blood against the walls of the arteries.

    i. Systolic pressure is the arterial pressure at the time of the contraction of the ventricles.

    ii. Diastolic pressure is the arterial pressure during dilation of the ventricles when relaxed between contractions.

    iii. The difference between diastolic and systolic is called pulse pressure.

  b. Average range for healthy adults is 120/80; pressure may change from hour to hour and day to day

  c. Blood pressure varies with age, sex, and muscular development.

It is usually lower in women than in men.

  d. Blood pressure can be measured at the brachial or popliteal artery, and must not be measured on an extremity with lymph node injury or a shunt.

  e. Hypotension: blood pressure lower than 100/60.

  f. Hypertension: blood pressure above 140/90.

  g. *Sphygmomanometer*: equipment used to measure blood pressure (stethoscope used to listen to the sounds).

2. Important points to remember:

  a. Blood pressure should be taken when client is quiet and relaxed.

  b. Seat client in a comfortable position (sitting or reclining) for a more accurate reading.

  c. Check sphygmomanometer and stethoscope before using them.

  d. Cuff size must cover 2/3 of extremity.

  e. Avoid applying excessive pressure on client's arm.

  f. Chart blood pressure on nurse's notes or graphic chart.

  g. Notify charge nurse of any change in client's pressure.

E. Height and weight

1. Weight is related to the body size and frame.

2. Elderly clients generally lose height due to osteoporosis.

3. These measurements are best done before breakfast and on the same scale each time.

4. Can be done standing, sitting in a chair, or lying on a stretcher, based on client need

Additional Resources Found on MyNursingLab

- Radial Pulse video

- Measuring Blood Pressure video

MODULE 2

Fundamentals

Submodule 2.7 Admission/Transfer/Discharge/Documentation

Learning Objectives

2.7.1 Discuss nursing responsibilities related to admission, transfer, and discharge.

2.7.2 Describe acceptable guidelines for documentation.

I. **Admission**

   A. Admission clerk gathers demographic information from the client. RN performs complete health history. LPN/LVN assists RN in collecting data.

   B. Requirements

      a. "Unit" refers to client's room furniture and equipment.

      b. Room should be at a comfortable temperature.

      c. Room should have adequate lighting.

      d. Room must be kept noise free.

      e. Room and unit must be cleaned and tidied daily.

      f. Room and unit must be kept safe with all equipment in working order, including proper functioning of call light.

   C. Client admission

      1. Treat new client like guest.

      2. Orient new client to hospital; explain hospital routine.

      3. Ensure that clothing (hospital gown) and ID bracelet are in place. ID bracelet has: ID number, date of birth (DOB), name, room number, doctor.

      4. Give admission bath if necessary and if hospital policy; ensure privacy

      5. Check clothing and valuables according to hospital policy.

      6. Report to charge nurse any medication brought in by client.

      7. Assist client into bed.

      8. Follow routine procedure of admission.

      9. Obtain data as ordered for initial assessment (including level of consciousness, vital signs, weight, mobility, and level of function).

      10. Chart time of admission, observations, vital signs, and other pertinent information.

II. **Transfer**

   A. Check doctor's orders for transfer.

   B. Provide information to client and family about the reasons for transfer; information helps reduce anxiety.

C. Document all treatments and medications to prevent duplication after transfer.

D. Call department prior to transfer to ensure room is prepared and client care will be continuous.

III. Discharge

A. Planning for discharge begins on admission.

B. Check doctor's orders for discharge; a written order is required.

C. Provide safe conveyance.

D. Prepare client for departure from hospital.

E. Check to see the business office has given release.

F. Return client's personal belonging and valuables.

G. Assist client in dressing.

H. Give discharge instructions.

I. Follow detailed procedure of discharge.

J. Chart time of discharge, method, observations, condition of client, and close chart.

K. If client leaves against medical advice (AMA), have the client sign the discharge form, inform the charge nurse, and inform the physician following facility policy.

IV. Documentation

A. Source-Oriented Record

1. Used in hospital and long-term care.

2. Each discipline has a special area in the chart to document.

3. The areas are: nursing notes, physician progress notes, history and physical, diagnostic tests, laboratory data, physician's orders, admission data, discharge data, graphic sheets, and rehabilitation therapy.

4. A disadvantage is that tracking client progress is fragmented.

B. Problem–Oriented Record (POR)

1. Documentation based on the client's problems

2. All disciplines documented in the same area of the chart.

3. Four areas of focus are data-base, problem list, plan of care, and progress notes.

4. The advantage is management of progress and problems, and collaboration among staff.

C. Narrative charting

1. Chronological: description of client experience and problems.

2. Charting can be by time or by events.

3. Documentation notes exactly what time an episode occurred.

4. A disadvantage is that it allows the charting of irrelevant information.

D. SOAP charting

1. Has been modified to use two other acronyms: SOAPIE and SOAPIER.

   a. SOAPIE monitors subjective data (information shared by the client), objective data, assessment, plan, intervention, and evaluation.

2. SOAPIER monitors subjective data, objective data, assessment, plan, intervention, evaluation, and response.

E. Problem Intervention and Evaluation (PIE)

1. Designed from the Problem–Oriented Record (POR)

2. Disadvantage of this charting format is that problems identified on admission become focus for charting.

3. Does not focus on the client as a whole or identify new problems.

F. Focus Charting (DAR)

1. Concerned with the client's problems

2. The data is documented in three columns: data, action, response

   a. The data column has the objective or subjective data derived from client assessment.

   b. The action column describes the implementation part of the nursing process.

   c. The response column describes the client response to treatment and reflects the evaluation phase of the nursing process.

   d. An advantage of focus charting is that it views the client holistically.

   e. A disadvantage is that it makes it more difficult to monitor client's progress.

G. Charting By Exception (CBE)

1. Views everything as progressing normally unless otherwise documented on flow sheets.

2. The contents of flow sheets vary by diagnosis or by medical specialty, such as neurological or gastrointestinal.

3. An advantage is that it is easily interpreted, conserves time, and reduces repetition.

4. A disadvantage is that it is task oriented and the checklist becomes routine, placing less emphasis on nursing judgment or critical thinking.

Additional Resources Found on MyNursingLab

MODULE 2

Fundamentals

Submodule 2.8 Comfort and Hygiene

Learning Objectives

2.8.1   List measures to promote comfort.

2.8.2   Discuss good physical care measures.

    I.   Comfort measures

        A. Position client for individualized comfort.

        B. Maintain quiet and darkness to help with sleep.

        C. Provide comfortable environment, including blankets or cooling as needed.

        D. Promote relaxation with a warm bath or back rub.

        E. Avoid overuse of prescribed sleep agents.

        F. Purpose of personal hygiene

            1. Cleanses, soothes, and refreshes client

            2. Stimulates circulation and movement, contributes to sense of well-being

            3. Frequency of bathing and shampooing may vary with cultures and individuals.

    II. Personal Hygiene Procedures

        A. Baths

            1. Bed bath is given to those confined to bed or with dressings.

            2. Showers or tub baths are given for clients who are up and without dressings.

            3. Room temperature should be 75° and free from drafts.

            4. Bath water should be 105°F and changed as often as necessary.

            5. Ensure privacy and talk to client about personal preferences.

            6. Avoid chilling.

            7. Begin by cleansing the face and neck, (use a separate part of the wash cloth for each eye), moving to the trunk and limbs, and ending with the groin and perineal area.

            8. Bath time is a good time to assess the condition of the client's skin.

        B. Oral hygiene

            1. Help keep client's mouth and teeth clean, healthy, and odor free.

            2. The mouth is cleansed to help prevent sores, surgical parotitis, and pneumonia.

            3. Brush teeth before (if necessary) and after meals.

            4. Use mouthwashes unless mouth ulcers or dry mucous membranes are present; alcohol-free mouthwashes are recommended to prevent drying of oral mucosa.

5. Routine or special mouth care is given daily.

6. Take care to keep fingers out of the client's mouth, in case the client clamps down.

7. For an unconscious client, the side-lying position is safest.

C. Care of removable dentures

1. Remove dentures to clean thoroughly and to examine gums.

2. Keep unused dentures in container labeled with client's name.

3. Use only cold water, brush, and dentifrice to clean dentures.

4. Dentures should be washed on a relatively soft surface. The bottom of the sink may be too hard and could damage dentures.

5. Remove dentures if client is having convulsions, is ready to sleep, is irrational, is unconscious, or is going to surgery.

D. Care of the hair

1. Comb hair daily and groom as needed.

2. Shampoo as needed.

3. Apply vinegar to hair to help remove tangles.

4. Braid long hair to prevent tangling.

5. Never cut a client's hair without permission.

6. Provide pediculosis treatment as needed. *Infestation of lice (parasites)*

E. Care of nails, hands, and feet

1. Care of nails, hands, and feet may be done as part of bed bath.

2. Good nail care helps to prevent transmission of infection.

3. Nail care includes cleaning beneath nails, and pushing back cuticles.

4. Toenails should be cut straight across to prevent infections and ingrown nails.

F. Skin care

1. Assess for reddened or broken areas.

    a. Document and report.

    b. Do not massage nonblanching, reddened areas or over bony prominences.

2. Keep bed linens clean, dry, and wrinkle-free.

3. Reposition client carefully to prevent shearing and skin breakdown.

G. Care of the incontinent client

1. Incontinence of urine or feces or both

2. May be temporary as in an acute illness or permanent

3. This condition causes embarrassment to clients.

4. Bathe buttocks, genitals, and back with mild soap and water.

H. Morning and evening care

1. A.M. or morning care

    a. Wash face and hands.

    b. Brush teeth.

        c.   Change client's position.

        d.   Adjust bed and bedclothes.

  2. Midmorning care

        a.   Give bath.

        b.   Care for nails.

        c.   Comb hair.

        d.   Change bedclothes and make bed.

        e.   Tidy and dust unit.

  3. P.M. care

        a.   Repeat all of the procedures of A.M. care.

        b.   Give back rub.

        c.   Comb hair.

        d.   The main objective is to get client ready to sleep.

I. Bed making

  1. Types of beds

        a.   *Occupied:* provides safety and comfort for client

        b.   *Open:* clean, safe, used by client who may be out of bed

        c.   *Closed:* clean, safe, made to receive new client

        d.   *Cradle:* made with linens over a piece of equipment that prevents linens from touching the body.

  2. Equipment

        a.   Linen must be tightly pulled to avoid wrinkling.

        b.   Do not shake out linens close to nurse's clothing.

        c.   Avoid holding linens close to nurse's clothing to prevent transmission of micro-organisms.

        d.   Complete one side of the bed at a time.

        e.   Use good body mechanics to avoid injury from straining.

Additional Resources Found on MyNursingLab

MODULE 2

Fundamentals

Submodule 2.9 Safety and Infection Control

Learning Objectives

2.9.1 Describe the infectious process.

2.9.2 Describe the body's defenses against infection.

2.9.3 List measures to prevent the spread of infection.

I. **Infectious Process**

  A. Infection occurs when pathogenic microorganisms successfully enter the body, then multiply and produce an adverse response.

  B. Two types of microorganisms: pathogens and normal bacterial flora.

   1. **Pathogens** are harmful microorganism that can cause disease.

     a. Examples of pathogens are bacteria, viruses, fungi, and protozoa.

     b. **Virulence** is the strength of the pathogen to overcome the body's defenses.

   2. Normal flora live in the gastrointestinal tract and vagina and on the skin.

     a. Their presence is beneficial; they prevent other types of opportunistic organisms from proliferating.

     b. In the gastrointestinal tract normal flora are important in the utilization and release of vitamins K and B.

     c. Normal flora have the potential to be harmful if they enter areas of the body where they are not usually found.

  C. Classification of infection

   1. **Local infection:** affects one region of the body.

   2. **Systemic infection:** pathogens invade the bloodstream or lymphatic system.

   3. Classifications of infections

     a. **Primary infection** is the first infection.

     b. **Secondary infection** occurs as a result of the primary infection.

     c. **Acute infections** have a rapid onset and short duration.

     d. **Chronic infections** have a slow onset and last for several weeks or months.

     e. **Latent infections** have very mild symptoms that may not be noticed initially. An example of a latent infection may be immunodeficiency viral infection.

     f. **Nosocomial infections** are hospital-acquired or healthcare-associated infections.

  D. Progress of infection

   1. **Incubation** is the stage between entry of pathogen and the onset of symptoms.

2. **Prodromal stage** is the stage from initial symptoms to more severe symptoms.

3. **Convalescent stage** produces active signs and symptoms of disease.

4. **Recovery stage** is the stage in which symptoms lessen and the client returns to a state of wellness.

II. **Levels of Defense Against Infection**

A. Primary defenses

1. Intact skin and mucous membrane are the first line of defense.

2. Hair found in the nostrils acts a filter to remove organisms.

3. The cilia lining the trachea and bronchi sweep organisms out of the gastrointestinal tract.

4. Coughing and sneezing help to expel organisms from the respiratory tract.

5. Tears in the eye contain enzymes that wash bacteria away.

6. Saliva contains the enzyme lysozyme that destroys bacteria.

7. Bile in the gastrointestinal tract inhibits the growth of microorganisms.

8. The acidic environment in the gastrointestinal tract destroys micro-organisms.

9. The urinary tract secretes mucus to inhibit microbes. Urine contains lysozyme to prevent bacterial growth.

10. The vagina has highly acidic mucous secretions to prevent bacterial growth.

B. Secondary defenses

1. Phagocytosis uses WBCs to engulf and destroy the pathogen.

2. Inflammatory response occurs when injury to phagocytes triggers basophils to release histamine.

   a. Symptoms of inflammation include swelling, heat, exudates, and pain as a result of pressure on the nerves.

3. Low-grade fever as a result of increased activity is a natural response and defense to pathogens affecting the body.

C. Tertiary defense:

1. This level of defense is an antigen-antibody response.

2. Two types of response are humoral and cell-mediated.

   a. Humoral immunity: pathogens invade, and in response macrophages stimulate B lymphocytes to produce antibodies, known as immunoglobulin.

   b. Cell-mediated immunity: destroys body cells that have been invaded by viruses.

3. T lymphocytes respond to the presence of antigens:

   a. **Killer (cytotoxic) T cells** kill infected body cells.

   b. **Helper T cells** regulate the production of antibodies.

   c. **Memory cells** recognize pathogens the body has fought off in the past; they respond and reproduce more quickly than the first time.

   d. **Suppressor T cells** turn off the immune response once the infection is controlled.

III. Measures to Prevent Spread of Infection

    A. Chain of infection

        1. **Pathogen:** cause of the infection

        2. **Reservoir:** where the microorganism can live and grow.

        3. **Portal of exit:** the way out of the reservoir

        4. **Mode of transmission**: the means of transmission (a tick, dirty linen)

        5. **Portal of entry**: the way into the reservoir

        6. **Susceptible host:** organism the pathogen can infect

    B. Infection control

        1. The responsibility for preventing the spread of infections belongs to all members of the healthcare staff, as well as to clients and visitors.

        2. The Centers for Disease Control (CDS) and Hospital Infection Control Advisory Committee (HICPAC) have established guidelines to prevent infection and the spread of disease-producing organisms.

            a. Hand washing

                i. Hand washing prevents the spread of microorganisms.

               ii. The nurse must use special protective wear to protect against contaminated substances.

              iii. Body substance isolation

              iv. Proper disposal of equipment, body waste

               v. Follow hospital or facility procedures.

        3. Types of precautions

            a. Standard Precautions must be used for all clients regardless of their diagnosis or infectious status.

                i. Gloves are worn for any contact with body fluids except sweat or saliva.

               ii. Gown and mask with goggles are worn if there is potential contamination from body fluids.

              iii. Separate disposal of sharps without breaking; do not recap needles.

            b. Types of isolation

                i. Neutropenic/Protective/Reverse Isolation: used with immunosuppressed clients.

                   (a) Private room

                   (b) Visitors wear gown, gloves and mask when entering room and do not bring items that might carry microorganisms (fruits, flowers, etc.)

               ii. Airborne Isolation: (sometimes called Respiratory Isolation) used with pathogens that are carried in the air.

                   (a) Private room, door closed

                   (b) Visitors wear specially fitted masks in the room.

                   (c) Negative air flow pressure filter

                   (d) Mask is worn by client when out of the room

PEARSON

        iii. Contact Isolation: gloves, gown, and proper disposal of drainage and articles from:

           (a) Drainage from wounds

           (b) Respiratory secretions

           (c) Body wastes

           (d) Blood

        iv. Droplet Isolation: used with respiratory organisms spread by droplet

           (a) Gloves worn for any contact with body fluids

           (b) Gown and mask with goggles worn if potential contamination from body fluids

           (c) Mask worn by client when out of the room

           (d) Disinfection, sterilization

4. Disinfection, sterilization

    a. Disinfectants

        i. May not kill all organisms but will check their growth; does not kill all spores. Examples: sunlight, fresh air, soap and water

    b. Hospital procedures may not kill all organisms but will check their growth.

    c. Organisms

        i. Enter body through:

           (a) Breaks in mucous membrane and skin

           (b) Respiratory system

           (c) Urinary and reproductive systems

           (d) Gastrointestinal system

        ii. Leave body through:

           (a) Vomitus and feces

           (b) Sneezing, coughing, and sputum

           (c) Mucus discharge and urine

           (d). Exudates from surface wounds

5. Medical aseptic techniques

    a. Procedures to control and prevent disease (such as handwashing)

    b. Destruction of organisms after they leave the body. Example: isolation

    c. General principles of medical asepsis

        i. Terms used to describe objects are "clean" and "contaminated."

        ii. Sterilization of equipment, inanimate objects. Terminal disinfection (after procedures or after client discharge) is part of routine nursing care.

        iii. When working in isolation, follow hospital policies to provide routine nursing care.

        iv. When working in isolation, follow hospital procedures regarding use of mask, gown, and handwashing.

6. Surgical aseptic techniques

    a. Destruction of all microorganisms

    b. Examples: sterilization

C. Dressing: General principles

    1. **Dressing** is defined as any material applied to a wound or incision to protect, promote healing, or absorb drainage.

    2. Dressings are always sterile to prevent introducing organisms into wounds.

D. Nurse's role

    1. LPN/LVN may be required to change dressing and assist doctor or registered nurse.

    2. LPN/LVN must know when to apply dressing that is sterile and clean.

Additional Resources Found on MyNursingLab

MODULE 2

Fundamentals

Submodule 2.10 Activity, Rest, and Sleep

Learning Objectives

2.10.1 Describe principles of good body mechanics.

2.10.2 Discuss problems associated with immobility and measures to prevent them.

2.10.3 Discuss measures to promote rest and sleep.

    I. Activity

       A. Body mechanics: general principles

         1. Means coordinating movements of the body

         2. With good body mechanics, the body can work smoothly with the least amount of strain.

         3. Use of good body mechanics is necessary to:

            a. Prevent strain or injury to client and nurse.

            b. Prevent fatigue to client and nurse.

            c. Maintain good body alignment for client and nurse.

         4. When nurse or client walks, sits, stands, or lies down, the body should be in the correct position required for the type of movement to be executed.

         5. Head and trunk must be kept erect when lifting or moving:

            a. Feet apart to width of shoulder

            b. Move object to be lifted close to body before lifting.

            c. Keep back slightly flexed.

            d. Contract abdominal and lumbar muscles during lifting.

            e. Use shoulder and arm muscles to pull.

            f. Flex knees slightly and then straighten as object is lifted; use strong muscles of the legs to reduce strain on the back.

            g. Base of support is the feet.

            h. Line of gravity is an imaginary line down the center of the body.

            i. Center of gravity is the pelvis.

       B. Body positions: general positions

         1. Client's body should be positioned in alignment and devices such as trochanter rolls used to support proper alignment.

         2. Special positions are necessary for clients.

3. The body must be moved correctly to prevent injury or pain.

4. Basic positions:

    a. *Standing:* necessary to observe neurologic and orthopedic conditions

    b. *Supine:* (horizontal recumbent) usually for physical examination

    c. *Prone:* position used for examination of spine or back

    d. *Dorsal recumbent:* desired position for rectal and vaginal examination

    e. *Sims' position:* used for rectal examinations and treatment of colon

    f. *Dorsal lithotomy:* preferred for rectal, vaginal, and bladder examinations

    g. *Trendelenburg position:* used when client is in shock

    h. *Fowler's position:* used following an operation when drainage from the upper part of the body is expected. This is one of the most comfortable positions and one that allows fuller expansion of the lungs

II. Mobility

A. Effects of immobility

1. Osteoporosis or atrophy of muscles; joint pain and stiffness

2. **Contractures**: permanent shortening of muscles

3. Diminished cardiac reserve

4. Orthostatic hypotension

5. Venous stasis, dependent edema, thrombophlebitis, and emboli

6. Pooling of respiratory secretions, pneumonia, **atelectasis** (lung collapse)

7. Loss of appetite

8. Urinary stasis, calculi, retention

9. Disruption of normal bowel habits

10. Skin breakdown.

B. When transferring the client from bed to chair or chair to bed, it is necessary to move or support the client without injury to client or nurse.

C. Precautions when transferring clients

1. Use proper body mechanics.

2. Check doctor's orders.

3. Lock bed.

4. Prepare chair or bed before moving client.

5. Prevent drafts.

6. Attach signal cord within easy reach of client.

7. Check client frequently.

8. Check patency of tubes, e.g., catheters.

9. If postop, administer medication for pain as ordered prior to transfer

10. Follow facility policy when assisting with ambulation.

D. Transferring client from bed to stretcher

1. Use at least two or three people.

2. Use draw sheet to move client.

3. Move client toward the edge of bed.

4. Adjust stretcher next to bed at level of bed.

5. Lock both bed and stretcher.

6. Reach across stretcher and use draw sheet to pull client toward you, first to edge, then to center of stretcher.

E. Assisting client from bed to chair

1. Lower bed to lowest position.

2. Move chair close to bed and firmly lock wheels.

3. Raise head of bed to sitting position, and help client to sit on side of bed with legs dangling.

4. Face client, maintain wide base of support, place hands around client's lower chest.

5. Keep client's knees between your legs to prevent falls.

6. Have client lean forward and place hands on your shoulders, not your neck.

7. Pull client to standing position.

8. Pivot client and lower into chair or wheelchair.

F. Positioning client up in bed

1. Adjust bed height to below your waist.

2. Position the client flat in bed.

3. Stand at side of bed with feet pointed in direction you are to move client.

4. Have client bend knees and use feet to push self up if possible.

5. For weaker client, reach under client's shoulders and back to move client without major lifting.

6. Use draw sheet, if possible, to avoid shearing force on client's back.

G. Turning client

1. Client should be turned every 2 hours while in bed to relieve pressure. Weak or unconscious clients may need to be turned more often.

2. Adjust bed to mid or upper thigh level.

3. Lower bed rail on the side where you are standing.

4. Cross client's arms over chest and cross client's legs.

5. Reach across client, placing your hands on the client's far shoulder and hip or use a draw sheet.

6. Turn client toward you using your whole body.

7. Put pillow(s) behind client's back and between legs; raise side rail.

H. Chart repositioning and transfers. Remember to document:

1. The procedure (bed to chair or chair to bed)

2. The length of time client stayed

3. Observations noted

I. Use of cane

1. To support balance and gait

2. Several types of canes exist.

3. Adjust height, allowing for a slight bend at elbow.

4. Client teaching:

   a. Hold cane on strong side.

   b. Move cane and weak side together.

   c. Weight bearing on strong side, then move the leg on strong side.

   d. Weight bearing is on cane and leg on weak side

5. Nurse is positioned to assist on the weak side.

J. Use of walker

1. Position walker in front of client.

2. Have client hold walker and move it 6 inches ahead.

3. Have client move the right leg forward first.

4. If one leg is weak, move the weak leg forward with the walker.

K. Use of restraints

1. Protective devices/restraints must have MD order.

   a. Use the least restrictive measure possible.

   b. Document need for restraints clearly on chart.

   c. Assess the client frequently for damage to tissue under restraint.

   d. Check every hour; remove for 15 minutes and reapply q 2 hours.

   e. Maintain restraint record per institutional policy.

   f. Reevaluate need for restraints frequently.

2. Measures used to avoid use of restraints

   a. Orientation to time, person, place,

   b. Monitor the client closely or use a chair alarm

   c. Special chairs

L. Range of motion (ROM) exercises

1. Types:

   a. **Passive**: movement of client's joints through complete range of motion when the client is unable to perform this activity independently.

   b. **Active**: client moves joints through complete range of motion independently.

2. Always exercise only to the limit of mobility or pain.

3. Support limb by cupping or cradling extremity to avoid stress on joints.

4. Often ROM exercises are done easily during bath.

M Continuous passive range of motion (CPRM)

1. Provided by a mechanical device used after joint surgery. Keeps joint mobile and speeds up recovery

2. Set for physician-prescribed number of movements per minute. Client may be premedicated against pain.

N. Muscle-setting exercises

1. **Isometric**: strengthen muscles of abdomen, gluteal muscles, and quadriceps.

2. **Isotonic**: done in cycles to maintain tone by tightening and releasing muscles

III. **Rest and Sleep**

A. Rest provides mental relaxation and feeling of well-being.

B. Sleep is a form of rest that occurs after a longer period of wakefulness

C. Sleep cycles vary with individual

1. Rapid eye movement (REM)

2. Non rapid eye movement (NREM)

D. Sleep deprivation – caused by stress, illness, and hospitalization. Sleep deprivation may lead to both physiological and psychological signs

1. Physical signs include:

a. Tremor

b. Decreased response time

c. Impaired memory and judgment

d. Cardiac arrhythmias

2. Psychological signs include:

a. Mood changes

b. Fatigue

c. Irritability

d. Agitation

e. Lethargy

f. Sleepiness

E. Measures to promote rest and sleep

1. Measures to promote rest include:

a. Quiet room

b. Comfortable temperature

c. Darkened room (soft light for infants)

d. Physical needs satisfied

2. Measures to promote sleep in the hospital include:

   a. Adhering to at-home patterns

   b. Quiet, comfortable environment

   c. Avoidance of caffeine, stress, and exercise just prior to sleep

   d. Empty bladder

Additional Resources Found on MyNursingLab

- ROM Exercise video

MODULE 2

Fundamentals

Submodule 2.11 Oxygenation

Learning Objectives

2.11.1 Describe nursing assessment of clients receiving oxygen.

2.11.2 Discuss nursing responsibilities for clients with airway problems.

I. **Oxygen and Oxygenation**

A. Oxygen is a colorless, odorless, and tasteless gas. Oxygen supports combustion and ignites around sparks or fire.

B. Exchange of O_2 occurs in the pulmonary capillary bed. Normal oxygen saturation is 97-100%.

C. Oxygen therapy must be ordered by a physician, specifying its concentration.

1. Must be humidified

2. Client needs frequent mouth care.

D. Safety precautions with oxygen use include:

1. "No Smoking" signs.

2. Use of grounded plugs for electrical devices.

3. Monitoring flow rate, concentration, and humidification frequently.

4. Securing O_2 equipment to prevent falling.

E. Signs and symptoms of oxygen deficiency **(hypoxia)**

1. Circumoral pallor (early symptom)

2. Restlessness, anxiety

3. Fatigue

4. Increased pulse rate

5. Decreased level of consciousness

6. Elevated blood pressure

7. Increased rate and depth of respiration followed by bradycardia

8. **Cyanosis** (blueish discoloration; late symptom)

F. Type of administration depends upon client's condition and availability.

G. Types of oxygen devices

1. Nasal cannula – delivers 24-44% oxygen at 1-6 L/min

a. Allows talking and eating

b. Very drying; must be humidified

PEARSON

2. Simple mask – fits over nose and mouth – delivers 40-60% at 6-10 L/min

3. Venturi mask – reliable with consistent O_2 flow 24-60% at 4, 6, or 8 L/min

4. Nonrebreather mask – delivers 90-100% at 12 L/min

II. **Nursing Responsibilities for Clients with Airway Problems**

A. Observe client's respirations for rate, depth, and character.

B. Document abnormal patterns, movement, or sounds.

C. Measure pulse rate frequently.

D. Check pulse oximeter.

E. Observe for signs of advancing hypoxia, cyanosis.

F. Observe for agitation and anxiety, as these will increase the body's need for oxygen.

G. Pulse oximetry

1. Measures amount of oxygen in the hemoglobin of the blood; normal oxygen saturation is 97-100%.

2. Cutaneous sensor is placed on top of fingernail (remove nail polish).

3. Report reading of less than 95%.

H. Oxygen therapy

1. Important functions of oxygen therapy

a. Increases oxygen concentration in the blood or reverses hypoxemia

b. Decreases the work of the respiratory system

c. Decreases the workload of the heart

2 Coughing and deep breathing

a. Done to effectively remove secretions from the respiratory tract

b. Improves oxygenation by preventing atelectasis

c. Method of effective coughing and deep breathing:

i. Sit client up in high Fowler's position.

ii. Splint abdomen or chest with pillows or hands to prevent incisional pain.

iii. Request deep inspiration through mouth several times.

iv. Bend client forward and instruct to contract thorax and abdomen to forcibly expel air.

d. Medicate for pain prior to coughing to improve effort.

e. Used for pre- and postoperative clients or those with decreased mobility.

3. Vaporizer/nebulizer

a. Provides air with a high humidity

b. Soothes irritated mucous membranes

c. Provides extra moisture to respiratory tract

d. Liquefies thick secretions

e. Loosens crusts on mucous membranes

    f. Administers medications directly to respiratory tract

    g. Administered by a wide variety of equipment

    h. Possibility of bacterial growth in warm water reservoir

    i. Monitor for bronchospasms and overhydration.

4. Inspiratory/incentive spirometer

    a. Helps client to breathe deeply, thereby expanding lung capacity

    b. Lips sealed over mouthpiece; client takes deep breath, holds 3 seconds, then exhales slowly.

    c. Encourage client to use spirometer hourly while awake.

5. Intermittent positive pressure breathing (IPPB) treatment

    a. Administers higher-than-ambient pressures and higher-than-client's normal tidal volume to force oxygen into respiratory tract; promotes deep breathing in clients

    b. Mobilizes secretions through stimulation of coughing

    c. Increases O_2 intake and CO_2 removal

    d. Produces mechanical bronchodilation

    e. Administers aerosol medications

    f. Prevents atelectasis by hyperinflation of alveoli

    g. Decreases work of breathing temporarily

    h. Should only be administered by trained personnel.

6. Postural drainage

    a. Positioning clients so gravity assists with drainage of secretions from lobes of the lungs

    b. May be combined with percussion, clapping, and vibration over affected areas of lungs

    c. Nurse should auscultate before and after postural drainage and record results.

    d. Drinking plenty of fluids between drainage sessions helps to loosen secretions.

7. Sputum specimen

    a. Performed to inspect sputum for infective agents or malignancy

    b. Best obtained in morning before breakfast

    c. Use proper container, sterile for culture, and with preservative for cytology.

    d. Have client breathe deeply to induce cough.

    e. Avoid contamination of inside of container.

8. Oxygen administration

    a. Used to treat hypoxemia, determined by blood gas analysis or pulse oximeter.

    b. Need physician's order.

    c. Can be given in many concentrations and through many devices.

    d. Various devices provide different concentrations; mask higher, nasal cannula lower.

    e. *Nasal cannula*: into nares ½ inch; can deliver 1 to 6 L/min.

  f. Oxygen mask: fits snugly over client's mouth and nose.

  g. A simple mask delivers 40-60% oxygen depending on liter flow rate.

  h. *Nonrebreather mask* has a one-way flap valve between bag and mask to prevent the dilution of the oxygen; delivers 0-95% oxygen at flow rates of 12 L/min.

  i. *Partial rebreather mask* without a one-way flap valve delivers 60-90% oxygen @ 8-11 L.

  j. *Venturi mask* can be adjusted to deliver 24-60% in precise concentration.

  k. Oxygen must always be humidified.

  l. Post signs against smoking because oxygen is highly combustible.

  m. Avoid high levels of oxygen in clients with chronic obstructive pulmonary disease (COPD) because high levels depress the breathing stimulus. Avoid high levels of oxygen over long periods of time for any client.

9. Suctioning

  a. Mechanical aspiration of secretions from tracheobronchial tree

  b. Tracheal suctioning is a sterile procedure.

  c. Oral or nasal suctioning is a clean procedure.

  d. Administer O_2 in high levels before and after suctioning.

  e. Apply suction while withdrawing the catheter. Withdraw catheter slowly with rotating motion.

  f. Do not suction for more than 10 seconds continuously (less with children).

  g. Suction pressure 80-110 mm.

10. Tracheostomy care

  a. Monitor client closely for signs of obstruction to tube.

  b. Suctioning and cleaning of tracheotomy is sterile procedure. Use hydrogen peroxide for cleaning the inner cannula.

  c. Monitor and maintain skin around stoma.

  d. Always provide humidified air.

Additional Resources Found on MyNursingLab

MODULE 2

Fundamentals

Submodule 2.12 Wound Care

Learning Objectives

2.12.1 Differentiate types of wounds.

2.12.2 Describe the process of wound healing.

2.12.3 Discuss staging of ulcers.

2.12.4 Describe nursing responsibilities for wound care and preventive measures.

2.12.5 List the principles and purposes in the use of hot and cold applications.

I. **Wounds**

    A. A wound occurs when there is an intentional or unintentional break in the integrity of the skin.

        1. Intentional wounds result from a surgical incision.

        2. Unintentional wounds occur by accident and result in abrasions, denuding cuts, or ulcers.

        3. Superficial wounds involve the epidermis only.

        4. Partial thickness wounds involve the epidermis and dermis.

        5. Full thickness wounds involved the epidermis, dermis, subcutaneous tissue, and possibly muscle and bone.

    B. Skin

        1. The skin is the largest organ in the body.

        2. It is divided into two layers, epidermis and dermis

            a. The outer thin layer of the skin (the epidermis) is made up of four layers of cells. Old cells shed and new cells generate and move to the top to replace them. The epidermis has no nerve or blood vessels.

            b. The inner thick layer is the dermis, which contains blood vessels, nerves, oil, and sweat glands.

        3. Functions of the skin

            a. Protective barrier to protect the internal body structure from invasion by bacteria and other harmful substances.

            b. Excretion of water through the skin allows some waste to leave the body to maintain homeostasis.

            c. Regulation of body temperature by acting as insulation or by cooling the skin through evaporation of water.

    d. Provide sensory sensations.

    e. The skin is open to threats from the outside influences.

C. Types of Wounds

    1. A wound can be open, such as a cut, or closed, such as a contusion.

        a. **Contusion** – wound resulting from forceful impact of object against the skin

        b. **Abrasion** – wound resulting from scraping of skin across a surface

        c. **Puncture** – wound resulting from object penetrating the skin

        d. **Laceration** – jagged wound resulting from a slicing object such as a knife

    2. Wounds can be acute, such as surgical wounds, made by an intentional incision, that heal in a few weeks; or chronic, such as pressure ulcers where healing take months or years.

    3. Ulcers

        a. Venous stasis ulcers are caused by congestion and decreased blood flow to the tissues.

        b. Arterial ulcers are caused by decreased blood flow to the tissues.

        c. Diabetic ulcers are caused by high levels of blood sugar in diabetic clients that result in changes in the vasculature.

        d. Pressure ulcers are caused by damage to the skin.

II. Wound Healing

A. Steps in healing

    1. Inflammatory process – first phase, involves **hemostasis** (stopping the blood flow. platelets and fibroblasts migrate to regenerate and repair tissue) and **phagocytosis** (WBC macrophages engulf microoranisms and debris). This phase lasts 3 to 6 days.

    2. Proliferative process – second phase, involves development of granulation tissue; lasts from about day 3 to day 21.

    3. Maturation process – third phase, new tissue becomes stronger and more structured, begins about day 21 and can last 1 to 2 years.

B. Classification of wound healing

    1. Primary or first intention, seen in surgical wounds. There is no tissue loss. The edges of the wound are approximated by use of sutures, clips, or a bonding agent. The wound heals with minimal scarring.

    2. Secondary or second intention. There is loss of tissue, such as in a pressure ulcer. The edges of the wound remain separated, granulation tissue is generated in the wound, and healing occurs from the inside outward. There will be scarring.

    3. Tertiary or third intention. The injury and repair of the wound occur at separate times. This is often seen after an infection where the wound may have been left open. At a later date, when the infection has resolved, the doctor sutures the area closed. Healing in this type of wound produces deep scarring.

III. Pressure Ulcers

A. Pressure ulcer is one of the most commonly occurring types of wounds. It results from impaired skin integrity. A client who may be developing a pressure ulcer has tissue ischemia (whitening) at the affected area, resulting from obstructed capillary blood flow

B. Risk factors

1. Decreased activity as a result of bed rest, paralysis, or state of consciousness

2. Poor nutrition; especially inadequate protein, vitamins and minerals, and fluid intake

3. History of pressure ulcers

4. Decreased sensation from cerebral and spinal cord injury, which increases the client's risk of injury and decreases the ability to identify signs of pressure

5. Poor circulation resulting from circulatory disease

6. Prolonged exposure to moisture, such as clients who have bowel or urinary incontinence

7. Medications that suppress the immune system or lead to side effects of pruritus and photosensitivity; these can alter the integrity of the skin.

8. The first sign that the skin is being injured is that the area is red and warm to touch. When pressure is applied to the area using the finger, blanching occurs. The reddening (erythema) occurs when blood vessels dilate to prevent tissue trauma. This can be corrected by relief of pressure.

9. The most common sites for pressure ulcer are over the bony prominences such as the sacral area, heels, elbows, shoulders, and the occipital area.

10. The client's risk for a pressure ulcer can be determined at the time of admission using one of several tests (e.g., Braden Scale).

11. The Braden Scale measures sensory perception, ability to communicate discomfort, moisture, activity, mobility, nutrition, and friction shear. A score indicates the client's risks and suggestions to improve client outcome.

C. Staging ulcers

1. Stage I

a. The skin is intact: the area is red, and when pressure is applied   with the finger over the reddened area, the color remains the same.

b. Injury may be resolved with pressure relief and protection.

c. In people with a darker skin hue, the area may not be reddened but may be a deep purple.

2. Stage II – There is redness with blistering or a break in the epidermis.

3. Stage III

a. The break extends to the subcutaneous tissue.

b. This is a full thickness tissue loss.

4. Stage IV – Break extends through muscle to the bone.

IV. **Nursing Responsibilities for Wound Care**

A. Prevention

1. Keep the skin clean, dry, and free of moisture.

2. Change position every 2 hours.

3. Use protective devices, such as air flow beds or air mattresses which will relieve some pressure.

4. Avoid **shearing,** which shifts the skin and subcutaneous tissue away from the bony prominence, and is caused by pulling the client up the bed rather than lifting, resulting in damage to the vascular bed.

5. Avoid friction that causes damage to the outer layer of the skin.

6. Provide adequate nutrition with supplemental vitamins and proteins.

B. Diagnoses and assessment of ulcers

1. Assessment of the ulcer

2. Wounds are diagnosed by the doctor or nurse specialist.

3. Diagnostic testing such as culture and sensitivity is usually ordered if an infection is suspected.

4. Routine chemistry profile is ordered along with a Doppler sonogram or arteriogram if the doctor must differentiate a venous stasis ulcer from an arterial ulcer.

5. Measure the wound width, length, and depth; document findings.

6. Color and appearance of the wound bed

    a. Granulating tissue is red and beefy indicating healing.

    b. Slough is yellow-gray, threadlike tissue

    c. **Eschar** (necrotic tissue) is black or brown indicating poor healing. Necrotic tissue or slough has to be removed to allow for healing.

    d. Presence of drainage exudates

        i.   **Serous** – clear, thin and watery

        ii. **Sanguineous** – containing blood

        iii. **Serosanguineous** – containing serum and blood.

    e. Appearance and consistency of the tissue surrounding the wound (called periwound).

    f. Client complaints of pain

    g. Presence of wound odor

    h. Vital signs, especially temperature.

C. Treatment

1. Use sterile technique when skin is broken.

2. Cleanse and irrigate wound.

3. Chemicals such as Accuzyme and Panafil derived from the enzyme papain are used only on necrotic tissue for debridement. They will break down and destroy healthy tissue.

4. The doctor can also surgically cut away necrotic tissue (manual or surgical debridement.)

5. Dressings can be simple dry sterile (to absorb drainage) or wet-to-dry (to provide mechanical debridement to get rid of necrotic or slough tissue). Wound may be packed with gauze.

6. Hydrocolloid dressings protect against friction and provide moisture to the wound, but they are not placed on delicate skin, a draining wound, or an infected wound. They conform to the wound and can stay in place for 3 to 5 days or until the seal is loosened.

7. Hydro gels keep the wound bed moist and soften slough and necrotic tissue.

8. Absorbers such as calcium alginates are derived from seaweed and can absorb a large volume of water from draining wounds.

9. Adequate nutrition and hydration are important for healing. Encourage client to increase protein intake.

D. Steps for nursing care of wounds

1. Wash hands.

2. Assemble sterile equipment and field.

3. Put on gloves. Remove old dressing.

4. Carefully note drainage for later charting.

5. Place old dressing in watertight container and dispose of it properly.

6. Carefully assess wound.

7. Put on sterile gloves.

8. Cleanse wound from clean area to dirty.

9. Apply sterile dressing.

10. Anchor dressing securely with tape or binder.

E. Types of dressings

1. Wet to dry dressings

   a. Similar to sterile.

   b. Done to cleanse wound and remove debris.

   c. Saline is used to wet the dressing when applied. The dressing is removed dry to help debride the wound.

   d. Avoid saturating dressing to avoid leakage.

   e. Cover with dry sterile sponges to increase wicking action.

   f. Secure dressing.

2. Bandages and binders

   a. Types of and uses for bandages:

      i. *Circular:* holds dressings in place.

      ii. *Spiral:* immobilizes part of extremity or decreases swelling.

      iii. *Figure of eight:* applies pressure, supports or immobilizes joint, shapes stump.

      iv. *Triangular:* creates sling to hold forearm immobile.

   b. Montgomery straps

      i. Consist of two large pieces of tape with cloth straps that tie over the dressing to immobilize it.

      ii. Used for frequently changed dressing to prevent constant retaping.

   c. Abdominal binders

      i. Apply tight enough to support chest or abdomen.

      ii. Avoid an overtight binder that prevents adequate chest expansion.

    d. T binders are used to secure rectal or perineal dressing.

    e. Antiembolic stockings (TED)

       i. Used for all postoperative clients

       ii. Support blood vessels in the legs to prevent blood clots

       iii. Should fit tightly but not cut off circulation

       iv. Circulation check should be performed periodically.

       v. Stockings are removed once each shift and skin checked.

       vi. Apply stockings before client gets out of bed.

       vii. Do not allow stocking to bunch up, as this will impede circulation.

V. Use of Cold and Heat

A. Cold applications

1. Dry cold

    a. Ice caps

    b. Ice collars

    c. Ice bags

2. Moist cold

    a. Colds packs

    b. Compresses

    c. More penetrating than dry cold

3. Effects

    a. Aid in prevention of swelling

    b. Help to control hemorrhage

    c. Prevent discoloration

    d. Prevent suppuration

    e Check process of inflammation

    f. Constrict blood vessels and reduce circulation of blood to particular area

    g. Help to relieve pain by blocking pain receptor sites

    h. May be very harmful when used on very weak or aged clients

4. Safety factors

    a. Observe condition of part of body where ice has been used.

    b. Remove cold application at frequent intervals.

    c. Cold applications should be used on doctor's order only.

    d. Observe infants, young children, or aged clients every 15-20 minutes when cold applications are applied.

    e. Observe condition of skin each time application is removed.

5. Cold compresses

    a. May be applied to eyes, head, or other parts of body

       b.   Wash hands and assemble equipment.

       c.   Explain procedure to client.

       d.   Change compresses every 15 to 20 minutes.

B. Hot applications

    1. Uses

       a.   Help localize infection.

       b.   Produce muscular relaxation.

       c.   Promote suppuration.

       d.   Relieve congestion and aid removal of waste from injured tissue (by dilating the blood vessels, thereby increasing the flow of blood locally).

       e.   May decrease pain

    2. Electric heating pads

       a.   Apply only when ordered by doctor.

       b.   Check to see if pad is in good order.

       c.   Set thermostat on low.

       d.   Cover pad.

       e.   Check skin periodically for redness.

    3. Hot compresses

       a.   Assemble necessary equipment before starting procedure.

       b.   Apply to eye or other areas of body only when ordered by doctor.

       c.   Determine correct temperature of solution.

       d.   Compresses should not cause discomfort or burning.

       e.   Observe client during procedure.

       f.   Record results.

Additional Resources Found on MyNursingLab

- Pressure Ulcers animation

MODULE 2

Fundamentals

Submodule 2.13 Nutrition, Fluids, Electrolytes, and Acid-Base Balance

Learning Objectives

2.13.1 Describe the elements that make up a nutritional diet and their sources.

2.13.2 Discuss fluid and electrolyte needs in the body and their relationship to acid-base balance.

2.13.3 Define the modifications seen in diet therapy, their purpose and objectives.

I. **Nutrients and Nutrition**

    A. Nutritional planning

        1. Food and nutrition are essential for the body to provide energy, build and repair tissue, and regulate metabolism. The most nutritious diet will contain a variety of foods.

        2. A balanced diet contains the essential nutrients: protein, carbohydrates, fats, vitamins, and minerals and meets the nutritional needs of the body.

        3. The United State Department of Agriculture (USDA) recommends daily allowances for all individuals.

        4. The daily allowances come from four basic four groups as a guide to maintaining good health.

        5. MyPyramid lays the foundation for sound nutritional practice for all age groups.

        6. MyPyramid recommends an allowance consisting of daily servings of:

            a. Grains – 6 ounces

            b. Vegetables – 2 ½ cups

            c. Fruits – 2 cups

            d. Milk – 3 cups; children 2-8 years, 2 cups

            e. Meat and beans – 5/12 ounces

        7. MyPyramid incorporates the need for physical activity along with sound nutritional practices.

        8. MyPyramid offers specific health food choices from which individuals can select for all the food groups.

    B. Nutrients

        1. Carbohydrates

            a. Primary source of energy in the body.

            b. Cheapest source of food and makes up the largest percentage of the American diet, especially among the poor.

PEARSON

    c. Carbohydrates are composed of carbon, hydrogen, and oxygen.

    d. One gram of carbohydrate yields 4 calories when metabolized.

    e. Carbohydrates are divided into three groups:

        i. **Monosaccharides** are simple sugars; require no digestion; are the most common form of sugar in the body.

            (a) Sources: fruits and vegetables

            (b) Glucose and fructose, which are fruit sugars

        ii. **Disaccharides** made from two sugar molecules

            (a) Sources: table sugar, sucrose, milk sugar from lactose

        iii. **Polysaccharides** are complex sugars

            (a) Sources: starches grains, vegetables, and fruits

            (b) Difficult to digest and add bulk, which aids peristalsis

    f. Functions of carbohydrates

        i. Aid in the production of energy and heat.

        ii. Spare protein: if carbohydrate intake is inadequate, the body will use protein for energy, which can result in muscle wasting.

        iii. Aid in fat oxidation

  2. Fats/lipids

    a. Composed of carbon, hydrogen, and oxygen and are insoluble in water.

    b. One of the largest parts of the American diet and are the most concentrated source of energy.

    c. Fats are easily stored in the body.

    d. One gram of fat yields 9 calories when metabolized

    e. Fats better satisfy hunger, add taste and texture to foods, and last longer in the stomach.

    f. Fats are classified as:

        i. Saturated fats: at room temperature remain solid.

            (a) Sources: usually animal fat

            (b) Trans fatty acids are found in processed forms of foods.

            (c) Hydrogen is added to oils such as vegetable palm oil to make them more stable and prevent spoiling.

            (d) These hydrogenated oils are high in cholesterol.

        ii. Unsaturated fats: at room temperature remains liquid.

            (a) Monounsaturated, such as olive oil

            (b) Polyunsaturated, such as soy oil

            (c) Fatty acids are essential in the body to avoid disease and to foster growth.

            (d) The essential fatty acids are linoleic acid omega-6 and linoleic acid omega-3.

3. Cholesterol

   a. Found only in animal tissue and belongs to a group of compounds called sterols.

   b. Cholesterol is a complex of bile that aids in fat digestion and formation of many hormones.

   c. Synthesized independently in the body during the metabolic processes.

   d. Sources of cholesterol: organ meats, egg yolks, milk

   e. High levels of cholesterol in the blood are unhealthy and cause heart disease.

   f. Lipoprotein molecules in the blood transport cholesterol.

   g. High-density lipoproteins transfer cholesterol from tissue to liver and are the good lipoproteins ("good cholesterol").

   h. Low-density lipoproteins transfer cholesterol from liver to tissue, causing atherosclerosis, and are harmful lipoproteins ("bad cholesterol").

4. Proteins

   a. One of the most important elements of all body cells

   b. Proteins are complex in structure and composed of carbon, hydrogen, nitrogen, and oxygen; made from amino acids.

   c. One gram protein yields 4 calories when metabolized.

   d. Protein is not stored in the body, but in severe deficiency the body can metabolize its own cellular protein.

   e. Proteins are classified as:

      i. Complete proteins: contain all the essential amino acids

         (a) Sources: usually from animals

      ii. Incomplete proteins: do not contain all the essential amino acids

         (a) Sources: cereals, gelatin, and vegetables

         (b) Two partial proteins can provide one complete protein.

         (c) Combining incomplete proteins allows vegetarians to have a healthy diet.

   f. Functions:

      i. Build and repair cells

      ii. Promote immune system function by aiding in production of hormones, enzymes, and antibodies

      iii. Combine with iron to form hemoglobin necessary to carry oxygen to tissue

      iv. Aids in regulation of fluid balance by keeping intracellular and intracellular fluids in their compartments

      v. Inadequate protein in the body leads to edema.

      vi. Aids in regulation of acid-base balance.

5. Vitamins

   a. Organic substances important in the metabolic processes to prevent disease

   b. Not manufactured by the body

   c. Present in most foods in minute amounts

  d.   Aid in building and maintenance of body tissue

  e.   Help the body fight disease by stimulating the immune system

  f.   Vitamins are classified as:

    i.   Fat soluble: vitamins A, D, E, and K

      (a)   Are stored in the liver and fatty tissue

      (b)   Sources: butter, poultry, and fish

      (c)   Can survive cooking

    ii.   Water soluble: vitamins B, C, folic and pantothenic acid, and biotin

      (a)   Excess amounts are easily excreted from the body because they are water soluble.

      (b)   Sources: fruits, vegetables, grains

      (c)   Are destroyed by cooking

6. Minerals

  a.   Minerals are inorganic compounds existing inside and outside of the body.

  b.   Major minerals are:

    i.   Calcium

      (a)   Most abundant mineral in the body, found mainly in the bones and teeth

      (b)   Aids in regulation of the heartbeat and muscle contraction and nerve response

      (c)   Aids in the formation of blood clots

      (d)   Sources: milk and milk products, vegetables, fruits, and fish

      (e)   Inadequate calcium intake causes bone to give up calcium and leads to osteoporosis.

    ii.   Iron

      (a)   Needed for the formation of hemoglobin, the oxygen-carrying component of red blood cells

      (b)   Sources: liver, kidney, enriched cereals, green leafy vegetables, and dried beans and peas

      (c)   Absorption increased in presence of vitamin C

      (d)   Need for iron increased during pregnancy and lactation

    iii.   Phosphorus

      (a)   Found in cells in small amounts

      (b)   About 1% of body weight

      (c)   Important for bone and teeth integrity

      (d)   Helps cells use carbohydrates, proteins, and fats

      (e)   Aids in regulation of acid-base balance

      (f)   Promotes functioning of muscles and nerves

      (g)   Sources: meat, fish, poultry, milk, and legumes

iv. Water

(a) Water is the most important and critical compound needed in the body.

(b) Water provides the transport needed to deliver nutrients to cells and remove waste from cells.

(c) Water provides the medium for chemical reactions in cells.

(d) Water supports acid-base balance.

(e) Water aids regulation of temperature in the body through the process of evaporation.

(f) The percentage of water in the body varies based on age:

(1) Infants 70-80%

(2) Adults 50-60%

(3) Older adults 45-50%

(g) Water is also proportionate to body fat. The higher the fat, the lower the water content.

(h) Maintaining water balance is essential since adults lose about 2500 mL/day through urine, feces, and insensible loss (respiration and perspiration).

(i) To offset water loss, the adult should drink 6 to 8 glasses of water each day.

(j) Water in the body is distributed into different compartments:

(1) **Intracellular** – fluid within the cell; ICF.

(2) **Extracellular** – fluid outside the cell or ECF; is divided into two types:

(a) **Interstitial** – fluid between the cells and tissue; accounts for 27% of body water content. Interstitial fluid is found in cerebrospinal fluid, gastrointestinal tract, and lymph.

(b) **Intravascular** – fluid in blood vessels (plasma); accounts for 7% of body fluid

(k) Intracellular and extracellular fluids are separated by a semipermeable membrane that allows fluid to shift back and forth.

II. Fluids and Electrolytes

A. Intake and output

1. Fluid loss must be made up by fluid intake.

2. Water loss can be replenished by foods, liquid, and metabolism.

3. Fluid is lost through the kidneys, skin, respiratory system, and gastrointestinal tract.

4. Intake: all fluids taken into the body, including foods that become liquid at room temperature.

5. The client needs an intake of at least 2,500 mL/day.

6. Output: all fluids leaving the body (including by vomiting, diarrhea, and drains exiting the body);

7. Fluids primarily leave the body through the kidneys, which excrete a minimum of 30 mL/hr.

8. Fluid balance is best evaluated by weight: 1 liter fluid = 2.2 lb.

9. Electrolytes move from one compartment to the other but each favors a specific compartment.

B. Common electrolytes

1. Sodium

   a. Mostly found in the extracellular fluid

   b. Helps maintain normal water balance and acid-base balance

   c. **Hyponatremia** (sodium deficiency)

      i. Assessment findings: headache, fatigue, apathy, confusion, muscle weakness, abdominal cramps, and postural hypotension

      ii. Interventions: provide oral or parenteral supplement.

   d. Sodium is restricted in hypertension, congestive heart failure, myocardial infarction, hepatitis, adrenocortical diseases, kidney disease, lithium carbonate therapy, cystic fibrosis, and conditions such as cirrhosis of the liver and preeclampsia, which cause persistent edema:

      i. Mild restriction is 2 to 3 g of sodium/day.

      ii. Moderate restriction is 1000 mg of sodium/day.

      iii. Strict restriction is 500 mg of sodium/day.

      iv. Severe restriction is 250 mg of sodium/day.

      v. Limit foods high in sodium, such as potato chips and other salted snack foods; canned foods; baked goods which contain baking powder or baking soda; cereals; seafood; beef; processed meats such as bologna, ham, and bacon; dairy products, especially cheese; pickles, olives, and condiments such as soy sauce, steak sauce, Worcestershire sauce, and salad dressings.

      vi. Encourage low sodium foods such as fresh fruits and vegetables, chicken, salt substitutes, and low sodium products.

   e. **Hypernatremia** (sodium excess)

      i. Assessment findings: flushed dry skin and mucous membranes, decreased urinary output, increased thirst and heart rate, restlessness, and convulsions

      ii. Interventions: increased fluid to hydrate, and salt-restricted diet

2. Potassium

   a. Most abundant electrolyte in intracellular fluid

   b. Helps to maintain water and fluid balance and acid-base balance

   c. Loss of potassium is seen after vomiting and diarrhea.

   d. **Hypokalemia** (potassium deficit)

      i. Assessment findings: muscle weakness, lethargy, nausea, vomiting, decreased bowel sounds, and cardiac arrhythmias

      ii. Interventions: oral or parenteral potassium supplement; increased intake of foods such as bananas and oranges

      e. **Hyperkalemia** (potassium excess)

          i.   Assessment findings: nausea, vomiting, diarrhea, irritability, anxiety, abdominal cramps, decrease urinary output, irregular pulse, and cardiac arrhythmias

          ii. Intervention: restrict potassium intake

  3. Calcium

      a. The most abundant electrolyte in the body

      b. Calcium promotes the transmission of nerve impulses and regular muscle contraction

      c. Essential in clot formation

      d. **Hypocalcemia** (low calcium)

          i.   Assessment findings: numbness, tingling, muscle cramps, tetany, and convulsions

          ii. Intervention: increased intake of calcium (PO or parenteral)

      e. **Hypercalcemia** (high calcium)

          i.   Assessment findings: nausea, vomiting anorexia, muscle weakness, constipation, polyuria

          ii. Interventions: hydrate to decrease calcium levels, may need dialysis

III. Acid-Base Balance

  A. The balance of hydrogen ions (H+) in the body fluid

  B. Acid base balance exists when the rate at which the body produces acids or bases equals the rate at which acids or bases are excreted.

  C. The measure used to indicate hydrogen ion balance is pH.

    1. A pH less than 7.35 is acidic, called **acidosis.**

    2. A pH greater than 7.45 is alkaline, called **alkalosis.**

    3. A pH of 7.35 – 7.45 is neutral.

  D. Arterial blood gas analysis determines acidosis or alkalosis by measuring blood pH.

  E. Normal acid-base balance is regulated by buffers (chemicals that travel through the body to neutralize acid, the respiratory tract, and kidneys.

  F. Acid-base disturbances

    1. Respiratory acidosis

      a. Occurs when normal ventilation changes and causes retention of CO_2.

      b. CO_2 retention results in a decrease in pH.

      c. Conditions that result in respiratory acidosis are pneumonia, drug overdose, head injury, drowning, or asphyxiation.

      d. Assessment findings: shallow respiration, headache, lethargy, sweating, confusion, increased pCO_2 levels.

      e. Interventions: correct ventilation, upright position, increased fluids, and bronchodilator may be ordered.

2. Respiratory alkalosis

   a. Caused by hyperventilating resulting in excess loss of CO_2, decreased respiration, and increased pH

   b. Caused by diseases such as pneumonia, anemia, severe blood loss, heart failure, fever, and drug overdose

   c. Assessment findings: increased heart rate, anxiety, lightheadness, dizziness, muscle weakness, numbness in fingers, fainting, and seizure

   d. Interventions: breathe slowly, correct the underlying cause.

3. Metabolic acidosis

   a. Increased acid, decreased base, decreased blood pH below 7.35 to 7.45, decreased sodium bicarbonate

   b. Causes: prolonged vomiting, nasogastric suction, use of excessive diuretics, and electrolyte disturbances

   c. Assessment findings: headache, lethargy, irritability decreased level of consciousness, confusion, shallow breathing; may have periods of apnea

   d. Interventions: daily weight, intake and output, correct cause, and administer sodium bicarbonate

4. Metabolic alkalosis

   a. Results from loss of acids or increase in sodium bicarbonate

   b. Assessment findings: dizziness, tingling in the extremities, decreased respiratory rate

   c. Interventions: correct problem, increase sodium-rich fluids

IV. Diet Therapy

A. The nurse must understand the principles of a normal diet and the modifications needed in certain diseases.

   1. Modifications according to client's ability to metabolize specific nutrients

   2. To relieve and rest specific body organs and resolve inadequacies in nutrition

B. Common diet modifications

   1. Clear liquid diet consistency modification

      a. Indicated for resting the gastrointestinal tract, maintaining fluid balance, immediately post-op, for diarrhea, nausea, and vomiting.

      b. Prevents dehydration and supplies simple carbohydrates

      c. Includes water, tea, broth, Jell-O, apple juice, popsicles. "Clear" refers to the relative transparency of the food or drink.

      d. Not nutritionally adequate, just helps to maintain energy level

   2. Full liquid diet consistency modification

      a. When clear liquids are tolerated well, progress to full liquids.

      b. Includes clear liquids plus fruit juices and milk and milk products such as custard, pudding, creamed soups, ice cream, and sherbet

      c. Can be nutritionally adequate, but should only be used for short time

3. Mechanical soft diet

    a. For clients who have problem chewing

    b. Includes full liquids plus pureed vegetables, eggs which are fried, tender meats, potatoes, and cooked fruit

    c. Carries a full range of foods but is poor in fiber

4. Bland diet consistency modification

    a. To promote healing of gastric mucosa by eliminating chemically and mechanically irritating food sources, including fiber

    b. Indicated for gastric and duodenal ulcers and postoperative stomach surgery

    c. Goal is to limit foods that stimulate production of gastric acids.

    d. Given in small frequent feedings to assist in diluting or neutralizing stomach acid. Protein foods are good at neutralizing. Fat has ability to inhibit the secretion of acid and delays stomach emptying.

    e. Foods usually introduced in stages with gradual addition of foods.

    f. Includes milk, butter, eggs which are not fried, custard, vanilla ice cream, cottage cheese, cooked, refined, or strained cereal, enriched white bread, Jell-O homemade creamed and pureed soups, baked or broiled potatoes

5. Low residue diet

    a. Indicated for ulcerative colitis, postoperative colon and rectal surgery, prep for X-rays and colon surgery, diarrhea, and regional enteritis

    b. Goal is to decrease peristalsis and prevent distention of colon.

    c. Encourage ground meat, fish, broiled chicken without skin, creamed cheeses, warm drinks, refined strained cereals, and white bread.

    d. Foods high in carbohydrates are usually low in residue.

    e. Avoid high-residue foods which have skins and seeds.

6. Low cholesterol diet

    a. Indicated for cardiovascular diseases, diabetes mellitus, high serum cholesterol levels

    b. Controls cholesterol levels by limiting cholesterol intake

    c. Limit high cholesterol foods such as egg yolk, whole milk products, shellfish, organ meats, bacon, pork, avocado, olives.

7. Modified fat diet

    a. Indicated for malabsorption syndromes, cystic fibrosis, gallbladder disease, obstructive jaundice and liver disease, and obesity

    b. Fat content in the diet is lowered:

        i.   To stop contractions of the diseased organs

        ii. When there is inadequate absorption of fat

        iii. To decrease fat storage in the body

        iv. To stop aggravation of diseased organs.

v.   To reduce fat intake, avoid gravy, fatty meats, and fish, cream, fried foods, rich pastries, whole milk products, cream soups, salad and cooking oils, nuts, and chocolate. Allow 2-3 eggs per week, lean meat, butter, and margarine.

vi.   For a fat-free diet, restrict all fatty meats and fat. Allow vegetables, fruits, lean meats, fowl, fish, bread, and cereal.

8.   Carbohydrate modification (diabetic diet or ADA diet):

a.   Principles of diabetic diet management:

i.   Attain or maintain ideal body weight.

ii.   Ensure normal growth.

iii.   Maintain plasma glucose levels as close to normal as possible.

iv.   Provide 30 calories per kg of ideal body weight.

v.   Provide ¼ of the calories at each meal and ¼ for snacks.

vi.   Provide 20% of calories as protein, 55-60% as carbohydrates, and 20-30% as fats.

vii.   Include unsaturated fats, high fiber, and complex carbohydrates. (Fiber helps lower blood glucose.)

b.   Allows clients to develop meal plans designed using exchange lists:

i.   Milk exchanges

ii.   Vegetable exchanges

iii.   Fruit exchanges

iv.   Bread exchanges

v.   Fat exchanges

vi.   Combination foods

9. Low protein diet

a.   Indicated for client with chronic and acute kidney disease and liver disease

b.   Objectives:

i.   Reduce work of the kidney by reducing waste production

ii.   Prevent the accumulation of waste products in the blood

c.   Reduce protein intake to 40-60 g/day, based on client weight.

d.   Decrease salt to reduce edema.

e.   Increase caloric intake to provide energy.

C.   Feeding clients

1.   Place tray so client can see food being served.

2.   If possible, raise head of bed.

3.   Prepare foods, but allow client as much independence as possible.

4.   Use straws for fluids.

5.   Offer food in small amounts.

6.   Vary foods being offered or ask clients what they want next.

7.   Alternate liquids with solid foods.

8. For a blind client, describe what foods are being offered and the position of foods on the plate.

9. Always strive to make mealtimes pleasant to promote a good appetite. This includes removing unpleasant odors.

D. Nasogastric (NG) tubes

1. Used to either drain gastric contents or administer tube feedings

2. Suctioning

a. NG tubes (Levin, Salem Sump, Miller-Abbot, and Cantor) to continuous or intermittent suction.

b. Check proper tube placement before irrigating:

i. Check pH of aspirated contents.

ii. Inject 10 mL of air into tube while listening with stethoscope for whooshing sound over stomach.

c. Irrigate with normal saline at intervals to prevent clogging.

d. Note and chart amount, color, and consistency of drainage.

e. Subtract irrigating solution for correct I&O.

f. Provide mouth care every 2 hours.

3. Tube feedings

a. Done through nasogastric or gastrostomy tube for clients unable to swallow

b. Done continuously or intermittently throughout the day and night

c. Prepared solutions available; also may be made by dietary department

d. Always serve feedings at room temperature to prevent cramping.

e. Give feedings by gravity infusion; never force the feeding under pressure.

f. Raise head of bed during feedings and maintain elevated position for 45 minutes following feeding.

g. Administer feedings slowly to prevent nausea and overdistention of stomach.

h. Follow feedings with prescribed amount of water.

i. Aspirate stomach contents 1 hour after feedings, or as ordered, to check for residual feeding left in stomach.

j. Provide client with emotional support.

k. Administer mouth care every 2 hours.

E. Vomitus

1. Observe and report symptoms associated with vomiting.

2. Save specimen of vomitus if it has any unusual characteristics.

3. Record amount and characteristics on chart.

Additional Resources Found on MyNursingLab

- Carbohydrates animation
- Lipids animation
- Acid-Base Balance animation
- Fluid Balance animation
- NG Tube animation

PEARSON

MODULE 2

Fundamentals

Submodule 2.14 Elimination

Learning Objectives

2.14.1 Describe normal characteristics of urine and feces.

2.14.2 Describe nursing responsibilities in assisting clients with elimination problems.

2.14.3 Discuss collection of urinary and fecal specimens.

I. **Normal Characteristics of Urine and Feces**

A. Urine

1. Urinary elimination: voiding or urine formed by kidneys

a. Average output 1,000 – 1,500 mL in 24 hours; at least 30 mL/hr

b. Fluid output should equal fluid intake.

2. Normal characteristics of urine

a. Color: yellow amber

b. Clarity: clear

c. Odor: aromatic

d. Volume: voiding between 200-300 mL

e. Specific gravity: 1.010 – 1.025

f. Specific gravity below 1.01 indicates overhydration; above 1.025 indicates dehydration.

g. Abnormal components: blood, protein, glucose, WBCs, calculi

3. Altered urinary elimination patterns

a. Frequency

b. Nocturia

c. Polyuria

d. Urgency

e. Dysuria

f. Incontinence

g. Oliguria

h. Enuresis

i. Retention (may be the result of narcotic analgesics)

j. Nocturia

k. Anuria

B. Feces

    1. Bowel elimination: stool formed by intestines

    2. Normal characteristics of feces

        a. Color – yellow-brown

        b. Consistency – well formed, cylindrical

        c. Odor – aromatic

        d. Abnormal components – fat (steatorrhea), blood (melena)

    3. Abnormal bowel elimination patterns

        a. Diarrhea

        b. Constipation

        c. **Fecal impaction** – hardened stool that allows passage of liquid feces

        d. Flatus

II. **Nursing Responsibilities for Altered Elimination**

A. Assisting with urinary elimination

    1. Offer bedpan or urinal at regular intervals or leave within client's reach.

    2. Provide client privacy.

    3. Encourage client to sit or stand to promote ease.

    4. If client has difficulty voiding:

        a. Run water in client's hearing.

        b. Pour warm water over perineum.

    5. Always wipe the client from front to back to prevent bacteriuria.

    6. Help client wash hands after voiding.

B. Urinary procedures

    1. Urinary catheters – types

        a. Foley

        b. Straight

        c. Suprapubic – surgical insertion

        d. 3-way Foley

        e. External (condom) catheter

    2. Purposes

        a. To obtain sterile urine specimens

        b. To relieve retention

        c. To keep bladder decompressed during surgery

        d. To measure residue urine following voiding

        e. To empty the bladder before surgery

        f. To keep the perineum dry after surgery

        g. To irrigate bladder use caution: withdraw no more than 800-1000 mL at one time.

PEARSON

3. Catheter insertion

    a. **Straight catheters** inserted for decompression and then removed

    b. **Foley catheter** inserted and left in for length of time ordered

    c. General principles of sterile catheterization:

        i. Use smallest size possible to avoid trauma.

        ii. Provide privacy;

        iii. Explain procedure to client before beginning.

        iv. Position client.

        v. Put on sterile gloves and set up sterile field.

        vi. Cleanse the urinary meatus front to back for women and in a circular motion for men.

        vii. Lubricate catheter well before inserting.

        viii. Insert catheter about 3-4 inches in women and 6-8 inches in men.

        ix. For indwelling catheter, fill balloon with 5-10 mL of sterile water.

4. Catheter removal

    a. Position client and provide for privacy.

    b. Withdraw water from balloon port with syringe to deflate the balloon.

    c. Release tape, have client take deep breaths, and remove catheter with steady, gentle pull.

    d. Monitor client for voiding within 8 hours after removal.

    e. Encourage fluid intake to improve output.

    f. Warn client that some burning may occur with first voiding.

5. Bladder irrigation

    a. Must be done using aseptic technique

    b. Can be done as manual irrigation using syringe or constant bladderirrigation (CBI)

    c. Done to clear catheter of obstructions, remove clots, or decrease bleeding

    d. Done without disconnecting catheter using a three-way Foley

    e. Amount and type of solution determined by doctor's orders

    f. Account for amount of solution on output record.

C. Assisting with bowel elimination

1. Offer bedpan as needed. Tell client not ignore urge to defecate, as this may result in constipation.

2. Reassure client about using bedpan; provide privacy.

3. Cover bedpan both before and after use.

4. Assist client as needed. Place client in Fowler's position unless contraindicated.

5. Record frequency, contents of bedpan; measure urine if output.

6. Aid and encourage normal bowel function.

    a. Assess each client's normal bowel pattern and attempt to maintain it.

    b. Encourage adequate intake of fluids and fiber to prevent constipation.

    c. Provide privacy.

    d. Offer the bedpan as needed.

    e. Position client comfortably and offer privacy while client defecates.

    f. Help cleanse client after defecation.

    g. Monitor amount, color, and consistency of stool.

D. Bowel procedures

1. Rectal tubes

    a. Insert to relieve distention due to flatus.

    b. Lubricate tube before inserting 2-6 inches into rectum.

    c. Position client in left lateral Sims' position.

    d. Tape in place and leave no longer than 30 minutes.

    e. Report and record results.

2. Enemas

    a. Types:

        i. **Cleansing enema** – given to relieve distention and remove feces

        ii. **Oil retention enema** – given to soften feces

        iii. **Emollient enema** – given to soothe irritated mucous membranes

    b. Cleansing enema

        i. Can be tap water, mixture of soap and water, or saline.

        ii. Temperature of solution 105°-110° F; children, 100°F.

        iii. Administer 500-1000 mL of fluid.

        iv. Position client in left lateral Sims' position.

        v. Hold fluid container about 1 inch above anus.

        vi. Lubricate tube and insert 3-4 inches.

        vii. If cramping occurs, lower the height of the enema bag.

        viii. Observe results and record amount of feces.

        ix. If ordered "until clear," return should eventually be free of feces

        x. Solution is hypertonic, so no more than three enemas unless specified by physician.

    c. Oil retention enema

        i. Given to soften feces in order to ease defecation

        ii. Oil heated to 100°F

        iii. Encourage client to try to retain enema for 30 minutes.

        iv. May require cleansing enema afterwards

        v. Commercially prepared prefilled enemas approximately120 mL

3. Manual extraction of fecal impaction is done only with physician's order.

    a. Apply gloves and adequately lubricate index finger.

    b. Position client in left lateral Sims'.

    c. Gently insert finger into hardened stool and break off small pieces.

    d. Assess client's condition throughout.

    e. Place client on bedpan following procedure to allow evacuation of remaining stool.

4. Colostomy irrigation

    a. Done to empty bowel and regulate the passage of feces and flatus

    b. Not all clients require irrigation procedure in colostomy management.

    c. Irrigation done daily or every other day

    d. Equipment and procedure same as for enema administration

    e. Irrigation done with warm normal saline or tap water

    f. Special ostomy pouch worn for irrigation to collect fecal drainage

    g. Record results of irrigation.

III. Collecting Urinary or Fecal Specimens

A. Rules for specimen collection

1. All specimens must be collected on time.

2. All specimens must be labeled correctly, double bagged, and sent to laboratory promptly.

3. Inside of container must not become contaminated.

4. Correct amount of specimen must be collected.

5. Medical and/or surgical asepsis techniques must be utilized.

B. Urine specimen

1. Sterile specimen collected by straight catheterization.

2. Voided specimen:

    a. Wash meatus or perineal area well first.

    b. Collect **midstream specimen** by having client start void, stop, and then restart the middle void into sterile container.

    c. Clean specimen or up to 24-hour specimens may be collected.

    d. Single specimen or up to 24-hour specimens may be collected.

    e. Container and preservative dependent on type of specimen collected.

    f. **24-hour specimen**; discard first void and record time; collect all urine for next 24 hours; keep refrigerated.

    g. Double-voided specimen: client empties bladder; collect next void.

C. Stool specimen

1. Important in disorders of GI tract

2. Laboratory examination of occult blood: client should not eat either meat for three days prior to the examination (may give a false positive for blood).

3. Important in inflammations and ulcerations causing bleeding in tract.

4. Microscopic examination for ova and parasites must be kept warm.

Additional Resources Found on MyNursingLab

- Enema animation

MODULE 2

Fundamentals

Submodule 2.15 Sensory Perception and Pain

Learning Objectives

2.15.1 **Describe sensory perception, changes in sensory perception, and nursing responses.**

2.15.2 **Discuss pain perception and modulation, and nursing management strategies for clients in pain.**

2.15.3 **List the components of a neurological nursing assessment, including levels of consciousness.**

2.15.4 **Describe some common procedures for organs in the sensory system.**

I. **Sensory Perception**

A. Sensory stimulation and awareness

1. Through our senses we perceive and interact with our environment.

2. The sensory system allows us to receive information from inside and outside our bodies.

3. Sensory stimulus relates to sight, sound, taste, touch, and pain.

4. Stimulus is transmitted via nerve endings from all over the body along nerve routes to the central nervous system.

B. Sensory receptors

1. **Thermoreceptors** in the skin allow the detection of temperature changes.

2. **Proprioceptors** in the inner ear allow a sense of balance or equilibrium; those in muscle, tendons, and ligaments enable walking.

3. **Photoreceptors** in the retina allow the detection of light and shapes.

4. **Chemoreceptors** in the taste buds allow us to taste and distinguish between sweet, sour, salty, or bitter; those in the nasal cavity allow smell and distinguish different odors.

C. Sensory perception

1. Occurs when the person is conscious of a stimulus and receives and interprets the information.

2. Impulse travels to the spinal cord and brain where special cells interpret the meaning of the impulse.

D. Sensory changes in the older adult

1. Affected by age, illness, medications, and stress

2. Senses affected: vision, hearing, tastes, and vision.

3. **Presbyopia** (farsightedness) starts at about age 40 to 45 – difficulty focusing on near objects.

4. **Presbycusis** – decrease in hearing – starts with a loss of high-frequency tones

5. Taste buds atrophy; difficulty experiencing tastes; as a result, food interest may decrease or shift to sweeter, saltier foods, affecting the person's nutritional status.

6. Atrophy of the olfactory nerve decreases the ability to smell, especially gas.

7. Ability to perceive touch, pain, and variations in temperature are reduced, leaving person more susceptible to burns and undetected injuries

E. Imbalance of sensory input

1. **Sensory deprivation** is seen in clients with neurological injury, dementia, depressed sleep, or central nervous system depressants.

2. **Sensory overload** can be internal or external; stimulus exceeds the client threshold.

 a. Noisy, unfamiliar surroundings such as the ICU can be especially difficult for the client.

 b. Pain can cause sensory overload.

3. Nurse can often make adjustments in the environment to provide more or less stimulation to the client.

 a. Provide distraction (conversation, TV, radio)

 b. Reduce noise, close curtains, dim lights, etc.

II. Pain

A. **Pain** is an unpleasant sensory or emotional experience; pain is subjective and it is whatever the client says it is.

B. Pain is one of the most common manifestations of illness and fear.

C. Theories of pain

1. **Gate control theory:** states that the dorsal horn of the spinal cords acts as a gate either to prevent pain impulses from reaching the brain or to allow pain impulses to reach the brain.

2. Pain results when nociceptors (pain receptors) respond to stimulus of damage from trauma, inflammation, or surgery.

3. **Transduction** occurs when pain stimulus in the nerve endings changes and becomes an impulse.

4. **Transmission** is the manner in which that impulse travels to the brain.

5. **Pain perception** is the brain's interpretation of the impulse as pain.

6. **Modulation** is stimulation of the body's natural responses to mediate the pain.

D. Types of pain

1. **Neuropathic pain** is usually chronic and results from injury to nerves; can result from a stroke or infection

2. **Cutaneous pain:** arising from the skin

3. **Visceral pain:** arising from the internal receptors deep in the organs such as gastrointestinal tract and gallbladder

4. **Radiating pain:** extending beyond the original location

5. **Referred pain:** appearing at a distance from the site of origin

6. **Phantom pain:** occurring after removal of a limb in the place the limb used to be

7. **Psychogenic pain:** arising from the mind

E. Duration and persistence of pain

1. **Acute pain:** shorter duration, rapid onset; can result from accident or surgery; can be mild or severe

2. **Chronic pain:** lasts for over six months; can be mild or severe, such as musculoskeletal pain or cancer pain

3. **Intractable pain:** usually chronic; resistant to any relief

F. Body's response to pain

1. Pain can cause loss of sleep, irritability, and decreased functioning.

2. Chronic pain can lower the person's self-esteem and disrupt family and interpersonal relationships. It can affect most of the body systems, including psychological responses.

3. Endocrine system: triggers the release of hormones such as cortisol, usually a part of a inflammatory response

4. Cardiovascular system: leads to increased cardiac workload, increased heart rate and oxygen demands, and hypercoagulation that can trigger chest pain and blood clots.

5. Musculoskeletal system: results in decreased muscle function, immobility, and decreased physical activity

6. Respiratory system: pain in the thoracic region interferes with respiratory efforts and could lead to atelectasis.

7. Genitourinary system: pain causes the release of catecholamines that can lead to urinary retention and edema.

8. Gastrointestinal system: pain decreases gastric motility and leads to loss of bowel function.

G. Pain assessment in the adult

1. Pain is the fifth vital sign; clients must be assessed for pain as a part of a vital sign assessment.

2. The nurse accepts the client's attitude and behavior in response to pain.

3. The nurse institutes measures of comfort and reassurance and correctly assesses the pain by asking the client to describe it in his or her own words.

4. Quality of pain: descriptors include throbbing, dull, stabbing, burning, intermittent, or constant.

5. Location of pain; note:

   a. Quality and intensity of pain

   b. Factors that precipitate the pain

   c. Factors that aggravate the pain

   d. Actions that relieve the pain

   e. How pain affects the person's daily activity

6. Pain scales are used to determine the intensity of the pain; commonly used scale is self-rating of pain from 0 (no pain) to 10 (worst pain imaginable).

H. Factors that influence pain. The nurse must understand factors that affect a person's response to pain are:

1. Past experience

2. Pain threshold

3. Culture and religious beliefs

4. Level of anxiety

5. Previous physical state

I. Methods of controlling pain

1. Choice of pain control must involve the client and be based on cause, history,and physician's decision.

2. Transcutaneous electrical nerve stimulator (**TENS**): electrodes applied to the area of the pain causes stimulation of sensory nerve fibers

3. Percutaneous electrical nerve stimulator (**PENS**): needles introduced through the skin over the area cause stimulation of sensory never fibers

4. **Acupuncture**: use of fine needles applied in different areas of the body using Eastern medical practices to reduce pain by restoring harmony

5. **Massage**: provides cutaneous stimulation to relax muscles and reduce pain

6. Topical application of heat and cold: has traditionally been used to relieve muscle pain by affecting circulation.

7. **Immobilization**: resting the body part using splints for relaxation and healing

8. **Distraction**: taking the client's attention away from the pain

9. **Imagery**: taking the client to some pleasant present or past images that they usually find relaxing

10. **Therapeutic touch**: the nurse uses his or her hands to reduce tension and stress.

11. Medication: given before pain becomes severe, at equal intervals to maintain a therapeutic level

    a. Nonnarcotic analgesics for mild to moderate pain such as aspirin, ibuprofesn, and acetaminophen

    b. Narcotic analgesics for moderate to severe pain, such as morphine oral, transdermal, parenteral by PCA pump, or epidural

    c. Adjuvants such as anticonvulsants and antidepressant agents are used to heighten the effect of the analgesic.

III. Neurological Assessment

A. Data collection

1. Pupil reactions:

   a. Normal pupils are equal, round, react to light with accommodation (PERRLA) and shape, speed of reaction to light

2. Eye movements, ability to follow finger movement, movement of extremities

3. Reflexes, normal responses equal on both sides of the body.

4. Vital signs

5. Level of consciousness

    a. Observe what client is doing or able to do.

    b. Assess orientation to person, place, and time.

    c. Assess mental status, behavior, appearance, speech, memory, and judgment.

    d. Test reflexes, especially deep tendon and superficial tendon reflexes.

    e. Document findings; avoid labels.

B. Descriptors for level of consciousness

1. **Alert:** follows commands

2. **Lethargic:** appears drowsy but easily roused

3. **Stuporous:** asleep, needs vigorous stimulation to obtain response

4. **Comatose:** no response to verbal or painful stimuli

C. Staging of coma

1. Glascow coma scale used, score based on:

    a. Eye response: eyes open spontaneously or to command or pain

    b. Motor response: response to verbal command or pain, reflexes are decorticate or decerebrate.

    c. Verbal response: oriented, disoriented, or no response

IV. Nursing Procedures Related to Sensory Organs

A. Eye irrigation

1. Uses

    a. Superficial irritation of the eye

    b. Discharge from eye

    c. Infection of the eye

    d. Inflammation of the eye

2. Procedure

    a. Temperature of prescribed solution should be 95 – 100°F.

    b. Tile the client's head toward the side that is to be irrigated.

    c. Administer solution so that it flows from inner canthus to outer canthus.

    d. Chart time of procedure, temperature, drainage, and client response.

B. Ear irrigation

1. Ordered by doctor to cleanse external auditory canal

2. Procedure:

    a. Temperature of prescribed solution should be 105-108°F.

    b. Type and amount of solution ordered by MD

    c. Client's head should be tilted in direction of ear to be irrigated.

    d. Do not direct flow toward eardrum

3. Chart
    a. Time of procedure
    b. Reaction of client to treatment

Additional Resources Found on MyNursingLab
- Pain Management video

PEARSON

MODULE 2

Fundamentals

Submodule 2.16 Death and Dying

Learning Objectives

2.16.1 **Discuss the client's physical and emotional changes as death approaches.**

2.16.2 **Describe Kubler-Ross's death and dying concepts.**

2.16.3 **Describe nursing responsibilities related to the dying client and postmortem care.**

    I. **Changes in Death and Dying**

        A. Physical changes of approaching death

            1. Facial muscles relax, cheeks become flaccid, dentures do not fit, speech becomes mumbling.

            2. Pale, ashen skin that is cool and clammy

            3. Sight gradually fails.

            4. Hearing is believed to be the sense retained longest.

            5. Muscles become flaccid.

            6. Respirations become irregular

                a. **Kussmaul respirations**: rapid, deep

                b. **Cheyne-Stokes respirations**: periods of apnea and of dyspnea

            7. Pulse becomes weak, irregular, and thready.

            8. Mental status varies from clarity to coma.

            9. Reflexes decreased or absent

          10. Bowel and bladder retention or incontinence

        B. Psychosocial changes in death and dying

            1. Client's need to know of impending death

            2. Nurse's attitude toward death influences care of dying

            3. Cultural or ethnic responses to dying vary.

            4. Client and family's ability to cope with dying

            5. Dying clients worry about becoming a burden.

            6. The client's reactions to dying is somewhat predictable, following a basic pattern described by Kubler-Ross (1975).

            7. Spiritual needs

                a. Provide clergy for client as appropriate.

                b. Allow client to participate in appropriate religious practices.

      c.   Provide for family comfort and time with client

II. **Kubler-Ross's Stages of Death and Dying**

    A.   Denial – "I feel fine"; "This can't be happening, not to me!"

    B.   Anger – "Why me? It's not fair!" "NO! NO! How can this happen?" This stage is difficult for nurse and family to handle.

    C.   Bargaining - "Just let me live to see my children graduate."; "I'll do anything, can't you stretch it out a few more years."

    D.   Depression –"I'm so sad, why bother with anything?"; "I'm going to die . . . What's the point?" This stage also difficult for LPN/LVN and family to handle.

    E.   Acceptance - "It's going to be OK."; "I can't fight it, I may as well prepare for it."

III. **Nursing Care of the Dying Client and Family**

    A.   Advance directives and planning

        1.   Living Wills

        2.   Durable Power of Attorney

        3.   DNR

        4.   Comfort measures only

        5.   Organ donation

        6.   Hospice

    B.   Dying client

        1.   All care directed at client comfort and safety.

        2.   Provide for relief of unpleasant symptoms.

        3.   Maintain good hygiene and oral care.

        4.   Turn client frequently and position for maximum comfort.

        5.   Keep linens fresh and dry.

        6.   Allow family sufficient time with client.

        7.   Support client and family as needed.

        8.   Continue pain medications and treatments as appropriate.

    C.   Postmortem care

        1.   Physician must pronounce the client's death.

        2.   Position client flat in bed in a natural position with one pillow under head.

        3.   Close eyes.

        4.   Return dentures to mouth as soon as possible and close mouth.

        5.   Clean body and remove all tubes per institutional policy.

        6.   Allow family time with body after it is prepared.

        7.   Wrap in shroud and label body per policy.

        8.   Remove body to morgue or funeral home per policy.

        9.   Pack all belongings, give to family, and document in chart.

        10. Complete institutional death record.

D. Care of the family

1. Offer support.

2. Allow for time and privacy with deceased.

3. Answer questions.

4. Respect beliefs.

5. Offer referral to clergy, social worker, or others.

Additional Resources Found on MyNursingLab

- Terminally Ill Patients video
- Care of the Dying video

MODULE 3

Medical-Surgical Nursing

Submodule 3.1 Inflammation, Immunity, and Infection

Learning Objectives

3.1.1 Differentiate between the inflammatory response and infection.

3.1.2 Discuss the nursing responsibilities in caring for clients with inflammation and infection.

3.1.3 Describe commonly used antimicrobial medication, nursing implications, and client teaching.

3.1.4 Compare natural and acquired, and passive and active immunity.

3.1.5 Describe treatment and nursing care for clients with altered immune responses.

    I.   **Inflammation, Immunity, and Infection**

        A. Organs Involved:

           1. The skin and mucous membrane

           2. The blood containing antiviral and antibacterial substances

           3. Liver

           4. Bones of the cranium and torso protecting vital delicate organs

        B. Defensive responses at a cellular level destroy and neutralize foreign agents.

           1. Leukocytes (white blood cells) increase in number in the presence of inflammation in the body. Different types of cells carry out specific functions.

               a. To produce enzymes and chemical substances to destroy foreign agents

               b. To aid in clearing debris and dead bacteria from inflamed areas

           2. Reticuloendothelial cells located at various points in the body serve to trap, surround, and destroy foreign particles.

               a. Macrophages engulf foreign invaders

               b. Lymphocytic cells deal with immunity.

        C. Inflammation is one of the most important body defenses against infection.

           1. This can be induced by chemical or physical injury, or by bacterial or viral infection.

           2. Changes occur both locally and systemically.

                a. Vasodilation with increased capillary permeability can cause leakage of tissue fluid, resulting in swelling or edema.

               b. Circulating leukocytes increase.

               c. Reticuloendothelial cells enlarge (become macrophages), then migrate to the inflamed area.

      d.   This activity results in the formation of pus which is composed of dead cells, debris, and tissue fluid.

      e.   Immune system becomes activated and antibodies and antitoxin are formed.

3. Sign and symptoms

      a.   Local signs: Heat, redness, swelling, pain, and loss of function

      b.   Systemic signs: Fever, malaise, anorexia, aching   *feeling of run down, discomfort*

4. Diagnostic tests

      a.   Complete blood count

      b.   Computerized tomography (site specific)

      c.   Sedimentation rate (increased)

5. Healing and repair of tissue

      a.   Occurs as the inflammatory process begins and waste products and debris are removed.

      b.   Outcomes expected can be resolution and recovery, necrosis, or degeneration and scarring.

6. Nursing interventions

      a.   Encourage rest and immobilization of the area using splints, etc.

      b.   Maintain adequate blood supply by avoiding constricting articles and pressure.

      c.   Relieve edema by elevating the affected area. Apply cold/warm as ordered.

      d.   Assist in exercise.

      e.   Encourage foods high in protein and vitamin C.

      f.   Maintain normal fluid balance.

      g.   Protect from further injury – handle gently.

      h.   Perform debridement, cleaning, and draining.

      i.   Observe for signs of infection – culture and sensitivity.

      j.   Using wound precautions, record the color, odor, and amount of wound drainage.

      k.   Take temperature every 4 hours.

      l.   Administer medication, including analgesics for pain, antimicrobials to treat any infection.

D. Immune response

1. The body's resistance to a specific foreign invader

2. Body's response to a foreign substance **(antigen)** causes the development of substance **(antibody).**

3. Two types of immunity – **humoral** and **cellular**

      a.   **Humoral immunity** is the formation of antibody.

         i.   Antibody originates from B lymphocytes sensitized to a particular foreign agent.

         ii.   B-lymphocytes arise from stem cells in the bone marrow.

         iii.   When mature, they migrate to lymph nodes.

      iv. When stimulated by an antigen, they become plasma cells.

      v. They secrete antibody in response to a specific antigen.

      vi. Some antigens stimulate B cells to become memory cells.

      vii. Memory cells can be activated when the foreign substance enters the body. Immunity last a few months.

   b. **Cellular** or **Cell-Mediated Immunity** is delayed response from sensitized lymphocytes.

      i. Functions in response to viruses and cancer cells and in tissue rejection after organ transplant.

      ii. T lymphocytes located in the thymus glands stimulate phagocytosis.

      iii. T lymphocytes are divided into helper T cells and suppressor T cells.

      iv. Memory T cells and sensitized killer T cells

   c. Classification of Immunity

      i. **Natural:** inborn through heredity

      ii. **Acquired:**

         (a) **Active:** long lasting; body makes own antibodies as result of disease, vaccines, or toxoids

         (b) **Passive:** temporary; ready-made antibodies given to individual by immune serum, breast milk/placenta

E. Acquired Immunodeficiency Syndrome (AIDS)

   1. Caused by Human Immunodeficiency Virus (HIV)

     a. HIV is a retrovirus.

     b. A retrovirus carries its genetic coding on RNA and can replicate itself in the host cell.

     c. T cells have a protein called CD_4 on their surface where the HIV virus attaches.

     d. The virus enters the host cell and begins to replicate itself.

     e. When cells are infected they are unable to perform their function, making the person more prone to opportunistic infections.

     f. Normal CD_4 count is 600 – 1200.

   2. Modes of Transmission

     a. Sexual contact from unprotected sex with an infected partner

     b. Sharing needles with drug users infected with HIV

     c. Occupational exposure from needlestick from a needle that contains HIV

     d. Maternal transmission via during delivery or by breast feeding

     e. Receiving blood or blood products contaminated with HIV donated by HIV-infected individuals

     f. Transplant from organs donated by HIV-infected person

     g. Transmission by contact with blood or body fluids containing the HIV virus. HIV virus is found in body fluids, blood, vaginal secretions, breast milk, etc.

3. Diagnostic tests (blood)

   a. Positive ELISA (enzyme-linked immunosorbent assay)

   b. A positive result from ELISA is confirmed by the Western blot test.

   c. In neonates a polymerase chain reaction (PCR) test is done to differentiate antibodies caused by the disease from antibodies transferred from the mother.

   d. CD_4 test shows count of less than 200 cell/mm^3; other tests performed: CBC, chemistry profile (SMA_{12})

4. Stages of HIV Infection

   a. Primary infection: client may present with flu-like symptoms occurring within three weeks of initial exposure; can be asymptomatic; or can have enlarged lymph nodes, fever, malaise, and skin rash, with a normal CD_4 count.

   b. Asymptomatic HIV: may remain asymptomatic for 10 years or more. CD_4 count increased 500 cells/mm^3 or higher.

   c. Symptomatic HIV: CD_4 count 200 – 500 cell/mm^3 with characteristic symptoms of HIV.

   d. AIDS: CD_4 count 200 or below and client has accompanying bacterial and viral infection.

5. Assessment

   a. Fatigue, weakness, anorexia, weight loss, diarrhea

   b. Fever, lymphedema, pallor, night sweats, malnutrition, joint pain, swelling, and skin rash

   c. Disorientation, confusion, dementia

   d. Opportunistic infection

6. Opportunistic infection

   a. Fungal infections: Candida of the oral cavity and vagina, histoplasmosis, cryptococcosis, meningitis, and *Pneumocystis jiroveci* pneumonia.

   b. Viral infections: Herpes simplex 1 and 2; herpes zoster; cytomegalovirus (CMV) of the eyes, GI tract, lungs, and brain; hepatitis B and C virus.

   c. Bacterial infections: Mycobacterium in and outside of the lungs resulting in *Mycobacterium aviu*m complex (MAC)

   d. Parasitic diseases: toxoplasmosis and cryptosporidiosis

7. Medical management

   a. High calorie diet with high protein, small frequent feedings, daily weights

   b. Fluid-electrolytes replacement

   c. Activity as tolerated/ROM

   d. Total parenteral nutrition (TPN) and transfusions as ordered

   e. Chest physiotherapy

   f. Vital signs and neurologic checks

   g. Standard precautions

PEARSON

8. Nursing interventions

    a. Maintain diet; take daily weight.

    b. Force fluids.

    c. Encourage incentive spirometer.

    d. Position in semi-Fowler's.

    e. Encourage client to maintain activity level.

    f. Decrease client anxiety.

    g. Administer medication as ordered.

    h. Provide health teaching and referrals.

    i. Monitor for infection and related disease.

9. Drugs

    a. Antiviral/Antiretroviral agents destroy, prevent, or delay the speed of viral infection by preventing viral replication. Drugs are used in combination to treat AIDS.

F. Hypersensitivity

1. Hypersensitivity is another type of immune response to the presence of normally harmless substances in the body.

    a. The presence of the allergen activates B lymphocytes to secrete antibody IgE.

    b. IgE binds to mast cells. Mast cells rupture and release histamine and other chemical mediators.

    c. These chemicals in the body result in vasodilation and bronchial constriction.

    d. Hypersensitivity reaction can be mild or severe.

    e. Allergens that can trigger hypersensitivity reaction are drugs, food, plants, insect bites, or contact with material such as latex and metals.

2. Allergens

    a. Allergens enter the body by inhalation, ingestion, injection, insect bites, and direct contact.

    b. Diseases can result when allergens enter the body: asthma, hay fever, and atopic dermatitis.

    c. Mild hypersensitivity is usually manifested as a skin rash.

    d. Severe hypersensitivity (anaphylaxis) occurs with a previous exposure to the antigen and can result in respiratory or cardiovascular collapse.

3. Signs and symptoms

    a. Vasodilation, resulting in tachycardia, palpitation, hypotension, syncope, shock, and cardiac arrest

    b. Skin: urticaria, pruritus, and sweating

    c. Respiratory system: bronchoconstriction, coughing (resulting in SOB and wheezing)

    d. Gastrointestinal system: nausea and vomiting and abdominal discomfort

4. Diagnostic testing: allergic skin test, blood for CBC and differential

PEARSON

5. Medical management depends on severity

   a. Treat symptoms.

   b. Support cardiac and respiratory function.

   c. Identify and limit allergen.

   d. Provide drug therapy.

   e. Provide desensitization therapy once the client's condition has stabilized.

6. Nursing interventions

   a. Teach client to decrease contact with allergen.

   b. Promote symptom relief.

   c. Provide respiratory and cardiovascular support.

   d. Provide emotional support.

G. Infection – caused by microorganisms; signs in body may appear locally or systemically

1. Type of organisms

   a. Bacteria

   b. Viruses

   c. Rickettsias

   d. Protozoas

   e. Fungi

2. Helminths

3. Signs and symptoms

   a. Fever, chills

   b. Tachycardia, tachypnea

   c. Anorexia, weakness, malaise

   d. Arthralgia and mental depression

4. Diagnosis

   a. Culture and sensitivity on exudates from involved area

   b. CBC

5. Treatment.

   a. Antibiotics, antipyretics

   b. Fluids, rest, and comfort measures

Additional Resources Found on MyNursingLab

- Drug Chart: Antibiotics

MODULE 3

Medical-Surgical Nursing

Submodule 3.2 Caring for Surgical Clients

Learning Objectives

3.2.1 Identify critical elements for preoperative nursing care.

3.2.2 Discuss nursing care during surgery and postoperatively.

3.2.3 Describe drugs used preoperatively, intraoperatively, and postoperatively.

I. **Surgical Risks Factors**

    A. Age

    B. Obesity

    C. Malnutrition

    D. Electrolyte imbalance or dehydration

    E. Cardiovascular disorders

    F. Respiratory disorders

    G. History of alcoholism or smoking

    H. Medications

    I. Diabetes

    J. Infection

    K. Kidney and liver disorders

II. **Client Assessment**

    A. Assess concerns and need for surgery – clients and family

    B. Cultural aspect and religious beliefs and practices

    C. Occupation

    D. Measures used to cope with stress

    E. Source of emotional support

    F. Present problems, previous hospitalizations, and prior experience with anesthesia

    G. Current medication and allergy history

    H. History of past or existing medical diseases

    I. Physical assessment

    J. Vital signs

    K. Skin examination for lesions

PEARSON

    L. Weight, nutritional status, and diet restriction (NPO status)

    M. Teach deep breathing, coughing, splinting, position changes, and exercises

    N. Lab tests: CBC, urinalysis (U/A) SMA12, blood type, cross-match if needed

    O. Informed consent

    P. Orient to environmental changes, ICU, and physical changes – tubes, etc.

    Q. Prep and shave surgical area as ordered (against the direction of hair growth)

    R. Bowel prep as ordered (enema, suppositories)

III. Day of Surgery

    A. Vital signs and records

    B. Remove and secure jewelry

    C. Remove dentures and secure them

    D. Remove all nail polish and makeup

    E. Remove hair pins, contact lenses, and any prosthesis

    F. Provide a gown

    G. Have client void, and record

    H. Give preanesthetic medication 1 hour before surgery or on call if ordered as such. Give exactly as ordered.

    I. Raise side rail and call bell

IV. Premedication

    A. Given to reduce anxiety

    B. Decreases oropharyngeal secretions

    C. Reduces side effects of anesthesia

V. Intraoperative Phase

    A. Client received in operative area

    B. Oriented by the nurse

    C. Verify right client, right procedure, and right anatomical site

    D. Verify signed consent

    E. Provide safety and positioning during anesthesia

    F. Monitor vital signs and report significant change

    G. Verify sponge count and instruments

    H. Correctly label specimen and transport to lab

VI. Postoperative Phase

    A. Prepare bed

    B. At time of arrival, record time and condition of client

    C. Patency of airway, gag, and cough reflex

    D. Level of consciousness

    E. Vital signs: color of nails, skin, lips, and mucous membranes; O_2 saturation

F. Skin characteristics

G. Dressings: amount and type of drainage; tube location and drainage

H. Intravenous type, rate, amount left in bottle (L.I.B.)

I. Bladder checked for distention

J. Oxygen as ordered

K. Assess pain level; manage analgesia in consultation with anesthesiologist

L. Provide warmth with heated blankets as needed

M. Monitor for potential problems

VII. Postoperative Complications

A. Obstructed airway and aspiration

B. Hemorrhage and shock

C. Pain

D. Pulmonary emboli

E. Thrombophlebitis – generally 7-14 days post surgery

F. Nausea, vomiting, and abdominal distention; paralytic ileus

G. Urinary retention

H. Fluid and electrolyte balance

I. Wound infection and healing. Wound infection often occurs 36-48 hours after surgery.

J. Dehiscence and evisceration

K. Atelectasis and pneumonia

L. Constipation

VIII. Anesthesia

A. Two major classes: general and local

B. General anesthesia: produces a state of analgesia, amnesia, and unconsciousness followed by loss of muscle reflexes and muscle tone. See Table 1.

Table 1. Stages of General Anesthesia

Stage #	Name	Assessment Findings
I.	Analgesia	Drowsiness and dizziness; auditory or visual hallucinations
II.	Excitement	Increased muscle activity/irregular breathing
III.	Surgical anesthesia	Unconsciousness/muscle relaxation
IV.	Medullary paralysis	No spontaneous breathing; may not have heartbeat

C. Drugs used for general anesthesia (see Adjuvants to Anesthesia drug chart)

1. Given by inhalation or injection

2. Inhalation agents are gases or liquids

    a. Gases

        i. Nitrous oxide

        ii. Cyclopropane

    b. Volatile liquids

        i. Halothane (Fluothane)

        ii. Enflurane (Ethrane)

3. Injection agents

    a. Barbiturates example

        i. Thiopental (Pentothal) intravenously

    b. Nonbarbiturates

        i. Propofol (Diprivan)

        ii. Midazolam (Versed)

        iii. Fentanyl citrate and Droperidol (Innovar)

4. Side effects

    a. Coughing, laryngeal spasm, bronchospasm, respiratory depression, and malignant hyperthermia (a fatal side effect whose cause is undetermined)

D. Drugs used for local anesthesia

    1. Local anesthesia: Anesthetizes a region of the body only

        a. Topical – applied directly to the skin to desensitize an area

        b. Infiltration – injection of agent into the skin, subcutaneous tissue of a specific area

        c. Nerve block – anesthetizes a specific nerve or nerve plexus

        d. Spinal anesthesia – produces a nerve block in the subarachnoid space

    2. Local anesthesia: Agents

        a. Nupercaine

        b. Lidocaine (Xylocaine)

        c. Side effects: hypotension, nausea and vomiting, headache, neurological: weakness, and paralysis of legs

Additional Resources Found on MyNursingLab

- Preoperative and Postoperative Care video
- Inserting and Maintaining the Nasogastric Tube for Gastric Decompression
- Drug Chart: Adjuvants to Anesthesia

PEARSON

MODULE 3

Medical-Surgical Nursing

Submodule 3.3 Clients with Cancer

Learning Objectives

3.3.1 Discuss the pathophysiology of cancer.

3.3.2 Discuss common signs of cancer and diagnostic tests.

3.3.3 Describe various treatment modalities and the related nursing care for clients with cancer.

    I. **Introduction**

       A. Cancer is a neoplastic disease, characterized by new growth of malignant cells. It is a type of tumor.

       B. Classification of tumors:

          1. **Benign** – encapsulated; do not spread to other parts of the body

          2. **Malignant** – not encapsulated; cells grow rapidly, spread easily, are referred to as cancerous

       C. Types of tumors

          1. **Carcinoma,** the most common form of cancer, is a solid tumor arising from epithelial tissue found in skin, glands, urinary, gastric, and reproductive systems.

          2. **Sarcoma** develops from connective tissue such as bone, cartilage, and muscle.

          3. Mixed tumors are found in both connective and epithelial tissue, such as Wilms' tumor seen in children.

       D. **Metastasis** – spreading of malignant cells to other parts of the body

          1. Routes by which metastasis occurs:

             a. By direct extension to neighboring tissues

             b. Via lymphatic vessels

             c. By embolism through lymphatic vessels or blood

             d. By invasion of fluid within a body cavity

       E. Cancer grading or staging

          1. Grading and staging help determine the extent of the spread of the tumor to other tissue.

          2. Grading and staging help to give a prognosis and guide selection of treatment.

          3. Tumor **grading**

             a. Grade 1 – confined to tissue of origin (called in situ)

             b. Grade 2 – spread limited to local areas

       c.   Grade 3 – tumor large and may have invaded surrounding tissue

       d.   Grade 4 – metastasized to other part of the body

    4.   **Staging** – done by the TNM system, using letters and numbers

       a.   T describes the primary growth beginning at 1, progressing through 2, 3, 4, and based on size

       b.   N indicates lymph node involvement ranging from 0 to 4.

       c.   M stands for metastasis, ranging from 0 to 1.

II. Etiology of Cancer

   A.   Specific cause unknown; probably multiple predisposing causes:

     1.   Chronic irritations of skin or mucous membrane

     2.   Benign tumor which has become malignant

     3.   Other factors such as sex, age, familial tendency, first-degree relative

     4.   Viruses called *oncoviruses,* i.e., human immunodeficiency virus, human papilloma virus, and Epstein-Barr virus

     5.   Chemicals and pesticides such as asbestos, benzene, and DDT

     6.   Lifestyle practices, smoking, alcohol

     7.   Radiation and radioactive material

     8.   Stress over long periods of time

     9.   Diet with high intake of smoked, salt-cured, and charred foods

   B.   Seven danger signs of cancer listed by the American Cancer Society. Symptoms persisting beyond several weeks should be reported to a physician:

     1.   Any unusual bleeding or discharge

     2.   A lump or thickening in the breast or elsewhere

     3.   A sore that does not heal

     4.   Hoarseness or nagging cough

     5.   A change in bowel or bladder habits

     6.   Indigestion or difficulty swallowing

     7.   Any change in a wart or mole

III. Diagnosis

   A.   Early diagnosis important in successful treatment

   B.   Special diagnostic tests:

     1.   Biopsy – removal of sample living cells from growth confirms diagnosis

     2.   Papanicolaou smear – technique for collecting samples of body secretions and cervical cells to examine for malignant cells. Especially helpful in early diagnosis of cancer of the cervix.

     3.   Tumor markers: special proteins, antigens, hormones, genes, or enzymes released from cancer cells that alter composition of body fluids (e.g., prostate-specific antigen [PSA] to diagnose prostate cancer and CA-125 to diagnose ovarian cancer)

     4.   Mammography: use of radiography of breast to diagnose breast cancer

5. Computed tomography (CT scan): noninvasive three-dimensional cross-section of tissue to locate tumor and determine size and density

6. Magnetic resonance imaging (MRI): Magnetic fields differentiate healthy and diseased tissue and blood flow patterns.

7. Ultrasound: noninvasive use of sound waves to detect abnormalities in tissue

8. Endoscopic examination: direct visualization of bronchus, colon, and bladder

IV. Treatment

A. Surgical removal – works well for tumors that are readily accessible; adjacent tissue and lymph nodes and vessels must also be removed or treated

B. Radiation therapy – the use of radiation to penetrate and destroy malignant tissue

C. Chemotherapy – use of chemical agents to destroy malignant cells.

V. Prevention

A. Monthly breast self-examination beginning at age 20; done one week after menses when hormone levels are at lowest point in cycle

B. Annual Papanicolaou smear for females

C. Annual proctoscopic exam in people over 40

D. Avoidance of smoking and excessive intake of alcohol

E. Reduced exposure to direct sunlight.

F. Diet and exercise to reduce obesity

G. Digital exam for men over 30 years

H. Assessment of skin lesions and removal of suspicious lesions

VI. Radiation Therapy

A. Methods of radiation therapy

1. X-ray therapy – high-voltage x-ray machines are used to aim the beam of radiation directly at the tumor. Done in a series of treatments.

   a. Purpose is to destroy malignant cells.

2. Methods of delivery

   a. External radiation or **teletherapy** – source of radiation is outside the body

   b. Internal radiation or **brachytherapy** – the radiation source is implanted or injected into the body

   c. Internal radiation can be sealed or unsealed.

   i. Sealed radioistotope is enclosed in a container and does not enter body fluids. Sealed radiation can be temporary or permanently inserted in a body cavity using needles, wires, and seeds. Bed rest is needed to prevent dislodgement. If radiation source is dislodged, use a long-handled forceps to place in lead-lined container and inform nuclear medicine department. Do not touch.

   ii. Unsealed radioisotope is given orally or by injection and circulates in the body fluids. Need body fluid precautions for 8 to 10 hours after last dose.

B. Radiation protection

1. Amount of radiation that nurse might receive from x-rays or radioactive substances depends on exposure.

2. Healthcare workers are more at risk from internal than from external radiation.

3. A film badge is worn by healthcare workers to measure the amount of exposure received.

4. Pregnant nurses, children, and visitors should not be near the radiation source.

5. The nurse uses these three types of precautions (distance, time, shielding):

    a. Distance between nurse and source or radiation

    b. Amount of time spent in actual proximity to source of radiation

    c. Degree of shielding provided

6. Long-term effects appear years after exposure and include shortening of the life span, predisposition to leukemia and other malignancies, and development of cataracts. When the radiation is directed at gonads, genetic mutations may arise.

7. Radiation sickness – a generalized systemic reaction to radiation. Symptoms are temporary.

C. Common side effects of radiation

1. Anorexia, nausea, and vomiting: Give antiemetic prior to treatment. Offer small, frequent meals of client's preference, diet high in protein and calories; increase fluids.

2. Diarrhea: Give antidiarrheal agent, fluid and electrolyte replacement when necessary.

3. Depression of bone marrow: Thrombocytopenia, leukopenia, and anemia are most serious side effects.

    a. **Thrombocytopenia** (decrease in number of platelets): Watch for abnormal bleeding as evidenced by petechiae and ecchymosis.

    b. **Leukopenia** (decrease in number of white blood cells): Protect from infection and watch for signs of infection. Record temperature q 4h; report if above 100°F.

    c. **Anemia** (decrease in number of red blood cells): Provide rest and administer oxygen as ordered.

4. **Alopecia** (loss of hair): Instruct client that hair will regrow a different texture or color; promote use of wigs, hats, etc.

5. **Cystitis** (inflammation of the bladder): Increase fluids, watch for bleeding, monitor vital signs.

6. Fatigue: Allow periods of rest; do not overtire.

7. **Stomatitis** (inflammation of oral mucosa): Offer bland foods, mouth rinse with normal saline; avoid commercial mouth washes which contain alcohol that will cause further breakdown. Inspect oral cavity for signs of infection.

8. **Xerostoma** (dry mouth): Keep mouth and lips moist; offer mouth rinses.

D. Care of radiation area

1. Keep the skin dry. Do not wash off mark; wash gently with warm water if no blisters. Do not apply lotion or cream. Avoid direct sunlight for 6 months to 1 year. All applications should be prescribed by the radiologist.

    E. Caring for clients with sealed radiation:

       1. The nurse organizes tasks to limit time spent with the client, usually a 10-minute block of time.

       2. Determine area of radiation or implant; stand 6 feet away; if implant is in lower abdomen, stand at head of bed.

       3. Do not change linens unless necessary.

       4. Place a radiation sign on the door.

       5. For other visitors, limit stay to 10 minutes.

       6. Have long-handled forceps and lead-lined container in the room in case radiation dislodges.

       7. Check position of radiation implant q4h.

       8. Instruct the client to perform active ROM to prevent thrombophlebitis.

       9. Soiled linen and trash stays in room and is specially removed.

    F. Caring for clients with unsealed radiation area:

       1. Prevent exposure to body fluids. Flush the toilet 3 times after use.

VII. Chemotherapy

    A. Administration of chemotherapy

       1. Administration of chemotherapy is a specialty area of nursing or medicine called oncology.

       2. The drugs are grouped together for maximum effect.

Additional Resources Found on MyNursingLab

- Drug Chart: Antineoplastic Drugs

MODULE 3

Medical-Surgical Nursing

Submodule 3.4 Disorders Affecting the Integumentary System

Learning Objectives

3.4.1 **Compare pathophysiology, symptoms, treatment, and nursing care for clients with common skin disorders.**

3.4.2 **Discuss classification, estimation, and treatment for burns.**

3.4.3 **Describe nursing responsibilities for clients with burn injuries.**

Note: **Prior to beginning this unit the student should review the anatomy and physiology of the skin and its related organs.**

    I. **Definitions**

        A. Dermatology – specialized study of diseases of the skin

        B. Dermatologist – one who specializes in treatment of disorders of the skin

    II. **Diagnostic Tests and Examinations**

        A. Visual Examination

            1. Physician examines lesions under a strong light and palpates lesions to determine whether they are raised or nodular.

            2. Classification of skin lesions (Table 1)

            3. Note color of skin, pale pallor, erythema, and jaundice.

        B. Skin Biopsy

            1. Taking a cone-shaped sample of a lesion to differentiate between benign and malignant tumors or find the causative organism in an infection.

        C. Scratch Test

            1. Definition – test of individual's sensitivity to specific substances

            2. Methods:

                a. Skin is scratched slightly and a sample of pollen, food, etc. is applied to the scratch.

                b. The sample is injected just below the first layer of the skin.

            3. Reaction – a small small-sized wheal appears at the site of contact.

        D. Culture and Sensitivity Tests – used in cases of infectious diseases, especially boils, carbuncles

        E. Blood tests – Chemistry profile and CBC

F. History

1. Must know when the individual noticed a change in the skin

2. Where the lesions first appeared on the body

3. Whether or not the client has had these lesions before

4. Under what conditions the lesions appeared (for example – every time a certain soap was used)

5. Distribution and size, measuring length, width, and depth

6. Photograph for historical record and follow-up.

7. Condition of skin around the lesion

8. Antibiotic or anticancer drugs in use

9. Nutritional practices, including food allergies

10. Lifestyle practices, hygiene practices

11. Skin products used for exposure to sun or weather

12. Family history of diabetes or other dermatologic disease

13. Presence of pruritus, pain, and burning

Table 1. CLASSIFICATION OF SKIN LESIONS

NAME OF LESION	EXAMPLE	DESCRIPTION
Macule	Freckle	A discolored spot or patch on the skin. Usually not elevated or depressed and cannot be felt
Papule	Present in measles	A solid elevation of skin. May vary from size of a pinhead to that of a pea. Usually red, resembling small pimples without pus
Pustule	Acne, smallpox	A small elevation of the skin or pimple filled with pus
Vesicle	Blister	A small sac containing serous fluid
Bleb	Common in pemphigus	A large elevation of the skin filled with fluid
Excoriation	Friction burn/chemical burn	An injury caused by scraping or rubbing away of a portion of skin
Wheal	Insect sting, hives, nettle reaction, rash	An area of local swelling, usually accompanied by itching

III. **Prevention of Skin Disease**

A. Cleanliness – delicate skin requires special care to prevent dryness and irritation; oily skin requires frequent cleansing.

B. Age – changes the skin and can quickly lead to irritation and breakdown.

C. Diet – adequate intake of vitamin and minerals, well-balanced diet

PEARSON

D. Factors to Be Avoided in the Environment

1. Prolonged exposure to chemicals

2. Excessive drying of the skin

3. Excessive burning of the skin by strong light

4. Excessive exposure to ultraviolet rays from the skin

E. General Rules in Care of Clients with Skin Disease

1. Bathing with soap and water is usually contraindicated.

2. Dressings should not be removed without an order to do so.

3. Do not attempt to remove crust and scales without a specific order to do so.

4. Observe skin carefully and record observations.

5. Avoid excessive rubbing of the skin.

6. Do not apply lotions without an order.

7. Note presence of exudates (amount, color, and odor).

8. Avoid extremes in hot or cold applications.

9. Note presence of scratch marks.

10. Assess texture of hair.

11. Note nail beds and characteristics.

12. Obtain past history of medical and surgical diseases.

13. Ask about use of medications, steroids, and hormones.

14. Ask before acting.

F. Changes in Skin Related to Aging

1. Loss of subcutaneous tissue

2. Decreased elasticity, increased wrinkling

3. Decreased skin turgor

4. Slower response to heat and cold extremes

5. Decreased sweat and oil gland production

6. Decreased melanocyte production

7. Hyperpigmentation

8. Hair and nail growth decreases, hair grays, and nails thicken.

IV. Therapeutic Baths

A. Used to relieve itching and cleanse the skin before application of topical medication. They also soften eschar tissue. They are used for weeping, crusted, reddened areas in clients with psoriasis, eczema, and burns.

B. Commonly used medicated baths are oatmeal or Aveeno. Otherwise, water with saline is used.

C. Temperature of bath water should be comfortable; hot baths must be avoided.

D. The bath should last no longer than 30 minutes to avoid chilling.

E. A bath mat should be used in the tub for safety.

F. Emollients such as Keri Lotion are applied after bath on damp skin.

V. Therapeutic Treatment for Skin Disease

A. Wet Dressing – applied to open wet lesions that are weeping or crusted

    1. This type of dressing is used to soothe inflammation in clients with dermatitis, etc.

    2. Recommended use is for 72 hours to prevent maceration of skin.

    3. It is recommended that compresses be applied for a brief period (5-10 minutes).

    4. The common solution used is Burow's Solution, normal physiological saline.

    5. These dressings are applied every 4 hr for 15 to 30 minutes.

VI. Decubitus Ulcer

A. Ulceration of the skin due to the deprivation of oxygen and essential nutrients to tissues, caused by prolonged pressure that occludes blood supply

B. Ulcer Staging

    1. Stage I: Redness that fails to return to its normal color after applying and removing pressure

    2. Stage II: Redness with blistering or skin tear

    3. Stage III: Break in skin that extends to subcutaneous tissue

    4. Stage IV: Break in skin to muscle or bone

C. Prevention

    1. Change position every 2 to 4 hours.

    2. Keep skin clean and dry.

    3. Do not massage reddened areas. Use protective devices such as sheepskin, egg crate, and air or water mattresses.

    4. Avoid shearing.

D. Treatment

    1. Use sterile technique when skin is broken.

        a. Stage I: Protect from shearing forces

        b. Stage II: Hydrocolloid dressing to contain moisture

        c. Stage III: Absorb exudates and maintain moisture

        d. Stage IV: Chemical enzyme to debride or mechanical wet to dry or surgical debridant

VII. Burns

A. Destruction of tissue by exposure to extreme heat, hot liquids, electrical agents, strong chemicals, or radiation

B. Burn injury is classified based on degree of tissue loss and surface area of body affected.

C. Classification

1. Superficial: partial thickness (1st degree); involves the epidermal layer

2. Dermal: partial thickness (2nd degree); involves the epidermal and dermal layers

3. Full Thickness – (3rd degree) involves epidermal, dermal, subcutaneous layer, and nerve endings

4. First degree (superficial) – erythema, edema, pain, blanching

5. Second degree (partial) – pain; oozing, fluid-filled vesicles; shiny and wet

6. Third degree (full) – eschar – edema, no significant pain

D. Percentage of area burned is based on rule of nines (see Table 2):

Table 2.   RULE OF NINES

Area of Body	Percentage of Body Surface
Head and Neck	9%
Anterior Trunk	18%
Posterior Trunk	18%
Upper Limbs	18%
Lower Limbs	36%
Genitalia and Perineum	1%

E. Burn care is divided into different stages

1. Emergent Phase– Initially the primary concern is to stop the burning, maintain an open airway, and control any bleeding. During the first 24 to 72 hours it is critical to assess for shock and respiratory distress.

   a. Thermal – remove person, extinguish source

   b. Flame – drop and roll

   c. Electrical – note victim's position as well as entry and exit points of electrical current

   d. Chemical – remove clothing, wash area profusely for 10-15 minutes, apply cold to decrease pain and sensation; wrap in a cool moist towel or sheet; maintain airway; prevent sepsis; transport to hospital.

2. Acute Phase- Begins with fluid shifting. Care involves treatment and prevention of complications.

   a. Fluid remobilization

      i. Fluid shift from interstitial spaces back to intravascular spaces, resulting in diuresis and possible fluid overload. Decreased cardiac output and hypoproteinemia

      ii. Maintain strict intake and output.

   b. Prevent Infection: using protective isolation; prophylactic antibiotic therapy may be ordered.

    c. Burn care: open or closed method

       i. Debridement of wound to remove eschar. See below.

       ii. Cover with biologic or biosynthetic skin.

    d. Provide adequate nutrition diet:

       i. High calorie, 5000+ calories per day, high protein, high carbohydrate, vitamin C to provide healing, and additional nutritional supplements

    e. Prevent contractures:

       i. Perform active and passive ROM exercise as tolerated.

       ii. Mobilize client once vital signs are stable and medical condition permits.

3. Rehabilitation Phase-Begins at the time of admission. The goal is to help restore the individual to the highest level of functioning possible.

    a. Skin grafting to allow wound closure; promote to optimal level of functioning using rehabilitation.

    b. Promote psychological well-being.

F. Admission Assessment

  1. Assess the degree of the burn.

  2. Obtain a history – time or burn, how injury occurred and cause

    a. Determine degree of burn – minor burns less than 10% (that doesn't involve face)

    b. Assess for airway involvement: singed nasal hairs, soot around and in nostrils, red swollen mouth, and dark mucous membranes

G. Treatment

  1. Fluid loss—sudden shift of fluid from intravascular to interstitial spaces

  2. Correct fluid loss -Start IV; administer colloids.

  3. Prevent shock, which occurs in first 48 hrs:

    a. Monitor for dehydration, decreased blood pressure, elevated pulse rate, thirst, decreased urinary output.

    b. Monitor for electrolyte imbalances (hyponatremia, hyperkalemia), low blood protein levels, and metabolic acidosis.

  4. Respiratory status: check if singing and soot in nasal hair

    a. Maintain patent airway and intubate if needed.

    b. Suction to keep the airway free.

    c. Monitor pulse oximetry and arterial blood gases.

    d. Administer oxygen as prescribed.

    e. Encourage use of incentive spirometer.

  5. Pain management: intravenous opiates

  6. Administration of tetanus toxoids as prophylaxis

  7. Wound care: cleanse and debride

  8. Insert Foley to determine hourly output. Maintain minimum hourly output 30-50 mL, NPO, NG tube to suction.

9. To prevent paralytic ileus, antacid prophylactic to prevent stress ulcer (Curling's ulcer). Prevent infection (which usually appears 3 days after initial injury).

10. Record intake and output (important because physician uses this information to determine need for additional fluids)

11. Baseline weight and daily weight

H. Complications

    1. Infection of wound or respiratory tract

    2. Contractures: may be prevented by proper positioning and adequate exercise

    3. Loss of fluid through burn area causing shock in first 48 hours

    4. Pulmonary changes from inhalation injury (look for singed nasal hair and soot)

    5. Renal changes: decreased urinary output, frequent UTI

    6. Gastrointestinal changes: distention, paralytic ileus, Curling's ulcer

I. Methods of Treating the Wound

    1. Open – wound is thoroughly cleansed and left uncovered and exposed to air

    2. Closed – wound covered with nonadherent, absorbent dressing

        a. Nursing precautions – guard against infection, use sterile sheets.

        b. Special unit is desirable.

    3. Surgical – wound is debrided naturally, mechanically, surgically, or enzymatically.

J. Skin Graft – Replacement of damaged skin with healthy skin to protect underlying structures

    1. Types

        a. Split thickness – half the epidermis removed by a dermatome

        b. Full thickness – removal of the outer epidermis

        c. Pinch/insert graft – small piece of skin removed with a needle

    2. Sources of Graft

        a. Autograft: uses client's own skin

        b. Allograft/Homograft: uses human skin usually from a cadaver

        c. Heterograft/Xenograft: obtained from animals such as pigs

    3. Preoperative care as usual, except donor site prepared by cleansing

    4. Postoperative care routine

        a. Avoid weightbearing on extremity with graft site.

        b. Elevate and immobilize graft site.

        c. Assess site for infection, hematoma; take antibiotic as prescribed.

        d. Keep donor site clean and open to air.

        e. Prevent damage or pressure.

        f. Protect from direct sunlight.

K. Antimicrobials for burns – used to prevent or treat infection; either open or closed method

VIII. Skin Disorders

A. Herpes simplex (fever blister)

1. Caused by herpes simplex I; virus embedded in nerve ganglion that intersects site of lesion

2. Symptoms – vesicles inside mouth and on lips with burning and itching

3. Treatment – warm compresses; contact precautions

4. Antiviral agents (Acyclovir, Zorvirax)

5. Famciclovir (Famvir) and valacyclovir (Valtrex)

6. Autoinoculation of virus to other part of the body is possible by direct contact

B. Herpes zoster (shingles)

1. Caused by herpes virus (varicella)

2. Symptoms – vesicles appearing on skin along spinal nerve path accompanied by pain, itching, and low-grade fever

3. Vesicles and lesions affecting one side of body or face

4. Drugs: systemic steroids, Famvir, Valtrex

C. Contact dermatitis: inflammation of skin due to exposure to a given substance

1. Types

   a. Irritant: from contact with agents such as wool, detergent, etc.

   b. Allergic –from hypersensitivity reaction from exposure to certain antigens (ivy, drugs)

2. Signs and symptoms: pruritus, erythema, vesicles

3. Treatment: wet dressing and soaks using Burow's solution to soothe

   a. Protect skin from scratching; keep nails short

   b. Identify allergens using patch test

D. Furuncles (boils) – Infection of hair follicle

1. Caused by gram-negative/positive bacteria such as Staphylococcus

2. Lesion occurs on face, neck area, groin.

3. Characterized by redness, pain, swelling, and yellow center; can rupture releasing pus; is painful

4. Treatment: hot, moist dressing; excision and drainage, dressing; isolation (hand washing, separate towels)

E. Psoriasis – chronic excessive skin cell reproduction and inflammation

1. Symptoms: papules forming skin elevation, redness, and scaling plaques which appear slowly

2. Cause

   a. Genetic predisposition or stress (environmental) or autoimmune

   b. Lesion occurs on elbows, scalp, trunk

3. Treatment: therapeutic baths

   a. Drugs: topical steroids and keratolytics; coal tar; ultraviolet light; anti-metabolites like methotrexate

   b. Promotion of adequate rest and coping strategies

F. Parasitic Infestations Parasites are organisms that live on the human body and use it to obtain nutrients to survive.

1. The two most commonly seen parasitic infestations affecting humans are pediculosis (lice) and *Sarcoptes scabiei* (scabies).

   a. Pediculosis – lice infect areas that have hair, including head lice (*pedis capitis*), body lice (*pedis corporis*), and genital lice (*pedis pubis*).

   b. Other areas infected: eyebrows, eyelashes, or beard

   c. Sign and symptoms: itching and scratch marks

   d. Treatment:

      i. Pediculicide drugs

      ii. Treatment of family and close contacts also

      iii. Isolation of personal clothing and toys

      iv. Washing clothes in hot water and hot air dryer

2. Scabies – Burrow into the skin

   a. Signs and symptoms: itching burrow marks

   b. Scratching over body and axilla and groin folds

   c. Treatment:

      i. Isolate clothing

      ii. Pediculicide

G. Acne Vulgaris

1. Skin eruption caused by inflammation of the sebaceous glands when the ducts become plugged with sebum

2. Seen most commonly from adolescence to middle age

3. Cause unknown

4. Factors that contribute to acne: overactive hormones, diet, heredity, stress, and hygiene practices

5. Signs and symptoms: lesions found on face, neck, back, and shoulders

   a. Comedone or blackhead (occlusion of a hair follicle and formation of pustules)

   b. The skin is normally oily, shiny; rupture of lesion leaves a scar.

   c. Acne rosacea- chronic lesions appear over cheeks and nose; marked erythema

6. Diagnosis: presenting symptoms and increased hormone levels

    7. Treatment

       a. Changes in appearance lead to psychological stress. Clients need emotional support.

       b. Provide client teaching.

          i. Identify and eliminate precipitating factors.

          ii. Keep skin clean to prevent infection and promote healing.

          iii. Wash skin with medicated soap 2-3 times daily to decrease oils.

          iv. Keep hair and clothing away from areas.

          v. Increase fluids and add protein and vitamins to diet.

       c. Drugs, systemic antibiotics such as tetracycline may be needed and vitamin A preparations such as isotretinoin.

       d. Surgical dermabrasion

H. Cellulitis: Infection of the Skin and Subcutaneous Tissue

    1. Occurs when bacteria enter the body from a break in the skin

    2. The causative organisms are Streptococcus or Staphylococcus.

    3. Conditions that place the client at risk are diabetes, compromised immune system, lymphedema, surgery, or poor peripheral circulation.

    4. Diagnosis is based on clinical appearance, Doppler ultrasound, MRI, CBC, and culture of open area.

    5. Signs and symptoms

       a. Lower extremities swollen with erythema; hot and painful to touch

       b. Limited motion in affected extremity areas; wet, oozing serous fluid along with elevated temperature, tachycardia, malaise

    6. Treatment

       a. Prevent spread of infection; provide antibiotic therapy.

       b. Treat pain with analgesics.

       c. Monitor and improve nutrition and maintain adequate hydration.

       d. Elevate extremity to decrease edema.

       e. Cleanse extremities; change dressing as prescribed with daily care.

I. *Tinea Pedis* – Athlete's foot: common fungal infection

    1. Symptoms: cracks between toes, foul odor, watery blisters, burning or itching

    2. Treatment: cleanse area well; dry skin in affected area well after washing; use antifungal medications

J. Cancer

    1. Types

       a. Squamous cell: malignant lesion usually located on face or arm; develops from preexisting skin lesion; will metastasize via lymph nodes

       b. Basal cell: skin nodule (opaque, light pink or tan); predominantly on hairy areas; seen frequently in people 40 years and older with light skin; usually becomes invasive

        c.   Malignant melanoma: serious type, occurs on pigmented skin cells exposed to sunlight (legs, head, neck); lesions vary in color, may be blue-black or yellow; irregular shape and pigmentation, frequently metastasize via lymph nodes to brain. Symptoms result in pruritus or soreness around lesion.

    2.   Treatment: surgical biopsy, excision, and removal followed by chemotherapy or radiation

K.   Lupus Erythematosus – a chronic inflammation of the connective tissue

    1.   Cause is unknown; possible autoimmune or viral; occurs mostly in young women

    2.   Risk factors: drugs, sunlight, family history

    3.   Signs and symptoms: butterfly rash on the nose and cheek; fever ; fatigue; weight loss; weakness; joint pain (arthralgias)

    4.   Diagnosis: positive LE cell reaction

    5.   Treatment: provide tranquility, curtail exposure to sunlight; anti-inflammatory medication and corticosteroids; ointment for rash, analgesic for pain; watch for organ involvement (heart, lung, kidney, CNS, blood vessels); support group

Additional Resources Found on MyNursingLab

- Drug Chart: Drugs Affecting the Skin

MODULE 3

Medical-Surgical Nursing

Submodule 3.5 Musculoskeletal Disorders

Learning Objectives

3.5.1 **Describe and compare pathophysiology, symptoms, treatment, and nursing care for clients with musculoskeletal injuries and fractures.**

3.5.2 **Compare pathophysiology, symptoms, treatment, and nursing care for clients with common musculoskeletal disorders.**

Note: **Prior to beginning this unit the student should review the anatomy and physiology of the musculoskeletal system (muscles, bones, and joints).**

I. **Diagnostic Tests for Musculoskeletal Disorders**

   A. Blood tests: blood count, rheumatoid factor (RF), antinuclear antibody (ANA), creatine kinase (CK), and culture and sensitivity.

   B. Radiography: X-ray, noninvasive; done to confirm fractures and   alignment of bone.

   C. Computed tomography (CT) – a series of cross-sectional pictures used to detect problems in the spine and skull bones and soft tissue disorders; can be used with or without contrast

   D. **Bone scan** – performed after injection using radioisotopes to detect tumor, metastasis, and degenerative disorders.

   E. **Arthrography** – X-ray outline of the joints and soft tissue using radiopaque substances

   F. Magnetic resonance imaging – a magnetic field that produces picture images of the internal structures to detects disorders of the musculoskeletal system

   G. **Arthroscopy** – visual inspection of the joint using a fiberoptic endoscope.

      1. Done for biopsy of suspicious tissue and for removal of loose tissue such as cartilage

      2. Client needs informed consent.

      3. Will undergo local anesthesia or deep sedation

      4. Performed as same-day surgery

      5. Client must ambulate same day.

      6. Safety with use of sedative is a major concern.

      7. Tissue swelling and bleeding is controlled with use of ice.

   H. **Arthrocentesis,** – removal of joint fluid to aid diagnosis of infection or inflammation of joints.

   I. **Electromyelogram** (EMG) – evaluates nerve-to-muscle transmission. Client needs consent; no caffeine or smoking for 3 hours before procedure

II. **Physical Assessment**

   A. Posture can help detect deformity in the skeletal system.

   B. Gait – When client ambulates, an unsteady gait can increase risk of falls.

   C. Mobility – Can client get out of bed and ambulate independently? Or, what level of assistance is needed, from person to assistive device, cane, walker, crutches, or wheelchair?

   D. Range of motion – Can the client perform these motions with upper and lower extremities?

   E. Appearance of the joints – Are they movable or immoveable? Is there any deformity or swelling?

   F. Neurovascular assessment – Check the femoral, popliteal, posterior, tibial, and pedal pulses for strength and rate.

   G. Check capillary refill.

   H. Check color and temperature of the extremities; compare extremities.

III. **Fractures**

   A. **Fracture** – a break or interruption in the continuity of a bone

   B. Types

      1. **Comminuted:** one in which the bone is broken and shattered into fragments

      2. **Closed** (simple): one in which there is no break in the skin

      3. **Open** (compound): one in which there is a break in the skin with fragments of bone protruding

      4. **Greenstick:** one in which the bone is partially bent and partially broken; common in children

      5. **Complete:** involves the entire width of the bone

      6. **Incomplete:** does not involve the entire width of the bone

   C. Signs and symptoms: deformity, pain, swelling, loss of function, numbness, crepitus, ecchymosis, muscle spasm

   D. Treatment: aimed at establishing a sturdy union between the broken ends of bones so that healing will restore the bone to its former state of continuity.

      1. **Reduction:** procedure of bringing two fragments of a broken bone into proper alignment

      2. Open reduction: procedure of bone reduction after a surgical incision has exposed the site of the fracture

      3. **Internal fixation:** pins, screws, immobilization by splinting fracture

   E. Healing the break in the bone results in swelling and hemorrhage

      1. When the blood clots, it forms a fibrin network between the two broken ends of the bone.

      2. The fibrin network granulates when osteoclasts in the blood clot proliferate.

      3. Calcium deposit causes a callus formation.

4. The callus holds the bone together.

5. Bone healing is slow and can take up to 1 year for bone to return to former strength.

F. Complications

1. Fat embolus

2. Infection (e.g., osteomyelitis)

3. Venous thrombosis

4. Gas gangrene

5. Tetanus

6. Compartment syndrome

G. Compartment syndrome may be caused by internal or external pressure and results in decreased blood flow.

1. Causes of internal pressure: excessive IV fluid or inflammation

2. Causes of external pressure: a pressure dressing or tight cast

3. Increased fluid places pressure on tissue, blood vessels, and nerves.

4. Signs and symptoms of compartment syndrome: edema, pallor, tingling, paresthesias, numbness, weak pulses, cyanosis, and severe pain

5. Can result in permanent loss of tissue and nerve function

6. Treatment: Report immediately and elevate the extremity. Ice pack as ordered, MD may bivalve the cast to relieve pressure.

7. Pain relief using analgesics

8. Surgical intervention: **fasciotomy,** a surgical incision into the fascia and separation of muscle

H. Principles of cast care

1. After application, allow 24 – 48 hours for drying; cast dries from inside out; plaster cast gives off heat when drying.

2. Do not handle with fingers; handle with palms of hands; pad edges as indicated.

3. Keep extremity elevated; turn client away from affected side.

4. Allow to dry; do not use heat because this may burn skin under the cast.

5. Frequent turning helps the cast dry.

6. Cast should remain uncovered until it is completely dry. Bed cradles trap moisture and hinder drying of the cast.

7. Important observations for possible complications:

   a. Sharp, localized pain may indicate excessive pressure under the cast.

   b. Observe protruding fingers or toes for cyanosis, coldness to the touch, and failure of the skin to blanch and then return to normal color after pressure is released.

   c. Elevated temperature or foul smell, heat, and pain may indicate the development of an infection.

      d.   Support the cast so that there is no undue pressure on any part of the body over a period of time.

      e.   Monitor visible blood on cast. Outline bloody area with a pen, and observe for increasing size.

  8. Daily care

      a.   Give special attention to the skin around the edges of the cast.

      b.   Avoid wetting the cast with bath water.

      c.   Elevate the head of the bed slightly when placing a client in a spica cast on the bedpan. The perineal area must be cleansed thoroughly each time the bedpan is used. Cover the edge of the cast around the perineal area to prevent soiling of the cast.

      d.   When the cast is removed, the underlying skin will be dry and scaly; the skin should be gently cleansed with soap and water and massaged with lotion or oil.

      e.   Never place any objects inside the cast.

I. Nursing care of the patient in traction

  1. Types of traction

      a.   Skeletal traction – pull is exerted directly on the bone with pins, screws, or wires and tongs (e.g., traction on Crutchfield tongs which have been inserted into the skull)

      b.   Skin traction – uses moleskin or some other type of adhesive bandage to cover the affected limb; traction is applied to the bandage (e.g., Buck's extension and Bryant's traction in children)

      c.   Balanced traction – uses a Thomas splint and special pins and wires to stabilize the fracture (e.g., Russell's traction)

  2. Purpose of traction is to exert a constant pull on a certain part of the body to maintain alignment. Used in the treatment of fractures and contracture deformities; used to relieve muscle spasm due to strain.

  3. Weight of traction ordered by doctor

J. General nursing care

  1. Special back care necessary to prevent breakdown of skin

  2. When changing the linen, the bottom sheets are changed starting on the affected side, or they may be changed from head to foot. The limb in traction may be covered with a small blanket in case the limb becomes cold.

  3. Trapeze bar over bed frame should be installed to allow the client to lift him- or herself and to move about in bed. The client is instructed to lift straight up toward the trapeze.

  4. Special observation:

      a.   Be sure the weights are always hanging free and ropes and pulley are in good condition.

      b.   The client's weight is counteracting the pull.

      c.   Observe bony prominences for signs of pressure.

      d.   Maintain position so that body is in good alignment.

5. Use fracture bedpan. This is smaller and easier for client to use.

6. Pin care – pins, screws, and nails must be given special attention. Cleanse daily according to MD orders.

IV. Disorders of the Musculoskeletal System

A. Rheumatoid arthritis – systemic inflammatory disease affecting the synovial lining. Occurs more often in women than men.

   1. Cause unknown; considered autoimmune, genetic, viral, or caused by direct injury

   2. Symptoms: fatigue, anorexia, elevated temperature; swollen, painful joints; usually worse in the morning; often periods of remission

   3. Diagnosis: x-ray, elevated sedimentation rate, and elevated WBC, and positive rheumatoid factor

   4. Treatment: relief of pain with:

      a. Heat or cold application; refer to therapist.

      b. Reposition for comfort and rest periods every 2-4 hours.

      c. Drugs – anti-inflammatory; could include hydroxychloroquine (Plaquenil) and methotrexate.

      d. Physical therapy to rehabilitate client and adaptive devices to assist in ADL

      e. Possible intervention: joint replacement – synovectomy

      f. Refer to Arthritis Foundation.

B. Osteoarthritis

   1. Osteoarthritis – degeneration of particular cartilage affecting weightbearing joints

      a. Cause: age, obesity, trauma

      b. Symptoms: pain and stiffness that increases in damp and cold; limited ROM

      c. Treatment: diet (reduced calories); applications of heat and cold; anti-inflammatory and analgesics; activity as tolerated; walker or cane as needed

C. Gout – inflammation of joint caused by deposit of uric acid crystals; common at 50 or older. The body produces a substance called purine during the metabolic process that results in increased uric acid levels.

   1. Symptoms: acute pain in joints, great toe, feet, ankle, or knee; swollen, red, and dusky or purple, malaise, headache.

   2. Treatment: low purine alkaline ash diet, increased fluids, bed rest in acute phase, monitor ROM, monitor pain; drugs – antigout and NSAIDs, colchicine, and allopurinol

D. Osteomyelitis – bacterial infection of bone and soft tissue

   1. Cause: *Staphylococcus aureus* or hemolytic streptococci, trauma

   2. Symptoms: malaise, pyrexia, bone pain, localized redness, muscle spasm

   3. Diagnosis: elevated WBC and erythrocyte sedimentation rate (ESR); bone biopsy and scan

   4. Treatment: diet therapy and bed rest; immobilize affected body part; alignment with cast or splint; drugs: antibiotics, analgesics for pain; wound irrigation; watch for fractures.

E. Osteoporosis – loss of bone mass leading to fragile and porous bone

1. Cause: calcium deficiency, lower estrogen level, hyperparathyroidism, lack of exercise

2. Treatment: diet with increased minerals, safe hazard-free environment; bed board or firm mattress, corset; encourage exercise (ROM)

3. Complication – possible fractures

F. Malignant tumor – Mostly invades the ends of long bones

1. **Multiple myeloma:** proliferation of plasma cells on bone and bone marrow; often affects the ribs, vertebrae, pelvis, or skull

2. Osteogenic sarcoma: has poor prognosis; metastasizes to lungs

3. Glial cell tumor: nonmalignant, affects distal radius, can become malignant

4. Diagnosis: bone scan and biopsy, increased alkaline phosphates, bone marrow aspiration

5. Treatment: surgery, chemotherapy

V. **Amputation – Surgical Removal of a Limb or Part**

A. Preoperative plan includes plans for fitting of prosthesis and for rehabilitation.

B. Postoperative plan includes stump care:

1. Stump is elevated on pillow and protected with plastic for 24 hours.

2. Observe for hemorrhage.

3. Have tourniquet at bedside.

4. Observe for **phantom pain** – severe pain where body part was located

5. Keep stump in alignment.

6. Rotate position to abdomen.

7. Prosthesis when indicated by doctor; use wool socks; position firmly in prosthesis socket; clean prosthesis socket daily with warm mild soap and water. Check shoes for uneven wear on unaffected side; strengthen muscles to use assistive device.

VI. **Joint Surgery**

A. **Arthrodesis** – surgical removal of cartilage with fusion of two bones

B. **Synovectomy** – removal of the synovial membrane

C. **Arthroplasty** – total joint replacement using a metal or plastic prosthesis

D. Routine preoperative care

E. Postoperative care

1. Maintain activity passive → active ROM to unaffected limbs

2. Isometric exercises as tolerated

3. Drugs: analgesics and stool softener

F. Hip replacement

1. Maintain hip abduction with abductor pillow.

2. Flexion no more than 90° when sitting

175

3. Turn to affected and unaffected side as ordered.

4. Avoid sitting in low or soft chair.

5. Do not cross legs.

6. Use an elevated toilet seat.

7. Incision care daily

8. Watch for complications – dislocation, hemorrhage, infection

9. Encourage cough, deep breathing, and use of incentive spirometer.

10. Early ambulation helps prevent complications such as atelectasis and deep vein thrombosis (DVT).

G. Assistive device – crutch walking – used for clients who have partial or no weight bearing; height of crutch 2-3 fingers below axillae; and grip at 30° flexion of the forearm

Additional Resources Found on MyNursingLab

- Movement of Joints animation
- Muscle Contraction animation
- Muscles animation
- Bone Healing animation
- Drug Chart: Drugs Affecting the Musculoskeletal System

MODULE 3

Medical-Surgical Nursing

Submodule 3.6 Disorders Affecting the Nervous System

Learning Objectives

3.6.1 Describe the diagnosis, treatment, and nursing care for common neurological injuries.

3.6.2 Describe the diagnosis, treatment, and nursing care for common neurological disorders.

Note: **Prior to beginning this unit the student should review the anatomy and physiology of the nervous system.**

I. **Common Neurological Terms**

   A. **Paraplegia** – paralysis of the lower extremities or lower part of the body; commonly associated with spinal injury

   B. **Hemiplegia** – paralysis of one side of the body; commonly associated with cerebral damage

   C. **Quadriplegia** – paralysis of all four extremities

   D. **Flaccid paralysis** – paralysis of all four extremities

   E. **Spastic paralysis** – paralysis in which the muscles are tense and rigid

   F. **Amnesia** – loss of memory

   G. **Aphasia** – loss of the ability to speak

II. **Special Neurological Examinations and Diagnostic Tests**

   A. Neurological examination – measures the ability of the body to perform certain motor and sensory functions

      1. Tests ability of the cranial nerves to control sensory and motor activities.

         a. Senses of taste, smell, sight, hearing

         b. Facial expressions

         c. Gag reflex

         d. Ability to move the eyes

      2. Tests groups of large muscles

         a. Evaluates client's gait while walking and running

         b. Checks posture while standing

         c. Tests strength of hand grip

      3. Tests **reflexes** – involuntary muscular contractions in response to a stimulus

B. **Lumbar puncture** – insertion of a hollow needle into the arachnoid space between the third and fourth lumbar vertebrae. Performed under local anesthesia. Informed content is needed.

1. Purposes:

   a. Check color of cerebrospinal fluid, which is normally clear

   b. Obtain a specimen of spinal fluid from the spinal cavity for chemical analysis

   c. Obtain a specimen of spinal fluid for microscopic examination

   d. Measure the pressure within the cerebrospinal cavities

   e. Determine if there is blockage of the flow of cerebrospinal spinal fluid

   f. Remove blood or pus from the arachnoid space

   g. Reduce intracranial pressure

   h. Provide spinal anesthesia

   i. Inject air for x-ray examination of the skull

2. Before procedure:

   a. Position client to side with head and neck flexed towards chest and knees flexed toward the abdomen.

   b. Client must lie still during the procedure.

3. After procedure:

   a. Client is usually kept flat in bed for at least 1 to 8 hours after a lumbar puncture to reduce headache.

   b. Check puncture site for signs of bleeding, leakage of cerebrospinal fluid, or infection.

   c. Check and record presence of sensation and movement in lower extremities.

C. **Electroencephalogram** (EEG) – test that records the activity of the brain tissues; can be used while asleep or awake

1. Electrodes are placed on scalp to record wave pattern.

2. Hair should be clean and dry.

3. No central nervous system depressant or stimulant drugs is given the night before the test

4. Restrict coffee, tea, caffeine, and alcohol for 24 to 48 hours before the test.

5. Used to diagnose strokes, cerebral tumor, seizure disorder, brain death, and infection of the brain

D. **Cerebral angiography**

1. Provides visualization of cerebral blood vessels to detect abnormalities such as an aneurysm, tumor, hematoma, and narrowing

2. Catheter inserted into common carotid artery

3. Radiopaque liquid injected through catheter and a series of films taken

4. Before test:

   a. Informed content

   b. Determine history of allergy to iodine or shellfish

   c. NPO for 8+ hours

   d. Preoperative sedation with antihistamine to decrease allergy

   e. Instruct client that there will be a flush feeling when dye is injected.

  5. After test:

   a. Maintain pressure dressing over puncture site if femoral artery was used.

   b. Assess for bleeding at insertion site.

   c. Assess pulse distal to the insertion site.

   d. Perform neurological check every 15 minutes for 1 hour, then taper.

 E. Brain scan:

  1. Injection of radiopaque isotope; wait for absorption; then a series of scans

  2. Radiopaque isotope will accumulate in affected tissue.

  3. Used to detect brain tumor abscess, hematoma, or aneurysm

  4. Determine iodine allergy before test.

 F. **Positron emission tomography (PET)**

  1. Determines damage to brain cells or death of brain cells

  2. Uses radioactive material to aid differentiation in areas of normal cellular activity

  3. Before test:

   a. Informed consent

   b. Insertion of two IV lines

   c. No central nervous system depressant drug

   d. Empty bladder

   e. Inform clients they will be asked to perform special tasks during the test.

 G. **Single photon emission computed tomography (SPECT)**

  1. Injection of radioactive isotope; series of images taken

  2. Used to track O_2 and glucose use by brain cells and blood flow

 H. **Doppler ultrasound**

  1. Noninvasive, painless test, used to study blood flow pattern

III. **Assessment of Clients with Neurological Disorders**

 A. Determine mental status:

  1. General appearance and behavior

  2 Memory – recent and remote

  3. Emotional status and thought pattern

  4. Language – check for presence of aphasia

   a. Inability to speak – **expressive aphasia**

   b. Inability to understand – **receptive aphasia**

  5. Difficulty in speaking – **dysarthria** (problem of motor function)

 B. Presence of abnormal muscle movements:

  1. Muscle tone

2. Check deep tendon reflexes.

3. Examine posture, gait, and balance.

4. Muscle coordination

C. Neurological checks – Used to monitor the nervous system to diagnose increased intracranial pressure (ICP).

1. Monitor level of consciousness:

   a. **Alert:** responds appropriately

   b. **Confused:** disoriented to person, place, or time.

   c. **Lethargic:** drowsy but easily roused.

   d. **Stuporous:** responds to stimuli by moaning

   e. **Comatose:** no observable response

2. More objective evaluation of LOC can be done using Glascow Coma Scale.

3. Optimal score is 15, meaning client is awake and oriented.

4. Lowest score is 3; means prognosis is poor and client is in a deep coma. Score of less than 8 indicates client is in a coma.

5. Does the patient follow commands and respond to stimulus appropriately?

6. Response to pain can be by posturing.

   a. **Decorticate posturing** is flexion of the elbow, wrist, and fingers; extension of the legs; and internal rotation of the arms.

   b. **Decerebrate posturing** is extension of the extremities, suggesting brainstem damage.

D. Pupillary response:

1. The pupils are examined under low light, and size is recorded in millimeters. Response to light can be brisk or sluggish.

2. An acronym for the parameters to respond to is **PERRLA,** which means:

   a. **P**upils are

   b. **E**qually

   c. **R**ound and

   d. **R**eactive to

   e. **L**ight and

   f. **A**ccommodation

E. Respiratory response

1. Airway, respiration, and breathing pattern – may need intubation and respiratory support

2. Monitor oxygen saturation (O_2 Sat) and arterial blood gases (ABG).

3. Common breathing pattern in neurological clients is Cheyne-Stokes, hyperventilation.

4. General nursing care of the client with a neurological disorder:

   a. Care of the skin:

      i. Keep skin clean and drug- and pressure-free.

  ii. Client must be turned frequently. With loss of motion of various parts of the body, there is also loss of feeling. The patient does not complain of discomfort from lying in one position too long because he or she does not feel any discomfort.

  iii. Intramuscular injections should not be given in the areas of the body that have no feeling.

  iv. All points of pressure should be massaged frequently to increase circulation.

  v. Air flow mattress to alternate pressure

 b. Providing for self-care:

  i. All clients with neurological disorders are not totally helpless; they should be encouraged to do as much for themselves as possible.

  ii. The furniture in the room should be arranged conveniently for the client.

  iii. Side rails should be applied to assist the nurse in turning the client.

  iv. A trapeze bar may help the client lift himself or herself onto a bedpan.

 c. Fluids and nutrition:

  i. Assess for signs of dehydration (skin turgor and mucous membranes).

  ii. Maintain fluid and electrolyte balance.

  iii. If NPO, client may need IV fluid and eventually nasogastric tube feeding.

  iv. Provide mouth care every 4 hr.

  v. Record a baseline weight and daily intake and output.

  vi. Self-feeding may be slow or clumsy for clients, but they should be allowed to feed themselves if possible.

 d. Eye protection to prevent corneal abrasion

  i. Obtain order for artificial tears and patch when ordered.

 e. Maintain client airway:

  i. Position on one side to prevent airway obstruction.

  ii. Suction as needed.

  iii. Auscultate breath sounds.

  iv. Check respiratory rate, depth, and quality.

 f. Cardiovascular

  i. Prevent thrombophlebitis: apply TED stockings or sequential compression device.

 g. Regulate temperature to prevent increased cerebral metabolism.

 h. Perform neurological checks at regular intervals.

 i. Avoid pushing clients into activities beyond their physical limitations.

 j. Proper handling of extremities will help prevent involuntary spasms of the muscles.

 k. Prevention of complications:

  i. Proper positioning of the client

  ii. Passive exercises and splinting to prevent deformities

l. Emotional aspects:

    i. Emotional disturbances and personality changes often accompany these disorders.

        (a) Outbursts of anger or depression are not uncommon.

        (b) Client may lose the will to live.

    ii. The nurse must help the client adjust to handicaps.

m. Rehabilitation

    i. In some cases, rehabilitation is limited to keeping the client occupied as the disease progresses.

    ii. If possible, rehabilitation should be planned so that the client is able to be an active member of the community in spite of the handicap.

n. Increased intracranial pressure

    i. Swelling of the brain due to injury or surgery, hemorrhage, tumor, or inflammation

    ii. Pressure against artery results in decreased blood flow and local tissue ischemia, herniation of the brain.

    iii. Normal ICP is 0-15 mm Hg.

    iv. Signs and symptoms: decrease in LOC, lethargy; increase in systolic pressure with diastolic pressure unchanged; decreased pulse rate slow and bounding; pupils unequal, sluggish, or dilated; breathing irregular and labored

    v. Intracranial pressure monitoring when indicated

    vi. Maintain patent airway.

    vii. Fluid restriction may be indicated.

    viii. Head position 30-45 degrees; do not flex hip or rotate neck.

    ix. Stool softener to prevent straining

    x. Antiemetic to prevent vomiting

    xi. Prevent coughing.

    xii. Maintain temperature.

    xiii. Monitor intake and output.

    xiv. Protect stomach from stress ulcer.

    xv. Order needed for proton pump inhibitor like lansoprazole (revacid)or H2 receptor block like nizatidine (Axid).

    xvi. Administer osmotic diuretic to reduce cerebral edema.

    xvii. Anti-inflammatory such as dexamethasone to lower cerebral pressure

    xviii. May need prophylactic antiseizure drugs (see section XII. Epilepsy)

    xix. Complication – diabetes insipidus, hydrocephalus, aneurysm, tumor, hematoma, and narrowing

IV. Head Injuries – Trauma to the Skull Bones

    A. Types

        1. Open penetration of the skull or fracture

        2. Closed injury caused by blunt trauma which can result in:

            a. **Concussion** – a head injury in which the brain is jarred or compressed by a portion of the skull which causes a temporary impairment of the brain tissue

            b. **Contusion** – more serious; the brain tissue is bruised and swelling occurs, pressing the brain tissue against the skull; can result in increased intracranial pressure.

            c. Hemorrhage, which can be:

                i. **Epidural hematoma** – blood collecting between the dura mater and skull; client may be alert, then lethargic, unconscious.

                ii. **Subdural hematoma** – blood collecting between the dura and subarachnoid space with progressive loss of consciousness

                iii. **Intracerebral hematoma** – blood collecting within the cerebrum with increased signs of ICP

    B. Symptoms

        1. Depend on severity of brain damage

        2. Vomiting, headache, vertigo, confusion, disorientation, delirium, and loss of consciousness can occur.

        3. Diagnostic tests:

            a. CT scan, MRI, skull x-rays, and EEG

        4. Nursing care:

            a. Maintain patent airway.

            b. Position head 30-45 degrees and position so head dressing can be easily observed.

            c. Observation and neuro checks are the most important aspect of care.

            d. Report changes in blood pressure, pulse, respirations, or fluctuations in temperature.

            e. Observe for extreme restlessness, abnormal posturing, or paralysis.

            f. Observe for deepening stupor, loss of consciousness.

            g. Headache which increases in intensity

            h. Presence of vomiting, especially persistent projectile vomiting

            i. Pupils that are unequal in size or unreactive

            j. Leakage of cerebrospinal fluid from nose or ears that looks clear, yellow, or pink tinged

            k. Inability to move one or more extremities

            l. Administer ordered drugs; dexamethasone to decrease brain swelling

            m. A hematoma will need surgical intervention – craniotomy.

C. **Craniotomy**

1. Surgical opening into the skull to evacuate blood clot or control hemorrhage, reduce ICP, or remove tumor.

2. Preoperative care:

   a. Shampoo hair if ordered prior to surgery.

   b. Insert Foley catheter, IV lines.

   c. Check for informed consent.

   d. Explain head will be partially shaved and bandaged.

3. Postoperative care:

   a. Facilitate breathing.

   b. Position head elevated 30-45 degrees; can be side lying on unaffected side

   c. Neuro check initially q 15 to 30 minutes

   d. Watch for signs and symptoms of increased ICP.

   e. Check dressing for drainage of CSF and report if present.

   f. Monitor for temperature changes or seizures.

   g. Instruct to breathe deeply but no coughing, bearing down, or vigorous suctioning.

   h. Intake and output; restrict fluid to 1500 mL/day; watch for signs of inappropriate ADH.

   i. Keep NPO until gag reflex returns.

   j. Administer ordered medication:

      i. Corticosteroids to decrease cerebral edema

      ii. Stool softeners to prevent straining

      iii. Prophylactic antiseizure drug to prevent seizures

      iv. Mild analgesic for pain once client is neurologically stabilized

V. **Spinal Cord Injury**

A. Results from motor vehicle crash, gunshot wounds, tumor, infection, or degenerative diseases

B. Damage to the spinal cord can be contusion or complete transection of the cord,

C. Outcome can be motor and sensory loss, depending on severity and degree of injury.

D. Initial injury to the spinal cord results in edema, which resolves in about one week to give the prognosis.

E. An injured person should be treated as a case of spinal cord injury until a definite diagnosis is made if:

1. Client complains of neck pain.

2. Client cannot move his or her legs.

3. Client has no feeling in his or her legs.

F. Spinal cord injury can occur in cervical, thoracic, lumbar, or sacral region.

G. Cervical injury affects innervation to the diaphragm.

H. Injury to L1- L2 causes paraplegia.

I. Immediate care – handle carefully avoid neck flexion.

1. Client must be transported to hospital on a stretcher or board.

2. The client's back must be kept straight; no pillow is used.

3. Respiratory assessment and management of patent airway; replace fluid.

4. Urinary catheter inserted to prevent bladder distention

5. Immobilization of spine may require traction.

J. The nurse is primarily concerned with prevention of:

1. Bowel or bladder dysfunction

2. Decubitus ulcers

3. Urinary complications

4. Orthopedic deformities

5. Emotional instability

K. Complications:

1. Infection of bladder or lung

2. Skin breakdown

3. Spinal shock

4. Autonomic dysreflexia

5. Orthostatic hypotension

6. Deep vein thrombosis (DVT)

L. **Spinal shock** (*arreflexia*):

1. Loss of all function below point of injury

2. Occurs 30-60 minutes after spinal injury; may last 1 week to months

3. Other symptoms: hypotension, bradycardia, and dry warm skin

M. **Autonomic dysreflexia** (*hyperreflexia*)

1. Sudden response of autonomic nervous system to stimulation

2. Seen in spinal cord injury above T6

3. Occurs suddenly at any time after spinal shock

4. Signs and symptoms:

    a. Vasoconstriction of arterioles causes increase in blood pressure, decrease in heart rate, pounding headache, flushing, sweating, goose bumps, nasal congestion, blurred vision, nausea, anxiety.

5. Causes:

    a. Distended bladder or bowel, use of rectal suppositories or enema, fecal impaction

    b. Skin pressure or breakdown

6. Treatment:

    a. Position 45 degrees.

       b.   Administer antihypertensive drugs.

       c.   Outcome if untreated: seizure, stroke, and death.

N. Ruptured intervertebral disk – A condition in which part of the fibrous cartilage disk prolapses and pinches the adjacent nerve root by pressing it against the bone.

    1. Symptoms: pain in lower back which radiates down the back of one leg to the foot; walking is extremely painful.

    2. Diagnostic tests:

       a.   CT scan, MRI, X-rays, electromyography

    3. Treatment and nursing care

       a.   Medical

          i.   Firm mattress with bed board

          ii.   Bed rest

          iii.   Hydrocollator pack or heating pad to reduce muscle spasm

          iv.   Pelvic traction may be applied

          v.   Use of specially designed corsets or back braces to maintain proper alignment of the spine

          vi.   Client should be "log-rolled" when turned:

             (a) Client folds arms across the chest

             (b) Client flexes knee opposite to the side to which he or she is to turn

             (c) Client is rolled over

          vii.   Drugs such as NSAIDs to reduce inflammation and pain; opioids may also be prescribed.

       b.   Surgical

          i.   **Laminectomy** (excision of the posterior arch of the vertebrae)

          ii.   Diskectomy with spinal fusion

          iii.   Removal of disk and bone graft

VI. Infection of the Brain and Spinal Cord

A. **Meningitis** – an inflammation of the membranous lining of the brain and spinal cord; may be caused by various bacteria and viruses

    1. Symptoms: severe and persistent headache; irritability; **photophobia** (sensitivity to light) chills, fever, malaise, vomiting, possible seizures

    2. Other characteristic symptoms are

       a.   **Nuchal rigidity** – pain and stiffness of the neck

       b.   **Kernig's sign:** Extension of legs with a flexed hip causes contraction of the hamstring muscle, resulting in pain in the calf.

    3. Diagnostic test: spinal tap

    4. Special treatment and nursing care: administer specific antibiotics; maintain strict isolation; keep room quiet and dimly lit; observe for signs of temperature elevation and convulsion. Cool compresses or an ice bag to the head may help relieve headache.

    a. Measures to lower temperature

    b. Monitor fluid and electrolytes.

    c. Vital signs and neuro checks

    d. Prevent mobility complications.

    e. Diet: high-protein, high-calorie

    f. Rehabilitation to optimal level

B. Encephalitis – inflammation of the brain tissue; most frequently caused by virus

    1. Symptoms: headache; fever, chills; lethargy; vomiting; weakness, mental confusion; visual disturbances; disorientation and seizures may be present.

    2. Special treatment and nursing care: administer specific antibiotic; constant attendance to prevent injury to self during period of disorientation; measures to lower temperature

C. Poliomyelitis – an acute inflammation of the anterior horn of the spinal cord; may be caused by three strains of viruses

    1. Prevention: immunization now available

        a. Salk vaccine

        b. Sabin vaccine

    2. Symptoms: upper respiratory infection; fever, severe headache, stiffness of the neck

    3. Special treatment and nursing care: application of heat to the muscles for relief of painful contractions; observe carefully for respiratory difficulties.

VII. Transient Ischemic Attack (TIA)

    A. TIA is a sudden, brief, temporary interruption of blood flow to the brain.

    B. TIA is a warning of an impending stroke. A large percent have stroke within 1 year.

    C. Symptoms are immediate and can last for a few minutes or up to 24 hours.

    D. When symptoms disappear, there is no residual deficit.

    E. Signs and symptoms:

        1. Lightheadedness, decreased vision, speech impairment

        2. Muscle weakness, numbness, impaired coordination, or paralysis on one side

        3. Confusion, decrease in level of consciousness

    F. Causes:

        1. **Arteriosclerosis** – narrowing and thickening of walls of blood vessels

        2. **Atherosclerosis** – deposits of fatty plaque causing narrowing of blood vessels

        3. History of diabetes or heart disease

        4. Hypertension can cause rupture of blood vessels.

        5. Medication, such as estrogen, used for hormone replacement or as contraceptive

    G. Diagnostic tests:

        1. Neurological examination

        2. Bruit on auscultation of carotid artery

3. Ultrasound or arteriogram of carotid artery revealing narrowing

4. MRI of the brain to rule out other neurovascular disorder

H. Treatment

   1. Medications are primarily used, especially antiplatelets.

   2. Surgical intervention is needed if there is narrowing of the carotid or plaque in the carotid artery.

   3. **Endarterectomy** is removal of plaque from the carotid artery.

   4. **Balloon angioplasty** to dilate the carotid artery

VIII. Cerebrovascular Accident (CVA) or Stroke

A. Prolonged interruption of cerebral blood flow

B. Depriving brain cells of oxygen for more than 3-7 minutes results in death of the cells.

C. Stroke is the third leading cause of death and first cause of disability.

D. Incidence of strokes is higher in males than in females.

E. There are three types of stroke:

   1. **Thrombotic stroke,** also called *ischemic,* is one of the common forms of stroke and results from obstruction in the artery that carries blood to the brain.

   2. **Embolic stroke,** also common, results from formation of a clot or debris in narrowed blood vessels.

   3. **Hemorrhagic stroke** results from rupture of cerebral blood vessels.

F. Causes

   1. Arteriosclerosis

   2. Atherosclerosis

G. Risk factors that can result in stroke:

   1. Hypertension

   2. Smoking

   3. High intake cholesterol or genetic predisposition to hyperlipidemia

   4. Consistent high blood sugar levels

   5. Excessive use of alcohol

   6. Decreased exercise or sedentary lifestyle

   7. Obesity

   8. Recreational drug use

   9. Heart disease

   10. Use of estrogen for contraception or hormone replacement

H. Diagnostic tests

   1. Neurological exam

   2. CT scan, cerebral angiogram

   3. MRI, EEG, and Doppler ultrasound

I. Signs and symptoms

1. Depend on area of brain affected

2. Brain cell injury on the right side of the brain affects the left side because the neurons cross over.

3. Numbness, weakness on one side of face, arms, or legs

4. Mental confusion

5. Difficulty speaking or understanding

6. Impaired walking and coordination

7. Severe headache

8. Emotions are labile; person cries easily.

J. Nursing care

1. Maintain patent airway.

2. Neurological check and vital signs; observe for increased ICP, hyperthermia, seizure, or shock.

3. Bed rest, head elevated 30-45 degrees; reposition every 2 hr.

4. Maintain fluid and electrolyte balance, using IV therapy, then nasogastric feeding.

5. Have client assessed for swallowing before resuming diet.

6. Promote skin integrity.

7. Passive ROM exercise every 4 hr.

8. Maintain elimination; may need Foley catheter.

9. Prevent constipation using stool softeners.

10. Establish communication mode with client.

11. Administer ordered medication:

   a. Corticosteroids to reduce cerebral edema

   b. Anticonvulsants to prevent seizures

   c. Anticoagulants or antiplatelets to prevent clotting

   d. Antihypertensives to maintain normal blood pressure

12. Long-term – need rehabilitation to optimal level

IX. Myasthenia Gravis

A. Myasthenia gravis – grave muscle weakness; affects more women than men

1. Caused by autoimmune process

2. The body is triggered to create antibodies that destroy acetylcholine at the neuromuscular junction.

3. Signs and symptoms: progressive muscular weakness of the skeletal muscles; the fatigue is relieved by rest, but soon returns.

4. **Diplopia** (double vision), **dysphagia** (difficulty swallowing)

5. **Ptosis** (drooping of eyelid) and masklike facial expression

6. Diagnostic tests:

    a. Tensilon test, when given by IV injection, symptoms immediately relieved but only for 10-15 minutes

    b. Electromyography

    c. Blood test

7. Treatment mainly drug therapy: neostigmine (Prostigmin), pyridostigmine (Mestinon)

    a. Promote nutrition, soft mechanical diet.

    b. Monitor respiratory status.

    c. Assess muscle strength.

    d. Plan rest periods.

    e. Watch for myasthenia crisis.

8. **Myasthenia crisis:** a period of severe weakness which may result in death because of weakness of the muscles that can lead to respiratory failure.

    a. Inability to swallow or speak

    b. Contributing factors:

        i. Sudden, abrupt withdrawal of medication

        ii. Physical or emotional stress

        iii. Infection

            (a) Nurse must be in constant attendance.

            (b) Throat and mouth must be suctioned frequently.

            (c) Nurse can reassure client by calm and competent manner.

            (d) A tracheotomy and artificial respirator may be necessary to maintain life.

            (e) Need increased dosage of anticholinesterase drugs.

X. Parkinson's Disease

A. Parkinson's disease – a degenerative disease of the nerve cells of the basal ganglia of brain

1. Results in degeneration in dopamine-producing neurons in the substantia nigra of the mid brain.

2. Signs and symptoms: tremor, most marked in the fingers, causing the individual to perform a constant "pill rolling" movement; rigidity of the skeletal muscles

    a. Stooped posture with slow, shuffling gait

    b. Masklike facial expression, decreased speech

    c. Increased salivation, drooling, sweating, constipation

    d. Depression and labile emotions

3. Treatment: medication that produces mild sedation and muscular relaxation; neurosurgical procedure that destroys certain areas of nerve cells and thereby eliminates the tremor and muscle rigidity.

4. Antiparkinson drugs: benztropine (Cogentin), trihexphenidyl (Artane), carbidopa-levodopa (Sinemet)

XI. Multiple Sclerosis

A. Multiple Sclerosis – a demyelinating disorder of the CNS causing plaques or patches of sclerosis in the brain and spinal cord, hindering neuromuscular conduction.

    1. Cause: unknown; may be linked to autoimmune response

        a. Genetics may predispose individuals to the disorder.

        b. Occurs more commonly in women than men between the ages 20-40.

    2. Signs and symptoms:

        a. Acute stage: edema around plaques

        b. Chronic stage: gliosis of the axons leading to permanent disability; characterized by periods of exacerbation and remission.

        c. Muscular weakness and stiffness, spastic paralysis, bowel and bladder incontinence

        d. Facial muscle weakness, paresthesias

        e. Nystagmus and ophthalmological problems

        f. Gait disturbances: ataxia and hypotonia

        g. Emotional lability

    3. Treatment and nursing care

        a. Administer steroids and biological modifiers and muscle relaxants.

        b. Provide symptomatic treatment for muscle weakness, stiffness, pain, respiratory problems, and bowel and bladder atony.

        c. Teach good health practices and nutritional needs to prevent complications.

        d. Refer client to physical therapy for gait training and muscle strengthening as needed.

        e. Provide counseling as indicated.

XII. Epilepsy

A. Epilepsy – Recurrent uncontrollable seizures in which the individual has muscle twitching and a temporary loss of consciousness

    1. Cause is unknown but it is believed that neurons in the brain become excited spontaneously.

    2. Seizures are classified as generalized or partial.

        a. **Partial seizures** are also called simple or focal seizures; these seizures involve one part of the brain.

        b. **Generalized seizures** affect both sides of the brain and are characterized by tonic-clonic contractions, incontinence, and loss of consciousness; also called *grand mal seizure*.

        c. Absence or petit mal seizures affect children 5 to 12 years old and disappear at puberty.

        d. **Petit mal seizure** is characterized by a brief lapse of consciousness; may go unnoticed and consists of a vacant stare (hence the name *absence seizure*) that lasts for a few seconds.

PEARSON

e. Seizures are often preceded by an **aura,** a specific warning which enables the client to sense that an attack is coming; examples – flash of light, dimming of vision, peculiar odor

f. Sequence of events in seizure:

   i. Usually heralded by a sharp cry

   ii. Muscles are held rigid and skin becomes cyanotic.

   iii. After a few seconds, jerking movements begin.

   iv. As the convulsion subsides, client falls asleep and usually awakens hours later with headache and depression; this is termed **postictal stage.**

g. **Status epilepticus** describes a state of prolonged partial or generalized seizures without a recovery period; can lead to irreversible damage to brain if not controlled.

h. Diagnosis

   i. Based on clinical findings such as an observed seizure, EEG, MRI to determine area of brain affected

i. Nursing care during a seizure:

   i. Provide for safety – pad side rails, protect client from falls, never use restraints or place tongue blade in the mouth.

   ii. Keep airway open; place head to side.

   iii. Loosen tight clothing.

   iv. Suction mucus from airway.

   v. Observe and record the sequence of symptoms.

   vi. Note and record presence of aura.

   vii. Note and record type of movements and affected parts of body.

   viii. Note and record presence or absence of incontinence of urine or stool.

   ix. Note and record level of consciousness.

   x. Note and record if patient sleeps after seizure.

   xi. Provide discharge teaching: wear or carry Medic-alert; comply with antiseizure medication

Additional Resources Found on MyNursingLab

- Brain and Brainstem animation
- Brain Scans animation
- Drug Chart: Drugs for Nervous System Disorders

MODULE 3

Medical-Surgical Nursing

Submodule 3.7 Disorders of the Eyes and Ears, the Sensory System

Learning Objectives

3.7.1 **Describe the diagnosis, testing, treatment, and nursing care for common eye disorders.**

3.7.2 **Describe the diagnosis, testing, treatment, and nursing care for common ear disorders.**

Note: **Prior to beginning this unit the student should review the anatomy and physiology of the sensory system.**

    I. Eyes

        A. Eye disorders can be caused by:

            1. Injury

            2. Disease

            3. Genetic predisposition

            4. The two diseases that contribute to most disorders of the eyes are diabetes and hypertension.

        B. Signs and symptoms:

            1. Headache, burning, itching, and redness of the eyes are symptoms of a visual defect and should be investigated by an ophthalmologist.

            2. Adequate diet and good nutrition play an important role in the conservation of sight, but no single type of food will improve the eyesight. Vitamin deficiencies (e.g., C and E) can produce visual defects.

            3. Visual defects should be corrected by prescription lenses.

        C. Eye care specialists

            1. **Ophthalmologist** or oculist – a medical doctor who specializes in the diagnosis and treatment of visual defects and diseases of the eye

            2. **Optometrist** – one who is trained to make glasses and optical instruments

        D. Diagnostic tests and examinations

            1. Visual acuity test uses **Snellen chart** and is the most commonly used test for determining a person's ability to see. It is read at a distance of 20 feet (6.1 m) and consists of rows of letters, each row smaller than the one above it. A normal reading is 20/20, meaning a person can see an object at 20 feet.

            2. Ophthalmoscopic examination

                a. Using a special instrument, the examiner visualizes the retina and interior aspects of the eyes through the pupils.

b. **Mydriatics:** drugs that dilate the pupils

c. Can diagnose disorders of the optic nerve and presence of tumors

d. Near-vision test uses **Jaeger's test** types – tests an individual's ability to see objects close at hand; uses different sizes of printer's type.

e. **Refraction test** – individual reads Snellen chart through various types of lenses; client chooses the lens through which the chart can best be read; these lenses are prescribed in glasses or contact lenses.

f. **Intraocular pressure** – measurement of the pressure within the eyeball; this is done with a tonometer and is used in the diagnosis of glaucoma.

g. Slit lamp biomicroscope:

   i. Examines the surface of the eye using a special microscope. A direct narrow beam of light illuminates a small section of the eye's anterior structure.

   ii. Used to identify corneal or conjunctival abnormalities; can detect floaters in the vitreous humor.

3. **Corneal staining** – a fluorescein dye is placed in the eye. The dye accumulates in the injured tissue and can help detect the presence of foreign bodies on the cornea or the presence of abrasion.

4. **Electroretinography** – electrodes embedded in a contact lens are placed in the eyes and measured. Electrical impulse given off by the retina is used to evaluate retinal function.

5. **Optical coherence tomography** – beams of light are directed into the eye to scan retinal structures.

6. **Ultrasonography** – a probe is placed into the eyeballs and sound waves are transmitted to detect changes in structure, presence of a lesion, or a foreign body.

7. **Amsler grid test** – The client focuses on the center of a handheld card with black lines; it is used to detect macular degeneration.

E. Common visual defects

1. Refraction errors are the most common type of defects. This means that the light rays entering the eye do not bend to focus properly on the retina; these errors may be caused by a number of structural defects in the eyeball.

   a. Normal vision – lens bends light rays so that they focus directly on the retina.

   b. **Hyperopia** – lens is too close to the retina; the light rays converge at a point beyond the retina; this is called *farsightedness*.

   c. **Myopia** – lens is too far from the retina; thus light rays converge before they reach the retina; this is called *nearsightedness*.

   d. **Astigmatism** – difficulty in focusing the horizontal and vertical rays as they strike the retina.

2. Treatment

   a. These conditions may be treated by wearing glasses in which the lenses have been shaped so the light rays are bought into proper focus on the retina.

   b. If the condition is slight, the eye will eventually accommodate by changing the shape of the lens.

      c. Surgical intervention – uses a laser or microsurgical instrument to alter the corneal curvature. The most common surgery is the laser-assisted in-site keratomileusis, or LASIK.

F. Injuries and infections of the eye

    1. Blunt trauma can cause swelling and bleeding into surrounding tissue, called a *black eye.* Initial treatment in first 24 hours is a cold compress, followed by a warm pack to increase absorption of blood in the tissues.

    2. Foreign bodies

        a. Irrigation of the eyes with clean lukewarm water or saline to prevent corneal abrasion.

        b. A speck in the eye can be removed with a moistened sterile swab.

    3. **Conjunctivitis**

        a. An inflammation of the mucous membrane lining that covers the eyelids and the front of the eyeball; also known as *pink eye.*

        b. May be caused by *Streptococcus, Staphylococcus,* or *Gonococcus, Rickettsia,* infection, or an allergic reaction

        c. Symptoms include redness, swelling, excessive tearing, purulent drainage.

        d. Treatment – antibiotics and steroids given systemically or applied locally in the form of eye drops or ointments. In addition, the eyes may be treated with hot or cold moist compresses and irrigation.

G. Stye (hordeolum)

    1. **Stye** – An infection of the small lubricating glands around the edge of the eyelids

    2. Redness, pain, burning, and itching of the eyelids are among the first symptoms. Later a small pustule forms on the lid.

    3. Treated with warm moist compresses to encourage rupture and drainage of the sty, plus a topical antibiotic. Surgical incision and drainage may be necessary.

H. Cataract

    1. **Cataract** – opacity of the lens resulting in blurring of vision.

        a. Cataract can be present at birth **(congenital cataract)**

        b. Most often occurs as a result of the aging process **(senile cataract)**

    2. Causes – Cataracts can be congenital or caused by injury by physical blow or exposure to sunlight, heat, chemical, radiation, infection, or drugs such as corticosteroids. Cataracts can also be caused by such disorders as diabetes mellitus or hypoparathyroidism.

    3. Other factors that are associated with cataracts are excessive smoking and alcohol intake.

    4. Signs and symptoms:

        a. Progressive decrease in vision with hazing, blurring, and diplopia, fading vision requiring increased light to read; may be painless.

        b. The pupils may be milky white in appearance.

        c. Increased sensitivity to glare

    d.   Poor night vision

    e.   Cataracts can develop in both eyes simultaneously.

5.   Diagnosed by examination with ophthalmoscope, Snellen visual activity test, slit lamp, or ultrasonography. Tonometry is useful to rule out glaucoma.

6.   Treatment:

    a.   Surgical removal of the affected lens is the only effective method of treatment; done when decreased vision interferes with activities.

    b.   One eye is done at a time. Surgery is performed under local anesthetic.

    c.   The two common surgeries are *intracapsular extraction* or *extracapsular extraction.* A small hole cut in the lens (**iridectomy**) can also be done during surgery or lens implant.

    d.   Preoperative care of the client having a cataract extraction includes familiarizing the client with the environment in the hospital so that he or she will not be frightened and confused after surgery when the eyes are bandaged.

    e.   Postoperative care:

        i.   Most important is teaching the client to avoid strain on the sutures, to keep the head elevated 30-45 degrees, and not to lie on the operative side. Coughing, sneezing, or sudden movements of the head must be avoided.

        ii.   Teach client not to bend, stoop, cough, or strain; not to rub or put pressure on the eyes.

        iii.   Instruct client to avoid lifting objects more than 15 lb.

        iv.   Amount of physical activity allowed the client depends on the desires of the surgeon.

        v.   Eyelids may be cleaned with compresses and saline irrigations. Remember that only the lids are cleaned; the eyeball is not disturbed. Eye shields are worn during the night, eyeglasses during the day.

        vi.   Medications:

           (a)   Mydriatics (e.g. epinephrine [Epifrin], Neosynephrine) and cycloplegics (e.g., cyclopentolate [Cyclogyl], atropine hydrobromide [Isopto Homatropine], scopalamine hydrobromide [Isopto-Hycosine]) for decreased spasm.

           (b)   Anti-inflammatory topical NSAIDs (e.g., Voltaren), corticosteroid (e.g., prednisolone Na) to decrease inflammation and scarring, and topical antibiotic to prevent or treat infection.

           (c)   Stool softeners such as Colace to prevent straining

I.   Glaucoma

    1.   **Glaucoma** – an increase in intraocular pressure. In the early stages, the individual does not realize that anything is wrong until permanent damage has been done to the eye and vision has been impaired.

    2.   Most commonly diagnosed as a part of a routine eye examination

    3.   Untreated glaucoma can lead to damage to the optic nerve.

    4.   Comes on slowly or abruptly can be present at birth or develop later in life.

    5.   Some individuals have a genetic predisposition or trauma.

6. Two types are seen: *open angle* or *closed angle;* can be acute or chronic

7. Danger signs of glaucoma include: blurred or hazy vision, difficulty in adjusting to darkened rooms, narrowing of vision at the sides of one or both eyes, seeing rainbow-colored rings around lights. Headaches most often occur in clients aged 40 years or older. It can be inherited or caused by disease such as diabetes mellitus, hypertension, trauma or inflammation of the eyes, or long-term use of corticosteroids.

8. Diagnostic tests – routine eye exam and tonometry with intraocular pressure (IOP) greater than 22 mm.

9. Treatment and nursing care – Objective is to decrease intraocular pressure.

    a. Drugs – Miotics (cholinergics) constrict the pupil and decrease intraocular pressure; pilocarpine (Isopto Carpine) and physotigmine (Neostigmine), carbonic anhydrase inhibitors (acetazolamide [Diamox]), mannitol (Osmitrol) decrease production of aqueous humor.

    b. Brief light pressure on inner canthus decreases systemic absorption of drug.

    c. Surgery may be performed in some cases to establish a means by which the aqueous humor may flow out of the eyeball when pressure builds up inside the eyeball.

J. Detached retina

1. **Detached retina** – hole or tear of the sensory retina; can be primary or secondary, traumatic or spontaneous; can have complete separation of retina that results in blindness.

2. Cause is sometimes unknown but is often due to trauma, inflammation, or secondary to diabetes, hypertension (HTN), and retinopathy. The tear allows the vitreous humor to seep out.

3. Signs and symptoms: floating spots, flashes of light, changes in vision (curtain over visual field)

4. Most commonly seen between ages of 40 and 70.

5. Treatment: bed rest, flat for 1 – 2 days, surgery; objective of treatment is to reseal the retina, photocoagulation laser. Retinal cryopexy, scleral buckling.

6. Postoperative care: eye medication such as antibiotics, steroids, mydriatics, and analgesics. Cold compresses to decrease swelling.

7. Client teaching: Avoid jerky movements and straining for 6 weeks. Restrict reading for 3 weeks.

K. Macular degeneration

1. Most common cause of vision loss in the aged. There are two types:

    a. *Atrophic* (dry) – the majority of cases

    b. *Exudative* (wet)

2. Factors that predispose to macular degeneration:

    a. Inflammation

    b. Some individuals have a genetic predisposition.

    c. Diseases that place client at risk for diabetes and hypertension (HTN)

3. Prevention

    a. Protect the eyes by wearing sunglasses

    b. Increase intake of vitamins, minerals, and antioxidants.

4. Signs and symptoms

    a. Inability to see details or color, blurring, and distorted vision

    b. Onset can be gradual, affecting both eyes.

    c. When condition is severe, a large dark spot on the pupils interferes with the ability to read.

5. Diagnosis

    a. Ophthalmoscopic exam of the retina giving findings of yellow exudates beneath.

    b. Tests: fluorescein angiography, optical coherence tonography, and Amsler grid test.

6. Treatment – Management aimed at slowing progression and maximizing remaining vision; depends upon the exact type of macular degeneration; may include laser therapy to seal leaking blood vessels, photodynamic therapy (PDT) or injections to seal or destroy affected blood vessels.

L. General principles in the care of the blind

1. Provide safety beep call bell near client.

2. Emotional aspects must always be considered. Depression and despair are to be expected until the individual adjusts to loss of vision.

3. Avoid shouting at those who are blind.

4. Speak to the blind person as you enter the room and do not touch the client until he or she is aware of your presence.

5. Leave doors completely open to avoid accidents. Be careful to keep the floor free from obstacles.

6. Do not pity the blind. They wish to be treated as normal people and prefer to ask for help rather than have someone do everything for them.

II. Disorders of the Ears

A. Introduction

1. Loss of hearing may be classified as sensorineural or conductive.

    a. **Sensorineural deafness** (nerve deafness) is brought about by a disorder of the eighth cranial nerve caused by infection or drugs.

    b. **Conductive hearing loss** occurs when there is a barrier in the canal, eardrum, or middle ear, and the sound waves are not conducted from the outside to the auditory nerve.

2. Loss of hearing affects one in every ten persons in the United States to some degree.

3. Signs and symptoms: inability to hear a whisper or watch tick; difficulty hearing with background noise

B. Diagnostic tests and examinations

1. Tuning fork test used to determine individual's ability to detect sound waves produced by vibration of the fork.

2. **Audiometry** – use of special machine to determine and measure sound perception.

C. Infections of the ear

1. **Otitis media** – inflammation of the middle ear. Usually a complication of an acute infection of the throat or sinuses. Can be acute or chronic.

   a. Organism responsible bacteria or viruses, streptococcal pneumonia; most commonly seen in infants and young children.

   b. Can also be caused by trauma

   c. Symptoms include pain in ear (children pulling and tugging ear), fever, feeling of fullness in head, or drainage of the ear.

   d. Treatment

      i. Use of analgesics to relieve pain and antibiotics to inhibit growth of the causative microorganism.

      ii. **Myringotomy,** or incision and drainage of the eardrum, may be done to relieve pressure inside the ear and to allow for drainage of exudates.

2. **Meniere's disease** – disease of the inner ear that affects the semicircular canals causing fluid to distend the labyrinth; may cause degeneration of vestibule or cochlear hair cells.

   a. Cause: unknown, possibly viral; seen in clients with upper respiratory tract infections (URTI), chronic ear disorders, and allergic symptoms.

   b. Signs and symptoms: headache, tinnitus, hearing loss, dizziness, **vertigo** (spinning sensation, nausea and vomiting, poor coordination caused by sudden movement of head or eyes).

   c. Diagnostic tests – ear examination and history

   d. Treatment

      i. Bed rest. Move slowly to prevent dizziness. Provide safe environment.

      ii. Drugs as prescribed, antibiotics, steroids, antiemetics, sedatives, meclizine (Antivert), Dramamine.

      iii. Diet salt free.

3. **Mastoiditis** – a bacterial infection of the cells of the mastoid bone.

   a. Most often occurs when infection is spread from the middle ear.

   b. Symptoms include earache and tenderness over the mastoid bone.

   c. Treatment

      i. Antibiotics are used to treat the infection.

      ii. Myringotomy is done to drain exudates and prevent spread of the infection.

      iii. **Mastoidectomy** (removal of necrotic bone cells from the mastoid) is necessary in many cases when the infection has become extensive and does not respond to antibiotic therapy.

D. Otosclerosis

1. **Otosclerosis**– destruction of the bones in the middle ear with formation of sclerotic bone cells. Bones become fixed and do not transmit sound waves to the auditory nerve. Mainly seen in females (teens to 20); can be hereditary.

2. Symptoms include a peculiar type of hearing loss in which the individual can hear his own voice clearly, but cannot hear others speaking unless they raise their voice.

3. Diagnosed by otoscopic exam.

4. Treatment

   a. May be treated with a properly fitted hearing aid or by surgery.

   b. **Stapedic fenestration** is surgical removal of the stapes and insertion of a prosthesis.

   c. **Tympanoplasty** – surgical reconstruction of tympanic membranes.

5. Postoperative care

   a. Flat in bed with affected side uppermost

   b. Change position slowly.

   c. Avoid coughing or sneezing.

   d. If must cough, open mouth to relieve pressure.

E. General principles in the care of the deaf and hard of hearing

1. Nurse should always be alert to signs of hearing loss:

   a. Listless expression

   b. Frequent requests for repetition of a statement

   c. Mispronunciation of words

   d. Inattention or failure to respond when questioned

   e. Tendency to avoid people

2. Nurse must remember that speaking slowly and distinctly to one with a loss of hearing is preferable to shouting.

3. Always remember to face the person with hearing loss when speaking.

4. Phrase your questions so that the client must answer with more than "yes" or "no."

Additional Resources Found on MyNursingLab

- Drug Chart: Drugs Affecting the Sensory System

MODULE 3

Medical-Surgical Nursing

Submodule 3.8 Endocrine System

Learning Objectives

3.8.1 **Describe common diagnostic tests and nursing care for endocrine disorders.**

3.8.2 **Describe medical and surgical treatment and nursing care for clients with pituitary, thyroid, and parathyroid disorders.**

3.8.3 **Describe medical and surgical treatment and nursing care for clients with pancreatic, adrenal, and other endocrine disorders.**

Prior to beginning this unit the student should review the anatomy and physiology of the endocrine system.

I. **Introduction**

    A. Endocrine glands are ductless glands and empty their secretions directly into the blood. Their secretions are called **hormones.** Hormones are chemical substances that regulate the various organs of the body.

    B. Diseases of the endocrine glands are concerned with oversecretion or undersecretion of the hormones. The prefix *hypo* refers to undersecretion; hyper refers to oversecretion of hormones.

        1. Pituitary gland

            a. Pituitary gland, regulated by the *hypothalamus,* is about the size of a pea; lies in the bony cavity of the sphenoid bone.

            b. Sometimes called the *master gland* as it secretes seven different hormones that control other glands and body processes.

            c. The pituitary gland consists of two main lobes- anterior and posterior. Hypothalamus controls the anterior portion of the pituitary.

II. **Disorders of the Pituitary Gland**

    A. Hyperpituitarism

        1. Excessive secretion of hormones from the anterior pituitary gland.

        2. Usually results from benign tumor growth or dysfunction of the hypothalamus.

        3. When the growth hormone is affected, the result is gigantism or acromegaly.

            a. Acromegaly is the overproduction of the growth hormone somatotropin after closure of the epiphyseal cartilage.

                i. In the adult, height is unchanged but the skeletal structure widens and grows outward, making the hands and feet large with protruding forehead and jaw. These body changes are irreversible.

      ii.   Signs and symptoms

         (a) Bone and joint enlargement resulting in impaired gait

         (b) Increased growth hormone causes internal organs, cartilage, and soft tissue to grow, leading to arthritis, muscle weakness, headache, and visual disturbances.

         (c) Early-onset heart failure leading to tachycardia, hypotension, and dyspnea

         (d) Males develop impotence and women experience menstrual problems.

         (e) Diabetes can occur as an outcome of this disorder.

      iii. Diagnostic tests

         (a) X-ray, CAT scan, and MRI to detect tumor

         (b) Ophthalmic examination

         (c) Bloodwork:

            (1) Increased level of growth hormone

            (2) Elevated levels in oral glucose challenge test

      iv. Treatment

         (a) Range of motion exercises to relieve joint pain and stiffness

         (b) Assistance with ADL

         (c) Do not overtire; provide rest periods

         (d) Soft diet; allow fluid with diet for easier swallowing

         (e) Emotional support because of body image changes

         (f) Medications: analgesic for pain, Bromocriptine (Parlodel) to inhibit growth hormone

         (g) Irradiation of the tumor to decrease size; removal of the tumor **(transsphenoidal hypophysectomy)** may be necessary

  b. **Gigantism** is an excessive secretion of the growth hormone when the epiphyseal cartilage is still open; it occurs in children.

      i.   Children can grow 7 feet or more in height

         (a) Causes: tumor of the pituitary gland or dysfunction of the hypothalamus

         (b) Signs and symptoms

            (1) Rapid growth of the skeletal structure that causes pain, headache, and muscle weakness.

            (2) High levels of the growth hormone cause enlargement of the heart and lungs.

         (c) Treatment

            (1) Pain relief, emotional support to help cope with change in body image.

B. Hyposecretion of the anterior lobe of the pituitary gland

  1. Decreased secretion of the growth hormone (somatotropin) causes dwarfism.

2. Affects children; typical growth pattern of 3 to 4 feet with a delay in sexual development.

   a. Cause: tumor of the pituitary gland

   b. Diagnostic test

      i. Bloodwork: decreased serum level of growth hormone

      ii. X-ray and CAT scan to locate tumor

   c. Treatment

      i. Replacement growth hormone (somatotropin) or surgical removal of the tumor

C. Hyposecretion of the posterior lobe of the pituitary gland

   1. **Diabetes insipidus** – Hyposecretion of the antidiuretic hormone from the posterior pituitary gland results in this condition.

      a. Diabetes insipidus

         i. A temporary or permanent metabolic disorder resulting from a decrease in the antidiuretic hormone (ADH).

         ii. Deficiency in ADH results in inability to concentrate urine.

         iii. Antidiuretic hormone aids in reabsorption of water from the distal tubules.

         iv. Absence of the antidiuretic hormone prevents the kidney from reabsorbing water, resulting in the excretion of a large amount of dilute urine.

      b. Cause: pituitary tumor, secondary to brain injury from stroke, or infection (meningitis, surgery).

      c. Signs and symptoms

         i. **Polyuria** – over 10 to 15 liters/day of urine; appearance of urine like water; urine specific gravity below 1.006; urine osmarlarity decreased; serum osmarlarity increased.

         ii. **Polydipsia** – excessive thirst, with dry skin and mucous membranes

         iii. Dehydration and electrolyte imbalance, usually high levels of sodium

         iv. Tachycardia, hypotension, fatigue, increased hemoglobin, hematocrit, and BUN

         v. Muscle weakness, pain, cramps, and ataxia

         vi. Untreated can lead to hypovolemia, shock, and death

      d. Diagnosis tests

         i. Urinalysis: decrease in urine specific gravity and increase in serum osmolarity

         ii. X-ray, CAT scan to locate tumor

      e. Treatment

         i. Monitor state of hydration, skin turgor, weight, intake and output, and urine specific gravity.

         ii. Encourage fluid intake to equal fluid output.

         iii. Decrease sodium intake and replace electrolytes.

         iv. Monitor cardiovascular and neurological status

        v. Medications: replacement of antidiuretic hormone, vasopressin (Pitressin), and chloropropamide

D. **Syndrome of inappropriate antidiuretic hormone** (SIADH)

    1. Excessive production of antidiuretic hormone when plasma osmolarity is low; leads to hyponatremia and water retention.

    2. Kidneys reabsorb more fluid than needed; leads to water retention, dilutes the blood

        a. Causes

            i. Medication, such as opiates, thiazide diuretic, oxytocin, antidepressants, and general anesthetic

            ii. Other factors such as stress factors, malignancies of the lung and pancreas, pulmonary disease, brain injury from strokes, trauma, or surgery

        b. Diagnostic test: Plasma or urine osmolarity and hyponatremia

        c. Signs and symptoms

            i. Nausea, vomiting, and anorexia

            ii. Decreased urine output, weight gain resulting from fluid overload

            iii. Urine specific gravity increased above 1.030

            iv. Tachycardia, hypertension

            v. Hyponatremia causing muscle weakness, fatigue, headache

            vi. Fluid overload causes cerebral edema, seizures, coma, and death.

        d. Treatment

            i. Baseline weight and daily weight

            ii. Intake and output

            iii. Restrict fluids and watch for water intoxication

            iv. Diet: encourage salty foods (potato chips, broth, tomato juice, and bacon) to increase sodium.

            v. Monitor level of consciousness and mental status.

            vi. Monitor cardiac and neurological status.

            vii. Medications: diuretics to remove excess fluid, infusion of hypertonic saline solution to correct sodium loss, and doxycycline to inhibit ADH production.

III. Thyroid Gland

A. Located in the neck; regulates metabolism of body cells by producing two hormones.

B. The principal hormones secreted are thyroxine (T_4) and triiodothyronine (T_3).

C. Diagnostic tests and examination

    1. Radioactive iodine uptake – Assesses function of the thyroid gland; readily absorbs and utilizes iodine in the production of its hormone, *thyroxine*. The overactive gland accumulates more radioactive iodine than the underactive gland. Amount of iodine absorbed is measured with a scintillation counter because the iodine has been made radioactive.

2. Thyroid scan – Client swallows radioactive iodine and a scintillation scanner is passed back and forth across the throat. The pattern of the scan shows concentration of iodine in the thyroid tissues. Used to determine size, shape, and activity.

3. Palpation of the thyroid gland may reveal an enlargement of the gland.

4. Blood test assesses the amount of thyroxine in the blood to evaluate thyroid function T_3 (total triidothyronine) and T_4 (total thyroxine). Thyroid-stimulating hormone measurements diagnose whether disease is from primary or secondary hypothyroidism.

D. Disorders of the thyroid gland

1. Simple **goiter** – an enlargement of the thyroid gland. One type is most frequently seen during adolescent and pregnancy. There is no increase in serum thyroxine levels.

   a. Caused by a decrease in the intake of iodine (endemic to certain areas)

   b. The cause of the second type of goiter is unknown.

   c. Symptoms include:

      i. Enlargement of the neck

      ii. Difficulty in swallowing when goiter presses on esophagus

      iii. Dyspnea when goiter presses on trachea

   d. Diagnosis made by history and physical examination and low to normal level of T_4 and radioactive iodine uptake test.

   e. Treatment includes administration of iodine preparations and inclusion of iodine in the diet (iodized salt most common form).

   f. Surgical removal of the gland may be necessary if it has enlarged to the point that it interferes with swallowing and breathing.

2. **Hyperthyroidism** – overactivity of the thyroid gland and excessive secretion of thyroid hormone. Also known as Graves' disease, toxic goiter. Seen more in females age 30-50.

   a. Cause unknown; related to emotional stress, physical stress, autoimmune process, or secondary to hormone replacement therapy.

   b. Symptoms include:

      i. Extreme nervousness

      ii. Increased appetite with loss of weight

      iii. Tachycardia, palpitations, and increased blood pressure

      iv. Heat intolerance and sweating

      v. Nervousness and insomnia

      vi. Irritability and agitation

      vii. **Exophthalmos** (protrusion of eyes) may be present

   c. Diagnostic tests:

      i. Elevated T_3, T_4, and radioactive iodine uptake test

      ii. Thyroid scan

PEARSON

    d. Treatment:

       i. May be medical or surgical-medical treatment

      ii. High-calorie, high-vitamin diet to help maintain normal body weight

     iii. Monitor weight daily and vital signs

     iv. Provide periods of uninterrupted rest; decrease stress

      v. Monitor for a **thyroid storm,** which is sudden, uncontrolled hyperthyroidism.

     vi. Perform eye care if exopthalmos is present; artificial tears to moisten, and sunglasses to protect eyes from sunlight.

    vii. Administer medication, antithyroid drug to block uptake of iodine and synthesis of T_3 and T_4

        (a) Administer beta-blocking agent to regulate blood pressure and heart rate.

        (b) Administer mild sedative to decrease restlessness.

        (c) Administer radioactive iodine as abalation therapy.

    e. Surgical interventions – removal of the thyroid gland **(thyroidectomy)** is necessary if medical treatment is not successful.

    f. Preoperative – assess weight and nutritional status.

       i. Administer antithyroid drugs to suppress production of thyroid hormone.

    g. Postoperative nursing care includes:

       i. Vital signs and intake and output

      ii. Placing client in Fowler's position as soon as he/she has reacted

     iii. Support the head with pillows to relieve tension on the sutures.

     iv. Keep client quiet and discourage talking.

      v. Observe carefully for bleeding, swelling behind the neck, or tightness of bandage, difficulty in breathing, difficulty in swallowing, and hoarseness.

     vi. Tracheotomy set should be kept at bedside.

    vii. Monitor for thyroid crisis and tetany. Tetany results from accidental removal of parathyroid glands and consequent decrease in blood calcium levels, resulting in twitching.

   viii. Tetany is treated with intravenous calcium.

3. **Hypothyroidism** – undersecretion of the thyroid gland. In children, it is called *cretinism;* in adults it is *myxedema.*

    a. Cause: Destruction of too many thyroid cells during ablation or surgery for treatment of hyperthyroidism. Can also result from genetic defect.

    b. Symptoms include:

       i. Mental retardation in children

      ii. Pronounced lethargy in older clients

     iii. Intolerance to cold, weight gain, constipation, anorexia

     iv. Bradycardia, hypotension

      v. Dry hair, dry skin, thick brittle nails

PEARSON

      vi.   Menstrual irregularity

      vii. Puffiness of the face

      viii. Decreased emotion; impaired memory

      ix.   Goiter may be present.

  c. Diagnosis

      i.   Decreased T_3 and T_4 and presence of T_4 antibodies

      ii.   Decreased radioactive antibodies, uptake test

  d. Nursing care

      i.   Daily weights, intake and output

      ii.   Monitor vital signs and watch for cardiovascular complications.

      iii. Provide warm environment.

      iv. Diet low in calories, increased fiber, increased fluids.

      v.   Avoid use of sedatives and narcotics; very sensitive to effects of these drugs.

      vi.   Prevent constipation; clients may need stool softener.

      vii. Administer medication.

      viii. Thyroid replacement drugs – thyroid USP, levothyroxine (Synthroid) returns patient to euthyroid state; side effects tachycardia and hyperthyroidism

VI. Parathyroid Glands

  A. The hormone parathormone, secreted by the parathyroid, helps maintain a constant calcium balance in the blood.

    1. A disturbance in the secretion of parathormone may be due to a tumor of the gland or to injury to the gland during thyroidectomy.

  B. Hyperparathyroidism – oversecretion of the hormone

    1. Causes

      a. Benign enlargement of the parathyroid glands or hyperplasia.

          i.   Hyperactivity of the parathyroid glands.

          ii.   Increased blood calcium levels result in depletion of calcium from the bones; they become fragile and painful and may break spontaneously.

          iii. Other symptoms result from excess of calcium in the blood and include the formation of kidney stones.

    2. Symptoms

      a. Dehydration, lethargy, confusion

      b. Nausea and vomiting (N&V), constipation, anorexia, weight loss

      c. Gastric ulcers

      d. Personality changes, depression

      e. Hypertension

    3. Diagnostic tests

      a. Elevated serum calcium and decreased phosphate levels

4. Treatment

    a. Correct phosphate and calcium imbalance.

    b. Prevent pathologic fractures.

    c. Monitor vital signs and report irregularity.

    d. Diet should be low in calcium, high in phosphate.

    e. Monitor fluids and electrolyte balance.

    f. Administer medications.

    g. IV fluids and diuretics to promote excretion of calcium.

    h. Administer phosphate to correct deficit.

    i. Administer calcitonin to decrease rate of calcium release from bones.

    j. Treatment may also consist of surgical removal of the tumor on the gland when one is present or removal of all but one of the parathyroid glands.

C. Hypoparathyroidism

1. Cause: atrophy or traumatic injury of parathyroid gland. This most often occurs when the parathyroid gland is accidentally removed during a thyroidectomy or irradiation of the thyroid glands.

2. Symptoms are the results of a deficiency of calcium in the blood. Outstanding symptom is **tetany** (muscle spasm, muscle cramps, mental changes). Tracheal spasms may produce dyspnea and cyanosis.

3. Treatment is administration of calcium and of vitamin D, which increases the absorption of calcium.

V. Pancreas

A. Diabetes mellitus

1. A metabolic disease resulting from an inability of the body to use and store glucose in a normal manner; primarily, this is due to insufficient production of insulin in the body.

2. Cause is not known. Heredity does play a part in the development of the disease. Or, may be autoimmune response or viral.

B. Types of diabetes

1. **Type I** or **insulin-dependent diabetes mellitus** (IDDM)

    a. Type I diabetes occurs when the body's immune system destroys the beta cells and as a result no insulin is secreted. Type I diabetes occurs early in life; since no insulin is produced, clients will need insulin replacement for life.

b. Table 1 lists types of insulin.

TABLE 1. TYPES OF INSULIN

Classifications	Types of Insulin	Appearance	Onset	Peak of Action	Duration (hours)
Rapid	Novolog Humalog Apidra	Clear	15 min	30-90 min	3 hr
Short Acting	Humulin Novolin	Clear	30 min-1 hr	2 -3 hr	6-8 hr
Intermediate	NPH Humulin N NPH Novolin N	Cloudy	1-2 hr	4-12 hr	24 hr
Intermediate	Humulin L Novolin L Lente	Cloudy	4-6 hr	12-24 hr	36 hr
Long Acting	Lantus	Clear	1 hr	No peak	24 hr

2. **Type II** or **non insulin-dependent diabetes**

a. Type II diabetes comprises the highest percentage of people with diabetes. It is caused by insulin resistance. The body cannot utilize insulin and, over time, the body will lose its ability to produce insulin.

b. Type II diabetes develops later in life but today an increased incidence is seen in children with poor nutritional practices and lack of exercise.

c. The highest incidence of diabetes appears in American Indians, African-Americans, and Hispanic Americans.

3. The third type of diabetes seen is **gestational diabetes,** which develops in pregnancy as a result of stress. After delivery a small percentage of women will go on to develop Type II diabetes.

C. Symptoms:

1. Elevation of blood sugar **(hyperglycemia)** and presence of sugar in the urine (see Table 2)

2. **Polyuria** – increased urinary output

3. **Polydipsia** – increased thirst

4. **Polyphagia** – increased hunger

5. Weight loss in Type I diabetes

6. Fatigue and muscle weakness

7. **Ketosis** – use of protein and fats as a source of energy when cells cannot utilize insulin to move glucose into cells. The end product of this metabolism leads to ketone bodies in blood and urine. Ketones depress the central nervous systems and can lead to a coma. Excess loss of fluids can lead to dehydration and electrolyte imbalance.

TABLE 2. SYMPTOMS OF HYPERGLYCEMIA AND HYPOGLYCEMIA	
HYPERGLYCEMIA	**HYPOGLYCEMIA**
➢ Gradual onset; may be more rapid in active children	➢ Sudden onset, begins abruptly
➢ Skin hot and dry, face may be flushed	➢ Perspiration; skin pale, cold, and clammy
➢ Deep labored breathing	➢ Shallow breath
➢ Nausea	➢ Hunger
➢. Drowsiness and lethargy	➢ Mental confusion, strange behavior
➢ Fruity odor of the breath	➢ Double vision
➢ Loss of consciousness	➢ Loss of consciousness, convulsions
➢ Urine containing sugar and ketones	➢ No sugar in the urine
➢ Blood sugar high (above 200 mg/dL)	➢ Blood sugar below 60 mg/dL

D. Diagnosis

1. Serum glucose level above 350, presenting clinical symptoms; special diagnostic tests, and examination.

    a. Urinalysis – testing the urine for sugar; when the level of sugar in the blood is high, some will spill over into the urine.

    b. Blood sugar – normal range of blood sugar is 80 to 120 mg per 100 mL of blood; an increase indicates improper utilization of sugar in the blood.

    c. Glucose tolerance determines the individual's ability to utilize glucose in the blood.

E. Treatment and nursing care

1. Aimed at control of the diabetes and prevention of complications; there is no cure for diabetes.

2. Diet is calculated on an individual basis, depending on amount of exercise, ability to utilize carbohydrates, and metabolic needs for building body tissue and producing energy. Diet usually is low in carbohydrate, high in protein, and contains a moderate amount of fat.

    a. Client is given a special diet with lists of foods to substitute for those restricted on this diet.

    b. Physical exercise is important to increase and improve circulation.

F. Complications of insulin administration

1. Diabetic coma and insulin reaction

    a. People with diabetes are susceptible to disturbances arising from poor blood circulation; they have a tendency to develop arteriosclerosis. Proper care and assessment of the feet is very important.

    b. Diabetics also have poor resistance to infections; meticulous skin care and prompt attention to breaks in skin are imperative.

c. Changes in vision may result from retinitis and cataracts, which are common in diabetics. Regular visits to an ophthalmologist are necessary to prevent visual defects or blindness.

d. Oral cavity – increased incidence of dental caries, periodontal disease, and candidiasis. Regular dental visits oral assessment, and care are needed.

2. Signs and symptoms:

a. Cardiopulmonary- rapid heart rate, hypotension

b. Urinary – increased incidence of urinary tract infections. Client must be monitored for signs and symptoms of renal failure. Edema of face and hands and decreased urinary output must be reported.

c. Gastrointestinal – Increased incidence of gastroparesis (slow and faulty absorption). Watch for vomiting.

d. Reproductive – menstrual irregularities; increased incidence of vaginal infections or possible impotence

3. Treatment

a. Type I diabetes client will need insulin replacement and diet modification

b. Type II diabetes client receives oral hypoglycemic drugs (see Table 3).

TABLE 3. ORAL ANTIDIABETICS

Classification	Action	Drugs	Side Effects
Sulfonylurea	Stimulates beta cells to produce insulin	Glucotrol Micronase	Increased weight, decreased blood sugar, allergy, rash
Meglitinide	Causes pancreas to produce insulin faster	Prandin Starlix	Decreases blood sugar
Biguanide	Reduces glucose released from liver	Glucophage	Nausea & vomiting, gas, decreased weight
Thiazolidinediones	Helps body utilize glucose better	Actos Avandia	Liver toxicity, increased weight, abdominal pain
Alpha glucosidase	Controls post-meal hyperglycemia	Precose Glyset	Gas, bloating, diarrhea, abdominal pain

VI. Adrenal Glands

A. Addison's disease

1. A disease caused by decreased function of the adrenal cortex; results in decreased secretion of the adrenal hormones (mineralocorticoids and glucocorticoids) and sex hormones.

2. Causes

a. Primary Addison's – idiopathic due to atrophy of adrenal cortex or tumor, inflammation, infection of the gland, or autoimmune origin

b. Secondary Addison's – results from failure of the pituitary gland to secrete adrenocorticotropic hormone (ACTH), surgical removal of pituitary gland, or sudden withdrawal of corticosteroid therapy

c. Iatrogenic Addison's – from prolonged used of corticosteroid therapy

3. Signs and symptoms

   a. Early symptoms include fatigue, muscle weakness, irritability, and loss of weight.

   b. Nausea and vomiting appear later and client may have severe dehydration, hypotension and circulatory failure, bronzing of skin, and decreased pubic and axillary hair.

4. Diagnosis

   a. Low cortisol levels

   b. Electrolyte imbalance, hyponatremia, hyperkalemia, hypoglycemia, elevated WBC

5. Treatment and nursing care

   a. Replacement of the adrenal hormones lacking in the body; cortisone and other steroids must be taken for the rest of the individual's life; moderation in all activities; provide periods of rest; good personal hygiene is essential; monitor for addisonian crisis.

   b. Diet, intake and output, daily weights

   c. Stress management

6. **Addisonian crisis** – sudden onset of severe general muscle weakness, hypotension, hypovolemia, and shock

   a. Treatment

      i. IV fluids, 5% dextrose and water with NaCl to prevent shock

      ii. IV corticosteroid or vasopressor

      iii. Check for infection as a cause and give antibiotic.

B. **Pheochromocytoma**

1. Rare tumor of the adrenal medulla. It results in secretion of high levels of catecholamines (epinephrine, norepinephrine) in the body. Occurs most commonly between 25-50 years old.

2. Signs and symptoms

   a. Headache, apprehension

   b. Hypertension

   c. Tachycardia, palpitations

   d. Nausea and vomiting, profuse sweating

   e. Hyperglycemia

   f. Cold extremities

3. Diagnostic tests

   a. Increased levels of catecholamines

   b. Hyperglycemia

   c. 24-hour urine for vanillylmandelic acid (VMA)

   d. CT scan, MRI to locate tumor

4. Treatment

    a. Monitor vital signs and drugs to control hypertension.

    b. Promote rest periods and decrease stress.

    c. Diet high in calories with decreased intake of stimulants

    d. Prepare for adrenalectomy

    e. **Adrenalectomy** – surgical removal of one or both adrenal glands

        i. Preoperative – routine preparation

        ii. Postoperative – routine care, plus:

            (a) Monitor fluids and electrolytes (disturbances more marked, disturbances of hormones, glucocorticoids, minerals, and corticoids)

            (b) Fingerstick and urine for glucose

            (c) Help client adjust to lifelong medication replacement.

            (d) Administer hormone replacement as ordered.

            (e) Teach client to recognize signs of hypoglycemia and hypovolemia.

            (f) Complications: shock, hypoglycemia, adrenal crisis

C. **Cushing's syndrome**

1. Disease results from excessive production of hormones from the adrenal cortex; occurs mostly in females between 30-60 years old.

2. Cause – Primary Cushing's – tumors in adrenal glands. Secondary Cushing's – increase in production of ACTH by tumors

3. Signs and symptoms

    a. Sodium and water retention, typical "moon face;" muscle weakness, abnormal sexual development, masculinization in women

    b. Menstrual irregularity, decreased libido

    c. Thinning of hair, "buffalo hump"

    d. Decreased resistance to infection

    e. Hypertension, edema, and osteoporosis

    f. Slow wound healing

4. Diagnosis

    a. Cortisol levels increased

    b. Mild electrolyte imbalance

    c. Hyponatremia

    d. Hypokalemia

    e. Hyperglycemia

5. Treatment and nursing care

    a. Attempts are made to find the underlying cause; client will have disturbances in water and electrolyte balance.

    b. Intake and output must be carefully measured and recorded.

PEARSON

    c.   Weigh daily; low-sodium, high-potassium, low-calcium diet; vitamin D may be ordered.

    d.   Severe mental depression is often present; clients must be prevented from injuring themselves or taking their own life.

    e.   Prevent infection. If disease is caused by tumor, prepare for surgery, adrenalectomy.

VII. Thymus: T lymphocytes located in the thymus glands stimulate phagocytosis.

VIII.Gonads

    A. Male: androgens (testosterone) produced by testes

    B. Female: ovaries produce estrogen and progesterone. (See submodule 3.12, Reproductive System)

Additional Resources Found on MyNursingLab

- Endocrine System animation
- Diabetes animation
- Drug Chart: Drugs Affecting the Endocrine System

MODULE 3

Medical-Surgical Nursing

Submodule 3.9 Respiratory System

Learning Objectives

3.9.1 **Describe common diagnostic tests and nursing care for common respiratory disorders.**

3.9.2 **Describe treatment and nursing care for common respiratory disorders.**

Note: **Prior to beginning this unit the student should review the anatomy and physiology of the respiratory system.**

    I.   **Diagnostic Tests and Examinations**

        A. Chest X-ray: film of the chest; no special preparation necessary

        B. Pulmonary function study: normal values vary with age, sex, height, and weight; test measures air flow volumes in the lungs

            1. **Inspiratory volume:** amount of air inhaled

            2. **Expiratory volume:** amount of air exhaled in one breath

            3. **Total lung capacity:** volume of air in lungs after maximal inhalation

            4. **Vital capacity:** the amount of air exhaled after maximum breath

            5. **Residual volume:** amount of air remaining in the lungs after forced exhalation

            6. **Tidal volume:** volume of air inhaled in an average breath

            7. Determines presence of lung disease such as COPD: can also be used to determine effectiveness of drug therapy such as bronchodilator. Document any drug used prior to the test. Client breathes through spirometer; nose clip is placed on nose; preferably done on an empty stomach.

        C. **Arterial blood gases:** assessment of tissue oxygenation and acid-base status. Prior to test, document O_2 being given. Assist doctor; apply pressure to puncture site for 5 minutes. Test measures:

            1. Partial pressure of oxygen (PaO_2); normal is 80-100 mm Hg

            2. Partial pressure of carbon dioxide ($PaCO_2$); normal is 35-45 mm Hg

            3. Hydrogen ion concentration (pH); normal is 7.35 to 7.45

        D. **Oxygen saturation** (pulse oximeter): noninvasive sensor placed on finger or ear.

            1. Measures percentage of hemoglobin saturated with oxygen. Can be measured at rest or exercise. Can be used to determine need for O_2.

            2. Normal values 95-100%. Below 95%, notify MD.

E. **Lung scan:** radioisotopes inhaled or by IV route, then scanned to diagnose vascular disease or pulmonary embolism, distribution of blood flow in lungs. Preprocedure, calm clients so they can sit still; postprocedure, watch insertion site for bleeding.

   1. Need consent, jewelry removed, check for allergy to iodine or technetium dyes.

   2. Instruct client of the need to hold breath for short periods during the scan.

F. **Pulmonary angiography:** used to outline pulmonary vasculature and diagnose embolus.

   1. Catheter introduced in right side of heart. Radiopaque dye injected, films taken.

   2. Consent needed; check allergy to dye.

   3. Instruct clients they will feel warm as dye is injected.

G. **Bronchoscopy:** a scope introduced through the trachea to the bronchus

   1. Provides visualization of lung tissue; can be used to diagnose tumors, remove foreign objects, do bronchial washing, and biopsy.

   2. Before the test:

      a. Consent is needed.

      b. Instruct client that the throat will be anesthetized prior to the procedure.

      c. Procedure will be done using light to moderate sedation for test. Food and fluids are withheld for 6-8 hours prior to test.

      d. Dentures removed

   3. After the test:

      a. Food and fluids are withheld until gag reflex returns, approximately 2 hours.

      b. Position side lying and maintain patent airway.

      c. Observe for edema, bleeding, difficulty swallowing or breathing; these must be reported promptly.

II. **Other Procedures**

A. **Thoracentesis** – removal of fluid from the pleural cavity

   1. Done to diagnose cancer or tuberculosis or to relieve breathing problems in clients with pleural effusion

   2. Consent needed

   3. Assist client in position sitting up, leaning over a padded bed table with arms crossed.

   4. Baseline vital signs prior to procedure; monitor respiration, color, and response during procedure.

   5. Post procedure: monitor vital signs, breath sounds. Report any abnormal changes and leakage of fluid from client.

   6. Document procedure, color, and amount of fluid removed; send specimens to the lab.

B. Gastric washing

   1. Done early a.m. on an empty stomach to find evidence of mycobacteria.

C. Skin test

   1. **Mantoux test** for exposure to tuberculosis to test for antibodies against mycobacteria.

      a. 0.1 mL of tuberculin serum is injected intradermally on the anterior aspect of lower inner arm.

        b. The site is read in 48-72 hours for induration. The degree of induration, using CDC criteria, determines exposure.

        c. A positive Mantoux test is followed by chest X-ray and sputum culture to confirm presence of mycobacteria.

D. Chest tube

   1. Purpose is to re-expand lung tissue and remove air, blood, and fluid; chest bottle or Pleur-Evac drainage system.

   2. After insertion, drains by gravity or suction up to 20 mL as ordered

        a. Keep below level of chest.

        b. Observe fluctuation.

        c. Keep clamps available at bedside.

        d. Position client in high Fowler's; ambulate client.

        e. Deep breathing and cough exercises

        f. Check dressing; check drainage color and amount.

        g. Check for subcutaneous emphysema and tension pneumothorax.

        h. Milk and strip tubing only if ordered by MD since it can cause negative pressure in the pleural space, which sucks up living tissue and causes damage.

        i. Check all connection for tightness or kinks.

        j. Keep vascular gauge at bedside if tube falls out.

III. Common Symptoms of Respiratory Diseases

A. Coughing: may or may not be beneficial depending on type of cough and condition of client. It is a reflex triggered by foreign substance in the airway.

B. Types of cough:

   1. **Nonproductive:** dry and harsh, no production of sputum, exhausting for client and of no benefit in removing secretions in bronchial tree

        a. Sedative cough mixtures (e.g., those containing codeine) depress the cough reflex and lessen the desire to cough.

   2. **Productive:** deep and moist, produces varying amounts of sputum; may be beneficial

        a. Care must be used in handling these clients because they can be highly contagious.

        b. Client is instructed to cough into a disposable tissue and discard the soiled tissue in a paper bag at the bedside; tissue is held so it covers both nose and mouth during episodes of coughing or sneezing.

        c. Copious amounts of sputum should be expectorated into a waxed sputum cup.

        d. If sputum is foul-smelling, client will need frequent mouth care, especially before meals.

        e. Cough mixtures: expectorant cough mixtures increase flow of secretions, making them easier to cough up (e.g. SSKI, Robitussin).

      f.   Teach to cough effectively in a sitting position.

          i.   Bend head and shoulders forward.

          ii.   Take deep breath and exhale slowly while coughing; repeat 3 times.

C. Respiratory distress

1. Fowler's or semi-Fowler's position facilitates breathing.

2. Air client breathes is kept moist to prevent further irritation of the mucous membranes.

3. Warm moist heat provided by vaporizer

4. Rest provided; avoid exertion, which will place an added burden on the respiratory system.

5. Warm or cool moist air for client to breathe

6. Antibiotics for bacterial type of infection

7. Postural drainage may help in removal of secretions in bronchial tree.

8. Treatment:

    a.   Enforce bed rest; increase fluids; maintain nutrition.

    b.   Humidify air to maintain moist secretions and aid expulsion.

    c.   Administer antibiotics based on infectious organism.

    d.   Provide bronchodilator or expectorants as indicated.

IV. Respiratory Disorders

A. Histoplasmosis

1. Lung infection caused by fungus; transmitted by inhalation of spores which are commonly located in contaminated soil, dust.

2. Signs and symptoms: elevated temperature and WBC, splenomegaly, dyspnea, chest pain, lung infiltrates on X-ray, and presence of organism in culture.

3. Treatment: systemic antifungal agents

B. Tuberculosis

1. An infection in the lungs caused by the tubercle bacillus *(Mycobacteria);* leads to inflammation and formation of nodules.

2. *Mycobacteria* are a slow-growing, acid-fast bacillus. Transmission: airborne droplets or dormant nodules activated when the body is under stress.

3. Once in the body, the bacteria mostly live in the lungs *(pulmonary)* or can travel in body fluid to other organs such as bones, joints, gastrointestinal or genitourinary tract *(extrapulmonary)*.

4. Tuberculosis is often discussed as either an infection or a disease.

    a.   *Tuberculosis infection* is the presence of the bacteria without clinical symptoms but with antibodies in the bloodstream on testing. Infection does not always progress to active disease.

    b.   *Tuberculosis disease* is the result of destruction of body tissues by the bacteria; in this instance, the client is symptomatic.

5. Tuberculosis is prevalent in areas with poor living conditions and poverty that leads to malnutrition.

6. An increasing number of people with AIDS are also infected with the tubercle bacillus.

7. Prevention: teach basic hygiene and good nutrition in areas with high incidence; prevention by use of *Bacillus Calmette Guerin* (BCG) vaccine

8. Diagnosis by positive Mantoux test (induration 5 to 15 mm in 48-72 hours); positive chest X-ray; and positive sputum for acid-fast bacillus

9. Confirmation of tuberculosis is ability to grow the *Mycobacteria* in the laboratory, which takes 4 to 8 weeks.

10. Sign and symptoms: in early stage, asymptomatic; later, productive cough with night sweats and chills; elevated temperature in the afternoon; later, hemoptysis and progressive weight loss

11. Treatment: isolation as indicated to decrease spread; instruct client to cover mouth and nose to sneeze, laugh, or cough; dispose of tissues in a bag.

    a. Isolation for tuberculosis in a room with negative air pressure (air flow in but out through a filter).

    b. The nurse uses a particulate respirator mask when providing care or in close contact; mask worn by client when out of room

    c. Client has increased nutritional needs.

    d. Medication as ordered in 2-3 combinations: isoniazid (INH), ethambutol, rifampin, etc; explain need for long-term use of medication; prevent peripheral neuropathy with INH.

C. **Acute rhinitis** (common cold)

    1. Inflammation of the nasal mucosa

    2. Cause: strain of cold virus

    3. Spread: coughing, sneezing, and talking

    4. Disease spreads 48 hours prior to first symptom

    5. Duration: normally 5 days to 2 weeks

    6. Signs and symptoms: fever, malaise, sneezing, coughing, nasal congestion, sore throat, or headache

    7. Treatment: rest and increased fluids

        a. Teach basic hygiene practices (coughing into tissues and bagging)

        b. Report fever of more than 2 days, bloody sputum in clients with chronic lung disease to prevent pneumonia

        c. Give drugs for symptomatic relief such as acetaminophen (Tylenol), ibuprofen (Motrin), vitamin C, antibiotic if secondary bacterial infection.

D. **Influenza** (flu)

    1. Causes: strains of influenza virus; most epidemics are caused by types A-B.

    2. Signs and symptoms: fever up to 39°C lasting 2-3 days, chills, headache, photophobia, muscle pain, cough lasting several days, sneezing, sore throat, nausea, and vomiting

    3. Complications: pneumonia, heart disease, encephalitis, and sinusitis

    4. Treatment: increased fluids, bed rest; keep room warm, avoid exposing others to infection

PEARSON

5. Prevention: yearly immunization and avoidance of crowds for older clients and those with chronic diseases or immunosuppression; immunization for healthcare workers.

E. **Sinusitis** – inflammation of the maxillary or frontal sinus

1. Condition can be acute or chronic

2. Cause: viral or bacterial infection or complication of upper respiratory tract infection or presence of nasal polyps

3. Signs and symptoms: constant severe headaches, pain and tenderness of the sinuses, purulent discharge, decreased appetite, nausea, and malaise

4. Treatment: antibiotics, nasal decongestants, warm steam

F. **Asthma** – Chronic obstructive airway disorder characterized by inflammation of the airways

1. Cause of asthma is not known; occurs in children and adults

2. Factors that contribute to the occurrence of asthma are:

   a. Infectious agents such as viruses

   b. Environmental irritants and allergens

   c. Emotional stress

3. Signs and symptoms

   a. Inflammation of airway, accumulation of mucus and edema resulting in bronchospasm, constriction, and limited air flow

   b. Onset is sudden with coughing, wheezing, tightness in the chest, dyspnea; attacks can be frequent or occasional.

   c. **Status asthmaticus** is an attack that persists for more than 24 hours; it is a medical emergency and can lead to death.

4. Diagnostic tests

   a. History and clinical symptoms

   b. Pulmonary function test, arterial blood gases, and chest X-ray

5. Treatment

   a. Relieve the obstruction, secretions, and irritation of airway.

   b. Prevent infection; control contact with allergens.

   c. Administer bronchodilator and anti-inflammatory drugs.

G. Chronic Obstructive Lung Disease (COLD)

1. **Chronic Obstructive Lung Disease (COLD)** – any condition in which the client has constant respiratory distress due to chronic pulmonary disease; also called COPD (chronic obstructive pulmonary disease); chronic bronchitis and pulmonary emphysema are nearly always characterized by the symptoms of COPD.

2. **Pulmonary emphysema:** destruction of the alveolar walls, which results in permanent enlargement of the alveoli and lack of elasticity.

   a. Enlargement of the alveoli results in the trapping of air and an inability to exhale fully.

   b. Overdistention of alveoli causes the heart to work harder to get oxygen to other body tissues and can eventually lead to right-sided heart failure.

3. Chronic bronchitis: results from repeated attack of acute bronchitis.

   a. Excessive mucus secretion and damage to the bronchial tree leads to decreased air flow and a productive cough, often described as a smoker's cough.

   b. Cough is more severe on rising and progresses to coughing up pus and blood-streaked sputum.

4. **Bronchiectasis** – condition in which bronchial walls become permanently distended.

   a. The changes began in early childhood and progress slowly.

   b. It is caused by infections such as influenza, sinusitis, pneumonia, tuberculosis, or cystic fibrosis.

5. Signs and symptoms

   a. Dyspnea, orthopnea, tachypnea, cough, and sputum production; rales, expiratory wheezes, bronchitis, barrel chest, cyanosis, clubbing of fingers. ABG shows hypoxemia; accessory muscles are used to breathe; anorexia, weight loss.

6. Treatment

   a. High Fowler's position, O_2 1-2 LPM as ordered; watch CO_2 narcosis; assist with respiratory therapy; instruct client in slow, diaphragmatic, pursed-lip breathing; provide restful environment; monitor intake and output; avoid overexertion; diet – high protein, high calorie, small and frequent meals

   b. Administer drugs as prescribed; bronchodilators, theophylline; albuterol (Proventil), ipratropium (Atrovent), etc; corticosteroids, mast cell stabilizers, antileukotrienes, antibiotics, nebulizers with mucolytics.

7. Complications

   a. **Cor pulmonale,** which is enlargement of the right side of heart from pulmonary hypertension and persistent hypoxia

   b. Acute respiratory failure; pneumonia if infection occurs; rarely, spontaneous pneumothorax

H. **Pleurisy** – inflammation of the pleural membranes surrounding the lungs

   1. Pleurisy with effusion means an increase in the amount of serous fluid within the pleural cavity.

   2. Causes: congestive heart failure (CHF), tuberculosis (TB), cancer, or trauma

   3. Signs and symptoms: sharp, stabbing pain in the chest, worse on inspiration, present when coughing and sneezing; fever and chills

   4. Diagnostic tests

      a. Chest X-ray showing presence of fluid in the pleura

      b. Thoracentesis to identify whether it is caused by infection and to check for presence of blood or pus

5. Treatment

    a. Bed rest and observation of respiratory infection

    b. Support chest wall

    c. Thoracentesis to remove fluid or chest tube

    d. Antibiotics as ordered

    e. Analgesic to relieve pain

I. **Pneumonia** – inflammation of the lung tissue with consolidation of lung tissue

1. General types

    a. Bacterial – most can be reduced by using pneumococcal vaccine given every 3 to 5 years after primary immunization to those at risk (older people and those with chronic lung disease).

    b. Viral pneumonia – caused by influenza virus

    c. *Pneumocystis jiroveci* (formerly *carinii*) pneumonia – caused by a protozoon; seen mostly in clients who are HIV positive with AIDS

    d. Aspiration pneumonia – seen when vomitus, fluid, or chemical irritant is aspirated into lungs.

2. Signs and symptoms

    a. Bacterial pneumonia has sudden onset with chills and fever.

    b. Viral pneumonia is more gradual.

    c. Sharp, stabbing pain in chest or side especially when coughing or taking deep breath

    d. Sputum characteristically rusty color

    e. Fever blisters (herpes simplex) often occur with pneumonia.

3. Treatment and nursing care

    a. Conservation of client's strength, absolute bed rest; treatment and nursing care scheduled so as not to disturb the client any more than necessary

    b. Relief of symptoms – force fluids to combat dehydration; provide mouth care; protect client from chilling and drafts

    c. Respiratory isolation of the client as indicated

    d. Observation of vital signs and respiratory effort is important.

    e. Encourage deep breathing and coughing; administer oxygen as ordered.

    f. Encourage oral fluids; measure intake and output.

    g. Diet: frequent, small meals

    h. Medications as ordered – antibiotics, bronchodilator

    i. Complications to prevent during the convalescent period include emphysema and congestive heart failure.

J. Acute bronchitis

1. Inflammation of the bronchial tree

2. Causes: mostly viral but can be from pollutant chemicals, fumes, dust, and smoke

3. Signs and symptoms

   a. Early: dry hacking cough

   b. Later: productive mucus, pus, dyspnea, wheezing, fatigue, anorexia, and weight loss

   c. Chest pain, fever, and chills

4. Diagnostic test – change in ABG values

K. Cancer of the larynx

1. Occurs as a result of excessive use of tobacco and cigarettes, chronic alcoholism, straining of voice, and family history

2. Most common type of cancer is squamous cell carcinoma.

3. Incidence is higher in men than women, and in people about age 55-70.

4. Signs and symptoms

   a. Pain radiating from the larynx to the ears

   b. Palpable lump at neck; lump in the throat leading to difficulty swallowing

   c. Discoloration of the tongue

   d. Persistent hoarseness of more than 2 weeks is one of the earliest signs.

   e. Difficulty breathing and hemoptysis

5. Diagnostic tests

   a. Presenting clinical symptoms, CT scan, MRI, laryngoscopy, and biopsy

6. Treatment

   a. Determined based on the tumor growth

   b. Usually radiation or surgery

      i. **Laryngectomy** - total or partial removal of the larynx with the formation of a permanent tracheostomy – usually due to cancer extending to one of the cords and into larynx

   c. Preoperative routine plus:

      i. Establish method of communication.

      ii. Prepare for change in body image.

      iii. Nutritional assessment

   d. Postoperative routine plus:

      i. Oxygen via humidifier, trach mask

      ii. Tracheal suctioning under strict asepsis

      iii. Watch color and consistency of sputum.

      iv. Provide speech therapy; 4-6 weeks to restore voice.

      v. Provide stoma care and watch for signs of infection.

      vi. NG tube feeding until oral feeding is allowed; resume normal eating in a few weeks.

      vii. Elevate head of bed to increase pressure on spine.

        viii. Teach that client might lose sense of smell (might need smoke alarm).

        ix. Face numb for 6 months

        x. Assess ability to swallow.

        xi. Watch for edema of the area or bleeding behind the neck.

        xii. Referral to support group for psychological support as a result of disfiguration

L. Lung cancer

1. Primary or metastatic lesion in the lung

2. Types:

    a. Squamous cell

    b. Adenocarcinoma

    c. Oat cell carcinoma

3. Precipitating factors: cigarette smoke; asbestos exposure

4. Signs and symptoms – early stages: rust-colored sputum; cough; dyspnea; hemoptysis; weakness; fever; chills; might be asymptomatic

5. Diagnostic tests: chest X-ray, bronchoscopy, sputum for cytology; CT scan; MRI, and PET scan

6. Treatment

    a. Vital signs, cough and promote sputum production to maintain client's airway

    b. Comfort and safe environment

    c. Medical management or surgical removal followed by chemotherapy or radiation

    d. **Lobectomy** – Surgical removal of one lobe of lung

    e. **Pneumonectomy:** surgical removal of lung

7. Preoperative teaching: chest exercise, chest tube placement

8. Postoperative care

    a. Assess cardiac respiratory status.

    b. Assist O_2 and respiration:

        i. Position client on back or side of surgery (for pneumonectomy)

        ii. Position on back or opposite side of surgery (for lobectomy).

    c. Instruct in active and passive ROM.

M. **Pneumothorax** – collapse of lung resulting from loss of negative intrapleural pressure in the pleural cavity

1. Types and terms

    a. Spontaneous, open: caused by an underlying lung disease

    b. Traumatic: resulting from a blunt or penetrating chest wound; chest surgery, CVP insertion, stab, or gunshot wound

    c. Open: air can enter and escape via an opening in the pleural space

    d. Closed: air collects in the space cannot escape

    e. Tension: when pneumothorax is closed and air builds up in the pleural space, it can cause a mediastinal shift.

2. Signs and symptoms

    a. Sharp pain that increases with exertion

    b. Diminished or absent breath sounds; shallow breathing and tachypnea; dyspnea

    c. Drop in blood pressure and tachycardia

    d. Loss of chest movement on the affected side

    e. Gradual change in LOC

3. Diagnostic tests

    a. Clinical findings and client history

    b. Chest X-ray and ABG.

4. Treatment: chest tube insertion

N. **Pulmonary embolism** – obstruction of the pulmonary blood vessel by fat, air, thrombus.

1. Most emboli originate in a deep vein of the lower extremities.

2. Complication: break off and travel to the right side of the heart and obstruct blood flow

3. Signs and symptoms

    a. Dyspnea; tachypnea, hypoxia; tachycardia, cough

    b. Sudden sharp pain that is worse on inspiration

    c. Increased temperature; increased WBC

    d. Hypotension, diaphoresis

4. Diagnostic tests

    a. X-ray, ABG, lung scan, MRI, CAT scan

    b. Pulmonary arteriogram

5. Risk factors: thrombophlebitis, postpartum, postoperative, prolonged use of contraceptive pills, congestive heart failure, and fracture

6. Treatment

    a. Check peripheral pulses and elevate extremities; apply TEDS or sequential compression device.

    b. Promote deep breathing and coughing to promote lung expansion.

    c. Oxygen as ordered

    d. Bed rest initially

    e. Tissue plasminogen activator to dissolve clot

    f. Anticoagulant therapy

Additional Resources Found on MyNursingLab

- Respiratory System animation
- Asthma animation
- ARDS animation
- Drug Chart: Affecting the Respiratory System

MODULE 3

Medical-Surgical Nursing

Submodule 3.10 Diseases of the Circulatory System

Learning Objectives

3.10.1 Describe diagnostic tests for common cardiovascular disorders.

3.10.2 Describe diagnostic tests, treatment, and nursing care for common hematologic and lymphatic disorders.

3.10.3 Describe treatment and nursing care for common cardiovascular disorders.

Note: **Prior to beginning this unit, the student should review the anatomy and physiology of the circulatory system.**

I. Diagnostic Tests

 A. Complete blood count – determination of the number of red blood cells and white blood cells per cubic millimeter.

 B. Hemoglobin test – determination of the amount of hemoglobin present in the red blood cells; normal is 14-18 g/dL in men, 12-16 g/dL in women.

 C. Microscopic examination of the blood to determine the size of erythrocytes and types and number of leukocytes.

 D. Sternal puncture – removal of cells from the bone marrow of the sternum or iliac crest to examine to determine abnormal development.

  1. Used to diagnose anemia, leukemia, and thrombocytopenia.

  2. Preparation: Verify informed consent; instruct client a needle will be inserted into the bone to aspirate marrow. Client will experience pressure and will be required to lie still.

  3. Post procedure: Observe area for swelling, bleeding, or signs of infection.

 E. Blood typing – Determination of the blood group to which the individual belongs

 F. MRI – Three-dimensional imaging of the heart

 G. ECG – Electrical activity of the heart from different views to show rate and rhythm and presence of injury

 H. Holter monitor – Records ECG for 24 to 48 hours to match symptoms with ECG changes

  1. Client wears a small ECG recorder while doing normal daily activities.

  2. The client may be asked to keep a diary of daily activities and not to get the electrodes wet.

PEARSON

I. Stress test – Measures effect of exercise on heart and circulation

    1. Instruct client for preparation: no heavy meal or caffeine for 2-3 hours prior to the test; wear walking shoes and clothes.

    2. ECG electrodes are placed on the chest.

    3. The client walks or bicycles or uses the treadmill.

    4. The test can be done using radio nuclide imaging.

    5. The client is instructed to report chest pain or extreme fatigue or dyspnea.

J. Echocardiogram – Transducer transmits sound waves that bounce off the heart to produce graphic images of blood flow.

K. Thallium imaging – Injection of thallium to evaluate cardiac blood flow; can be combined with stress test.

L. Cardiac catheterization – A means of measuring fluid pressure in the chambers of the heart and of analyzing the O_2 and CO_2 content; catheter inserted through a vein into the heart.

    1. Need informed consent. Food and fluid withheld. Allergies to iodine determined.

    2. After removal of catheter, pressure dressing is placed; check for bleeding. No heavy lifting for 3 days.

M. Doppler ultrasound: a noninvasive test used to detect a clot in a blood vessel and the degree of obstruction.

N. Angiogram – detects obstruction in the blood flow caused by aneurysm or embolus in the brain, heart, or lungs.

    1. Preparation: Informed consent, NPO, groin prep, check allergy to dye.

    2. Instruct client that the catheter is threaded into an artery and the dye is injected; then x-ray films are taken.

    3. Post test: Bed rest until awake, no bending leg, flexing, or hyperextension for 8 hours.

    4. Pressure will be applied to groin of femoral artery used. Watch for bleeding.

    5. Monitor vital signs and peripheral circulation.

O. Technetium pyrophosphate scan and multiple-gated acquisition scan (MUGA):

    1. Used to determine area and extent of myocardial infarction.

    2. The dye is injected and several scans are taken within 1 ½ to 2 hours.

P. Hemodynamic monitoring (Swan-Ganz) is a catheter inserted in the pulmonary artery to determine pressure and oxygen flow in the cardiovascular system.

Q. Cardiac enzyme test – blood test to determine the type and extent of injury to heart muscle.

    1. CK-MB is a fraction of the enzyme that is specific to heart muscle damage.

    2. LDH1/LDH2 may indicate damage to heart muscle.

    3. Troponin T – Quicker and more accurate test for muscle protein

II. Disorders of the Blood

A. **Iron deficiency anemia** – an abnormal reduction in the number of circulating red blood cells in the bloodstream; result is a lack of hemoglobin to carry oxygen to tissues.

1. Types of anemia (three main groups)

    a. Resulting from acute or chronic blood loss

    b. Resulting from decreased production of red blood cells

    c. Associated with excessive destruction of red blood cells

2. Diagnostic tests

    a. Serum iron – markedly decreased

    b. Total iron binding capacity (TIBC) – below normal

    c. Hemoglobin and hematocrit – markedly decreased

    d. Serum ferritin level – decreased

3. Signs and symptoms

    a. Skin pale, chronic fatigue, headache, dizziness, shortness of breath on slightest exertion

    b. Tachycardia, palpitations, insomnia

    c. Anorexia, dyspepsia, and dysphagia

    d. Brittle hair and nails, sensitivity to cold

4. General treatment and nursing care

    a. Rest – absolute bed rest may be necessary in acute anemia. Client should take periods of rest during the day if B/P is low to prevent exertion. Best position is lying flat in bed without a pillow in order to increase flow of blood to the brain.

    b. Warmth – clients with anemia suffer from lack of warmth due to inadequate circulation. Extra warmth in the form of warm clothing and additional blankets is preferred.

    c. Diet –encourage foods rich in iron, protein, and vitamins B and C because these are used in the production of red blood cells. Adequate roughage is needed.

        i.   Client may need education in food values and the importance of eating a well-balanced diet.

        ii. Poor appetite is quite common in anemic patients; sore mouth and gums often contribute to anorexia; highly spiced foods and extremely hot or cold foods should be avoided in these cases.

    d. Special mouth care – often necessary because of sore gums that bleed easily. Toothbrushing may have to be discontinued and the mouth cleansed with a tooth swab dipped in normal saline.

    e. Blood transfusions

        i.   Used in both acute and chronic anemia; given to replace or maintain adequate blood elements

        ii. Nursing care – client must be carefully observed for signs of reaction or sensitivity to the transfused blood. Signs include rash, itching, chills, and fever; in more serious cases, client may have dyspnea, and restlessness may result.

    f. Medications – oral or parenteral iron

B. **Pernicious anemia** –anemia that occurs because of lack of the intrinsic factor

    1. Erythrocyte growth and maturity are decreased; RBCs become large and fragile and rupture easily.

    2. Signs and symptoms

        a. Weakness, pallor, fatigue, fever

        b. Dyspnea, hypoxia

        c. Weight loss, constipation or diarrhea, jaundice

        d. Burning of tongue, sore mouth, dyspnea, flatulence, and nausea

        e. Tingling in hands and feet and mental depression

    3. Diagnosis

        a. Schilling test positive, showing decreased absorption of vitamin B_{12}

        b. Bone marrow aspiration revealing abnormally developed red blood cells

        c. Gastric analysis to determine if there is a decrease in free hydrochloric acid and cause of vitamin B_{12} deficiency

    4. Treatment

        a. Encourage diet high in protein, vitamins and iron; avoid very hot foods.

        b. Special mouth care with soft toothbrush

        c. Provide warmth; extra blanket may be needed.

        d. Provide periods of rest; do not overtire the client.

        e. Administer ordered vitamin B_{12}; vitamin will be needed to make intrinsic factor for the rest of life.

        f. Administer packed cells as ordered.

C. **Aplastic anemia** – anemia with bone marrow depression affecting granulocyte, platelets, and erythrocyte production

    1. Cause: probably autoimmune or toxic substances such as benzene and insecticides; or drugs like antineoplastic drugs, gold compounds, sulfonamides, chloramphenicol, and radiation

    2. Signs and symptoms

        a. Fatigue, pallor, dyspnea, fever

        b. Abnormal bleeding (bleeding gums, epistaxis, ecchymosis, gastrointestinal and genitourinary)

        c. Depression of bone marrow and WBC leads to increased susceptibility to infection.

    3. Diagnosis – bone marrow aspiration

    4. Treatment

        a. Provide care to minimize risk of infection

        b. Monitor for bleeding.

        c. Prepare for bone marrow transplantation.

d. Administer blood transfusions as ordered.

e. Administer immunosuppressive therapy.

D. **Hemolytic anemia** – anemia in which there is an increase in the destruction of red blood cells

1. Some clients have a genetic predisposition to disease, or it can be acquired after incompatible blood transfusion and end-stage renal failure.

2. Diagnosis: CBC and appearance of red blood cell on smear

3. Signs and symptoms – signs of anemia plus abdominal discomfort, nausea, vomiting, diarrhea

   a. Abnormal bleeding in stool or urine; enlarged spleen and/or jaundice

4. Treatment

   a. Rebuild blood with transfusions and iron.

   b. Support respiratory effort.

   c. Provide skin care.

E. **Leukemia** – a malignant disease of the blood cells; white blood cells increase in number and fail to function normally.

1. Cause: not fully known but could be genetic, viral, or related to exposure to chemicals such as drugs and radiation.

2. Types

   a. Usually classified by cells affected (for example, lymphoid or myeloid)

   b. Can also be classified as acute or chronic

3. Acute leukemia has an increased number of immature cells in the bone marrow. Acute leukemia is divided into two types:

   a. Acute lymphocytic leukemia (ALL) – mostly seen in children

   b. Acute myeloid leukemia (AML) – seen more in adults

   c. Characteristics

   i. A rapid onset with high fever, extreme pallor, tendency toward hemorrhage, swelling of the lymph nodes, fatigue, malaise, bone pain, recurrent infection.

   ii. Increased WBC, decreased platelets, decreased hematocrit and hemoglobin (HCT and HB), decreased appetite, mouth ulcers

4. Chronic leukemia – mature cells decrease in number; abnormal cells increase in number. Chronic leukemia is divided into two types:

   a. Chronic lymphoid leukemia (CLL) – usually discovered with routine check-up

   b. Chronic myeloid leukemia (CML) –white blood cells are mature but malignant; the progression of disease is slower

   c. Characteristics – has more gradual onset with increase in white cell count, anemia, fatigue, night sweats, and swelling of the lymph nodes, spleen, and liver. Sometimes there is a tendency toward hemorrhage. It usually occurs in persons over 45 years of age. Decreased weight, SOB, and tenderness over the sternum.

   d. Diagnostic tests: WBC, bone marrow biopsy showing immature leukocytes, chest x-ray revealing mediastinal nodes, and biopsy of lymph nodes

    e. Treatment

        i.   Objective is to increase survival and reach remission.

        ii. There is no known cure for leukemia in children; the disease ALL is most responsive to treatment in adults; the disease progresses slowly.

        iii. Treatment is aimed at the relief of symptoms, prevention of infection, maintenance of a normal level of blood cells, and providing nutritional support.

    f. Nursing care

        i.   Protect the client from infection; nursing care similar to that of clients with severe anemia. Proper positioning important when neck glands are swollen and breathing is difficult.

        ii. Bone marrow suppression can increase risk of spontaneous bleeding. Monitor carefully.

        iii. Provide emotional support.

        iv. Administer ordered treatment (blood transfusion, antineoplastic drugs, radiation) or prepare for bone marrow transplant.

F. **Malignant lymphoma** – group of malignancies originating from stem cells in bone marrow.

    1. Hodgkin: origin unknown; trigger may be viral, genetic, autoimmune, or environmental; incidence greater in young males

        a. Characterized by painless enlargement of lymphoid tissue affecting cervical nodes and spleen

        b. The disease is staged based on number of lymph nodes affected on both sides of the diaphragm, bone marrow, and liver.

    2. Non-Hodgkin: malignancy of lymphocytes that invade other tissues outside the lymphatic system; may be caused by autoimmune process or viral infection; common in males after 60.

    3. Signs and symptoms

        a. Night sweats, fever, weight loss, enlarged lymph nodes, increased WBC, increased ESR.

        b. Anorexia, abdominal discomfort, and anemia

    4. Diagnostic tests

        a. Lymph node biopsy to identify Reed Steinberg cells

        b. Chest x-ray showing mediastinal mass

        c. Bone marrow biopsy

        d. CT scan and ultrasound

    5. Treatment

        a. Based on staging; Hodgkin disease curable if discovered early

        b. Splenectomy, chemotherapy, radiation, and stem cell transplant

G. **Sickle cell disease** – a group of hereditary disorders related to the presence of curved (sickled) red blood cells

    1. In sickle cell disease, the RBCs exposed to O_2 become crescent shaped.

2. In carriers of the sickle cell trait, only about 35% of the total hemoglobin is affected, and most persons with the trait have no symptoms.

3. Sickle cell disease is caused by a recessive inherited genetic pattern predominantly seen in African-Americans.

4. Diagnostic tests

    a. Electrophoresis

    b. Sickledex test

5. Signs and symptoms

    a. Caused by clumping of red cells and obstruction of blood flow leading to poor oxygenation of tissues

    b. Anemia is present as are periodic joint pain; swelling of the hands, feet, and abdomen; and jaundice.

6. Factors that lead to sickle cell crisis:

    a. Stress (physical or emotional)

    b. Dehydration, overexertion, or infection

    c. Exposure to cold

    d. Alcohol intake or smoking

7. Treatment: primarily symptomatic and prevention of crisis

    a. Severe anemia is treated with folic acid and other nutrients essential to the formation of blood elements.

    b. Encourage client to drink plenty of fluids to make blood less viscous, to eat a well-balanced diet, and to avoid upper respiratory infections.

    c. Teach to avoid high altitudes and vigorous exercise.

    d. Provide adequate rest periods and avoid overexertion.

    e. Provide pain relief with analgesics; high doses may be needed.

III. Cardiac Dysrhythmias

A. **Dysrhythmia** is a disturbance or irregularity in the rate or rhythm of the heart.

B. **Normal sinus rhythm (NSR)** is the heart's normal rate and rhythm.

1. Normal sinus rhythm originates from the sinoatrial node (SA node).

2. Impulse passes to the atrioventricular node (AV).

3. The atrium of the heart contracts, represented by a P wave on electrocardiogram (ECG).

4. Impulse passes from the AV node to the bundle of His and the Purkinje fibers in the ventricles, and the ventricles contract (represented as QRS wave on ECG).

5. The heart muscle recovers; this is the T wave on the ECG.

6. In normal sinus rhythm, atrial and ventricular contractions are regular at a rate of 60 – 100 beats per minute (BPM).

C. Dysrhythmias are diagnosed by 12-lead ECG.

1. Tachycardia: atrial and ventricular rate is between 100-180 BPM.

    a. Rhythm can be regular or irregular.

b. Can compromise cardiac output

c. Treatment depends on underlying cause.

2. Bradycardia: Atrial and ventricular rate are regular at less than 60 BPM.

   a. This can be a normal heart rate for some clients such as athletes. Athletes can have a heart rate of 40–60 BPM; this is normal if they are asymptomatic.

   b. Symptomatic bradycardia is treated with O_2 administration PRN.

   c. Drugs such as atropine sulfate increase heart rate.

   d. Transcutaneous or permanent pacemaker may be inserted.

3. Atrial fibrillation/flutter: contraction and depolarization of heart; rhythm is disorganized.

   a. Quivering of the atrium slows circulation, decreases cardiac output, causes blood to pool, leading to thrombus formation.

   b. Atrial rate is usually rapid and irregular; no visible P waves.

   c. Treatment

      i. Administer O_2 as needed.

      ii. Drugs: anticoagulants to prevent thrombus formation

      iii. Antiarrhythmic drugs to slow down the heart rate

      iv. Cardioversion to change the rhythm

4. Premature ventricular contractions (PVC): early contraction of ventricles; as a result, blood cannot be pumped from the atrium.

   a. This pattern repeated for 6 or more times per minute can trigger ventricular tachycardia.

   b. Treatment

      i. Immediate notification of MD

      ii. Administration of oxygen as needed

      iii. Correction of electrolyte imbalance

      iv. Antiarrhythmic drugs such as lidocaine to slow the heart

5. Ventricular tachycardia: life-threatening; caused by rapid depolarization of ventricles

   a. Ventricular rate can be 140–200 BPM.

   b. Blood cannot leave the atrium to move into ventricles.

   c. Cardiac output decreases; peripheral pulses may be difficult to find.

   d. Wide QRS complex

   e. Can lead to cardiac arrest

   f. Treatment

      i. Administration of antiarrhythmic drugs: amiodarone, lidocaine, procainamide

      ii. Oxygen administration

      iii. May need cardioversion to convert rhythm

6. Ventricular fibrillation: cardiac emergency; quivering of ventricles in a disorganized pattern

    a. No cardiac output

    b. Cardiac arrest imminent if not terminated in 3-5 minutes

    c. Treatment

        i. Begin CPR, defibrillation

        ii. Oxygen administration

        iii. Administer antiarrhythmic drugs, epinephrine, vasopressin.

7. Complete heart block: atrial and ventricular rates are uncoordinated.

    a. Blood is not flowing from atrium to ventricles.

    b. Markedly decreased cardiac output

    c. Rhythm can be so slow heart can stop.

    d. Treatment: pacemaker insertion

D. **Pacemaker** – a device for electrical stimulation of the heart

    1. Atrial synchronous (or demand) pacemaker senses the heart's rhythm and fires only if the rate falls below a preset rate on the pacemaker.

    2. Asynchronous pacemaker fires at a fixed rate regardless of heart rate.

    3. Can be temporary or permanent

    4. Temporary pacemaker is transcutaneous, meaning electrodes are placed on the chest wall connected to an external generator.

    5. Permanent pacemaker: the generator is surgically implanted in the subcutaneous tissue below the clavicle.

    6. Electrodes are introduced via the subclavian vein into the right side of the heart.

    7. Pacemakers are powered by lithium batteries that last 10 years or by nuclear batteries that last 20 years.

    8. Pacemaker function can be checked via telephone or in a doctor's office or a clinic.

E. Implantable cardioverter defibrillation (ICD)

    1. Detects and terminates episodes of ventricular tachycardia and ventricular fibrillation

    2. Delivers 25 to 30 joules 4 times when triggered

    3. Electrodes placed in right atrium and ventricle

    4. Generator implanted in the left pectoral region

F. Client teaching for pacemaker and IDC

    1. Wear loose clothing over the site of generator insertion.

    2. Avoid contact sports; they could dislodge the device.

    3. Keep ID in wallet or wear Medic-Alert stating presence of an implanted device.

    4. Keep a log of episodes when shock was needed from the IDC and activities being performed at that time.

    5. Instruct client and family to report signs of infection such as fever.

6. Client should sit or lie down if episodes of SOB, faintness, extreme dizziness, weakness, or fatigue occur; report episodes to MD.

7. Report edema of extremities or chest pain.

8. Precautions: avoid electromagnetic fields; keep a distance 4 to 5 feet away from them.

9. If MRI is needed, client and family must inform the technician about the presence of an implantable device.

10. Client must be instructed not to operate electrical devices (including cell phones) directly over the implantable devices.

11. These devices can interfere with functioning of pacemakers and an ICD.

12. When traveling, must inform airport security of presence of an implantable device, because it can set off security alarms.

IV. **Diseases Affecting the Heart**

   A. **Angina** – chest pain caused by inadequate oxygen supply to the myocardium

   1. Causes: arteriosclerosis; atherosclerosis; hypertension, activity or disease that increases the heart's demand for oxygen, and spasm in the coronary artery

   2. Risk factors that are nonmodifiable: gender, with males having a higher risk initially and females' risk increasing after menopause

   3. Risk factors that are modifiable: high blood cholesterol levels, hypertension, diabetes, obesity, decreased physical activity, stress, and smoking

   4. Precipitating factors: physical exertion, heavy meal, exposure to cold, smoking, and emotional factors

   5. Signs and symptoms

      a. Substernal crushing; pain radiating to arm, jaw, back, neck, wrist, or shoulders, lasting 3-5 minutes

      b. Precipitating events of exercise, sudden temperature changes, anxiety

   6. Diagnosed by ECG changes, performance on stress test, coronary arteriogram

   7. Treatment

      a. Diet therapy and lifestyle changes; oxygen as needed; rest and decreased activity; reduced stress

      b. Drugs – nitrates, beta-blockers, calcium channel blockers.

      c. Failed control of angina with medication may result in need for:

         i. **Percutaneous transluminal coronary angioplasty (PTCA)** – insertion of a balloon in the artery to open the vessel and increase the diameter

         ii. Coronary artery bypass graft (CABG) surgery

   B. **Myocardial infarction** – necrosis of myocardial tissue due to complete obstruction of blood flow and oxygen supply to an area of the myocardium

   1. Causes: atherosclerosis, coronary artery constriction, or spasms; coronary embolism or thrombosis, shock, or hemorrhage

   2. Complications: cardiogenic shock, ventricular aneurysm, dysrhythmias, congestive heart failure, pericarditis, pulmonary embolism, papillary muscle dysfunction, interventricular septal rupture, ventricular rupture

3. Signs and symptoms

    a. Chest pain; location is similar to angina (substernal) and may radiate to other sites.

    b. Description may be a feeling of tightness, heaviness, squeezing, crushing, severe chest pain, pain not relieved by rest or nitroglycerin.

    c. Duration can be 30 minutes or more.

    d. Precipitating factors may be stress, exercise, rest, exertion; predisposing factors include blood loss, respiratory tract infection, pulmonary emboli, and hypoxemia.

    e. Alleviating factors – it is not relieved with rest or nitrates.

    f. Psychological – client verbalizes feelings of fear, impending doom, weakness, apprehension, denial, or depression.

    g. Respiratory changes such as dyspnea, orthopnea, and presence of rales or rhonchi

    h. Vital signs – changes in heart rate, decrease in blood pressure, narrowing pulse pressure

    i. Nausea and vomiting, absence of high-pitched bowel sounds

    j. Skin changes – may be warm and dry or cool and clammy, diaphoretic, pale

    k. Fever – most clients develop fever up to 101° F over the first 24-48 hours after onset of MI.

4. Diagnostic tests

    a. ECG changes – Q waves, ST segment changes; dysrhythmias

    b. Laboratory tests

       i. Rise in leukocyte count

       ii. Rise in sedimentation rate

       iii. CPK enzyme peaks 12-18 hours after onset with CPK-MB elevated 2-4 hours after onset.

       iv. SGOT peaks 24-36 hours after onset.

       v. LDH elevated 24 hours after onset

       vi. Triponium elevated within 1 hour after injury

5. Treatment

    a. Provide supplemental oxygen for first 24-48 hours; observe for respiratory distress.

    b. Keep client on bed rest for the first 24-48 hours.

    c. Administer sedatives as prescribed, such as diazepam (Valium).

    d. Provide quiet and calm environment by explaining all equipment, tests, and procedures; help client identify effective coping strategies.

    e. Relieve chest pain with prescribed medications such as morphine sulfate or nitrates.

    f. Monitor vital signs every 1-2 hours.

    g. Monitor heart rhythm for dysrhythmias such as premature ventricular contractions, atrial fibrillation, or ventricular tachycardia.

h. Maintain intravenous line of D_5W for quick access of medications.

i. Report changes in vital signs or dysrhythmias to physician.

j. Administer prescribed drugs to decrease the risk of complications (see box below): digitalis, antiarrhythmics, anticoagulants, thrombolytics, vasodilators, vasopressors, diuretics, potassium, and stool softeners.

Complications of MI
Cardiac dysrhythmia Congestive heart failure Pulmonary edema Pericarditis Cardiogenic shock

i. Monitor pulmonary–artery catheter readings for cardiac function.

ii. Monitor intake and output.

iii. Monitor for signs of congestive heart failure.

iv. Assist with and monitor progressive activity level when condition is stable.

v. Educate client regarding lifestyle modifications: diet, activity, stress, and risk factors, etc.

vi. Cardiac rehabilitation

C. **Shock** – insufficient tissue perfusion or cardiac output depriving tissue of oxygen and nutrients

1. Types of shock

a. **Cardiogenic shock** – occurs when heart fails to pump enough blood to perfuse the tissue; caused by:

i. Myocardial infarction (most frequent cause)

ii. Congestive heart failure

iii. Cardiac arrhythmias

iv. Cardiac tamponade

v. Severe valvular disease

vi. Massive left ventricular aneurysm

b. **Hypovolemic shock** – occurs from loss of fluid within the vascular space, which leads to decreased circulation of blood volume to tissue; caused by:

i. Excessive blood loss

ii. Excessive loss of fluids other than blood

iii. Fluid shift from vascular space into another space (third spacing) as seen in burns

c. **Neurogenic shock** – occurs from acute vasodilatation and pooling of blood within the peripheral blood vessels, leading to tissue hypoperfusion

i. Caused by inability of the sympathetic nervous system to maintain vasomotor tone, as in spinal anesthesia and spinal cord injury

2. Signs and symptoms

   a. Restlessness

   b. Confusion

   c. Lethargy, can progress to coma

   d. Rapid, weak, thready pulse

   e. Blood pressure normal initially, then drops

   f. Cold, clammy, pale skin seen in cardiogenic and hypovolemic shock

   g. Low urine output due to decreased renal perfusion

   h. Decline in level of consciousness

   i. Increase in respiratory rate (shallow), dyspnea, cough

   j. Low PaO_2

   k. Decreased or absent bowel sounds

3. Treatment

   a. Monitor oxygenation status (deep breathing exercise, ventilator support).

   b. Administer prescribed fluid replacement with caution in cardiogenic shock, such as blood products and intravenous fluids.

   c. Administer prescribed vasoactive drugs.

   d. Monitor vital signs closely.

   e. Monitor urinary output.

   f. Keep client warm.

   g. Provide emotional support to reduce anxiety.

   h. Provide safe environment for the client with alterations in consciousness, such as keeping side rails up and call bell near, turning client every 2 hours to prevent skin breakdown.

   i. Monitor for signs of infection.

   j. Allow client to rest.

   k. Assist in comfort measures.

D. Congestive heart failure

1. The heart is unable to maintain adequate circulation to meet the metabolic needs of the body because of impaired muscle function, leading to decreased pumping ability.

2. Heart failure is one of the major causes of chronic disease.

3. Causes: myocardial infarction, hypertension, mitral valve disease, inflammation, anemia, diabetes, dysrhythmias, atherosclerosis, arteriosclerosis, and fluid overload. To compensate, the ventricles dilate and hypertrophy, and the heart becomes enlarged.

4. Diagnostic tests

   a. Chest x-ray showing enlargement

   b. ECG to diagnose dysrhythmias

   c. Echocardiogram to determine ejection fraction

      d.   Exercise stress test to determine activity tolerance

      e.   Cardiac catheterization to detect abnormality

      f.   Blood test to check electrolytes

      g.   B-type natriuretic peptide (BNP)

5.   Assessment – history of CAD, fatigue, dyspnea, anxiety, restlessness, exercise intolerance. Heart failure can be categorized based on degree of severity as right-sided or left-sided failure (see Table 1).

      a.   Left-sided failure occurs when the left ventricle is unable to pump adequately; signs and symptoms include dyspnea on exertion; orthopnea, productive cough with frothy sputum; pallor/cyanosis, rales on auscultation; and tachycardia.

      b.   Right-sided failure is caused by failure of the right ventricle to pump; signs and symptoms include pitting, dependent edema, ascites from portal hypertension, distended neck veins, or tenderness in the upper right quadrant.

      c.   When one side of the heart fails, eventually the other will.

Table 1. Right-Sided versus Left-Sided Heart Failure Manifestations

RIGHT-SIDED	LEFT-SIDED
Dependent edema (sacrum, ankles, feet)	Dyspnea
Enlarged liver	Orthopnea
Ascites (collection of fluid in the abdominal cavity)	Wheezing
	Cough
Weight gain	Pink frothy sputum
Distended neck veins	Tachycardia
Nocturia	Restlessness
Nausea	Anxiety
Anorexia	Confusion
Weakness	Pulmonary edema

6.   Treatment and nursing care

      a.   Position in high Fowler's position; elevate extremities; oxygen as ordered; provide quiet environment; conserve energy and prevent fatigue; monitor for electrolyte imbalance; take daily weight; monitor intake and output.

      b.   Administer prescribed drugs such as digitalis, diuretics, stool softeners, ACE inhibitors, and beta blockers.

      c.   To increase heart's ability to pump, client may have insertion of left ventricular access device (LVADs).

      d.   Short-term support of myocardial function with placement of an intra-aortic balloon pump (IABP)

      e.   Heart transplantation as a last resort

E.   Acute pulmonary edema

1.   Extreme case of left-sided heart failure resulting in collection of fluid in the lungs. It is a medical emergency.

2.   Causes: MI, valvular heart disease; congestive heart failure; fluid overload

3.   Signs and symptoms: tachycardia, restlessness, anxiety, jugular vein distention

4.   Diagnosis: symptoms and chest x-ray, ABG, and ECG

5. Treatment

    a. Bed rest, high Fowler's position; supplemental oxygen as needed; reassurance and calm; rotating tourniquet

    b. Drugs: analgesics (i.e., morphine), bronchodilator, diuretic, digitalis as needed

F. **Hypertension** (called the silent killer) – a continued increase in systolic and diastolic blood pressure

  1. Normal blood pressure: 120 systolic or less, 80 diastolic or less

  2. Prehypertension: systolic 120-139, diastolic 80-89

  3. Stage 1 hypertension: systolic 140-159, diastolic 90-99

  4. Hypersensitivity – characterized by elevated peripheral vascular resistance from constriction of arterioles, which may be caused by a sympathetic response and stimulation of the renin-angiotensin-aldosterone feedback system.

  5. There are two types of hypertension – secondary and primary (also called essential); etiology unknown; associated with atherosclerosis and CHF and is responsible for the largest number of cases.

  6. Risk factors that are modifiable: smoking, diet, obesity, occupational stress, increased sodium intake, caffeine, nicotine, and female hormone replacement

  7. Risk factors that are not modifiable: age and family history

  8. Signs and symptoms: mainly asymptomatic; initially numbness or tingling in the extremities; headache, blurred vision, dizziness; chest pain, SOB, fatigue, epistaxis, hematuria, proteinuria, retinal changes, anxiety

  9. Treatment

    a. Calm, quiet atmosphere; reduced anxiety

    b. Diet with restricted sodium, decreased alcohol and cholesterol intake; weight loss, exercise, stress management; avoid smoking

    c. Drugs as indicated: diuretics, beta blockers, calcium channel blockers, sympatholytics, ACE inhibitors, sedatives

G. Inflammatory diseases of the heart

  1. **Endocarditis** – inflammation of the inner lining of the heart, considered autoimmune

  2. **Pericarditis** – inflammation of the outer sac of the heart

  3. **Myocarditis** – inflammation of the muscle of the heart

  4. **Rheumatic heart disease** – an inflammation involving one or more parts of the heart; most often affecting the endocardium and the heart valves; follows acute rheumatic fever and occurs most often in children and young adults

    a. Causative organism: most commonly beta hemolytic streptococcal organism

  5. Signs and symptoms depend on the location of the inflammation in the heart.

    a. Changes in the rate and rhythm of the heartbeat and heart failure may result from myocarditis.

    b. Heart murmurs, fatigue, and hematuria may occur with endocarditis and involvement of the valve; subcutaneous nodules on fingers and toes

       c. Pain over the heart, increase in the heart rate (tachycardia), and dyspnea present in pericarditis.

       d. Mild fever, rash on trunk, joint pain and swelling, tachycardia, and heart murmur in rheumatic heart disease

6. Diagnostic tests

    a. Increased sedimentation rate

    b. Elevated C –reactive protein

    c. Blood cultures to identify organism

    d. Antistreptolysin O titer

    e. Electrocardiography showing valvular changes

7. Treatment and nursing care

    a. Aimed at decreasing the workload of the heart and preventing extensive damage to the heart tissue

    b. Rest and stress reduction are most important.

    c. Antibiotics are given to prevent bacterial infections and repeated attacks of rheumatic fever.

    d. Well-balanced diet is necessary to improve client's general health.

    e. Instruct client in need for prophylactic antibiotic before invasive procedures such as dental work.

    f. Surgical repair of damaged mitral valve (**commissurotomy**) done in some cases.

V. Peripheral Diseases

A. **Thrombophlebitis** – inflammation of the vein with clot formation

    1. Occurs in any vein but mostly those of the lower extremities

    2. Causes

        a. Decreased circulation related to inactivity

        b. Compression or injury to vein

        c. Intravenous administration of drugs causing irritation of vein

        d. Use of oral contraceptives, especially when combined with smoking

    3. Types

        a. **Intermittent claudication** – pain in extremities at rest, diminished or absent pulse; cold, pallor, or cyanosis; ulceration in the extremities; relief on ambulation; skin thin, shiny, and easily injured

        b. **Buerger's disease** – inflammation of blood vessels in the extremities, resulting in obstruction

            i. Incidence higher in men than women

            ii. Characteristic hard, painful areas along the blood vessel tract

            iii. Purple-reddish discoloration of extremities when dangling, and very pale when raised

        iv. In advanced stage, circulation becomes increasingly poor.

        v. Pain at rest; ulceration, infection, gangrene possible

  c. **Raynaud's disease** – spasm in the blood vessels of the extremities often affecting fingers more than toes

        i. Higher incidence in young women

        i. Characteristic acute episodes of cold, pale, sweaty, numb, and painful digits

        iii. When warmed, area becomes red and flushed.

        iv. See comparison of Buerger's and Raynaud's in Table 2.

Table 2. Comparison of Buerger's Disease and Raynaud's Disease

BUERGER'S DISEASE	RAYNAUD'S DISEASE
Cold and numbness in fingers, toes Weather related Intermittent claudication becoming more severe Ulceration, gangrene of extremities	Color change, fingers and toes from white, blue, to red Edema in extremities Numbness

        v. In advanced stages: attacks become more frequent and bluish discolor persists.

        vi. Poor circulation can lead to ulceration or gangrene.

4. Risk factors:

  a. Smoking

  b. Atherosclerosis

  c. Spasm in blood vessels

5. Diagnostic tests: Doppler studies, arteriography, blood lipids

6. Treatment

  a. Diet therapy, isometrics, and ROM exercise; neurovascular monitoring; bed cradle use.

  b. Avoid exposure to cold.

  c. Keep extremities warm.

  d. Instruct client not to wear restrictive clothing around extremities.

  e. Protect the skin from injury.

  f. Instruct client not to smoke.

  g. Drugs: aspirin, analgesics, vasodilators, anticoagulants, thrombolytics, antibiotics

  h. Surgical treatment: sympathectomy

B. **Aortic aneurysm** – ballooning in the wall of the blood vessel due to weakness; most commonly occurs in the aorta and cerebral blood vessel.

1. Aneurysm can rupture spontaneously and is often the cause of sudden death.

2. Causes: congenital defect; trauma; atherosclerosis, arteriosclerosis

3. Symptoms based on location; most times asymptomatic

4. Diagnostic tests: angiography and x-ray

5. Treatment: medical regimen or surgery to clamp or remove or graft aneurysm

C. **Varicose veins** – weakening of the valves in the vein resulting in pooling of blood in the vein of the legs or rectum (hemorrhoids)

1. Causes: heredity, prolonged standing, multiple pregnancies, obesity, tumors, hypertension, liver and kidney disease, thrombophlebitis, wearing constrictive clothing around extremities

2. Incidence is higher in women 30-50 years than in men.

3. Diagnostic tests: clinical symptoms and history; Trendelenburg test, Doppler ultrasound

4. Signs and symptoms

   a. Tortuous veins, veins are prominent on standing with pain, heaviness, and cramping in the extremities.

   b. Veins are more prominent in hot weather and at high altitude.

5. Treatment

   a. Elevate affected extremity q 2-3 hours for a few minutes.

   b. Avoid prolonged standing.

   c. Instruct client not to wear restrictive clothing on extremities.

   d. Use support hose to promote venous return.

   e. Surgical interventions: ligation and stripping or injection of sclerosing solution in small veins

D. Deep vein thrombosis

1. Diagnostic tests

   a. Venography

   b. Doppler ultrasound

2. Signs and symptoms

   a. Pain in calf of the leg that is aggravated by flexing the ankle (**positive Homan's sign**); elevated temperature, and increased pulse rate, local area of redness and swelling along the affected vein

   b. Anorexia, fatigue, and malaise

3. Prevention

   a. Early ambulation after surgery

   b. Passive and active range of motion

   c. Prophylactic low dose anticoagulants and antiplatelets for high-risk clients

4. Treatment and nursing care

   a. Medical treatment consists of relief of symptoms by proper support of the vessels with elastic stockings, removal of causative factors.

   b. Bed rest with gradual ambulation

   c. Passive range of motion exercises

   d. Warm moist packs

e. Extremity elevated to decrease swelling

f. Intravenous heparin based on severity followed by oral anticoagulants for 3-6 months

g. Stool softeners to prevent straining on defecation

Additional Resources Found on MyNursingLab

- Electrocardiogram video
- Lymphatic System animation
- Sickle Cell animation
- Ventricular Contraction animation
- Heart and Major Vessels animation
- Angina animation
- Shock animation
- Drug Chart: Drugs Affecting the Cardiovascular System

MODULE 3

Medical-Surgical Nursing

Submodule 3.11 Gastrointestinal Disorders

Learning Objectives

3.11.1 Describe the etiology and common diagnostic tests related to gastrointestinal disorders.

3.11.2 Describe treatment and nursing care for clients with gastrointestinal disorders.

Note: Prior to beginning this unit, the student should review the anatomy and physiology of the gastrointestinal system.

I. **Laboratory and Diagnostic Tests**

    A. X-ray examination – uses radiopaque substances, i.e., barium

        1. **Upper GI series** – barium swallow– visualizes esophagus, stomach, and small intestine

            a. Preparation

                i. Explain procedure to client, withhold fluids and food 6-8 hours prior to test.

                ii. Purpose – diagnosing obstruction, ulcers, and growths

            b. Post procedure

                i. Client must expel barium; use laxative and fluids to prevent impaction.

                ii. Explain stools will be chalky-colored until barium is expelled.

        2. **Lower GI series** – barium enema– x-ray of lower intestine

            a. Preparation

                i. Explain to client; give laxative night before; give enemas until clean on morning of exam.

                ii. Restriction of fluid and food after midnight before test

                iii. Purpose – diagnose tumors, ulcerations, obstructions, and abnormalities of lower intestine

            b. Post test: laxative is given to aid expulsion of barium.

    B. **Gastroscopy** and **esophagoscopy** – direct visualization of internal GI structures by passing a fiberoptic scope through mouth, esophagus, stomach, and duodenum

        1. Used to diagnose tumors and ulceration of the esophagus and stomach and to perform biopsy

            a. Preparation

                i. NPO 6-8 hours prior to test

      ii.   Informed consent; sedative administered to calm client

      iii. Explain the need to gargle or be sprayed with a local anesthetic agent

  b. Post test

      i.   The client is NPO until gag reflex returns – about 2-4 hours.

      ii.   Observe vital signs for signs of bleeding.

      iii. Use warm normal saline gargle once gag reflex returns to relieve soreness.

C. **Proctoscopy** and **sigmoidoscopy** – direct visualization of internal wall of rectum and lower intestinal tract

  1. Used to diagnose tumors and polyps of the lower intestinal tract

  2. Allows for removal of tissue for testing

  3. Preparation

    a. Enemas the evening before to clear lower bowel; informed consent required

    b. Explain to client there is cramping when scope is inserted.

  4. Post test: observe for signs of bleeding, extreme distention, and tenderness.

D. **Colonoscopy** – visualization of the lining of the large intestine to identify abnormalities; flexible scope is inserted rectally; can remove polyps or biopsy tissue.

  1. Preparation: liquid diet 24 hours, NPO after midnight, bowel prep – Go-LyTely night before; prior informed consent

  2. During procedure: conscious sedation; left side lying, knees bent; scope passed and air instilled to keep visualization

  3. After procedure, monitor for bleeding.

E. **Gastric analysis** – laboratory analysis of fasting contents of stomach

  1. Preparation: nasogastric tube inserted, sample of gastric contents taken, histamine given, more specimens taken and examined for amounts of HCl

  2. Instruct client to be NPO after midnight.

  3. Client should not smoke or use anticholinergic drug for 24 hours prior to test.

F. Stool analysis

  1. Occult blood – **guaiac test** or **Hemoccult test**

  2. Used to detect hidden blood in feces caused by trauma, benign or malignant tumor, inflammation, or ulceration

  3. Source can be upper or lower gastrointestinal tract.

  4. Preparation: diet free of red meat for 24-48 hours

  5. Stool specimen obtained in a stool container

  6. Wearing gloves, the nurse transfers the stool to the paper using a tongue blade.

  7. Test can be done at home or hospital.

  8. Specimen is labeled and sent to laboratory.

G. Parasites

  1. Stool specimen collected x3, transported to laboratory within ½ hour

H. Blood and serum studies – to evaluate GI function

1. Albumen-globulin ratio – decreased levels with malabsorption and malnutrition

2. Alkaline phosphatase – elevated levels in liver disorders

3. Bilirubin – elevated levels in impaired biliary excretion or with increased RBC production

4. Cholesterol – indicates liver metabolism

II. **Gastrointestinal Disorders**

A. **Gastritis**

1. Inflammation of the mucous membrane lining the stomach

2. Caused by ingestion of drugs, alcohol, smoking, or stress

3. Diagnosis: stool for occult blood, CBC, electrolytes, endoscopy

4. Signs and symptoms: nausea, vomiting, pain, tenderness, diarrhea, anorexia, hematemesis

5. Treatment and nursing care

   a. Acute gastritis – withhold PO fluids, administer IV fluids, drugs to decrease peristalsis

   b. Chronic gastritis – bland diet, drugs to coat and reduce spasms

B. **Appendicitis**

1. Inflammation of the vermiform appendix

2. Cause: bacteria in the lumen or accumulation of fecal matter

3. Appendix becomes inflamed, distended, can contain pus.

4. Can cause rupture of the appendix and leakage of the content into the peritoneal cavity leading to peritonitis.

5. Symptoms: pain in the lower right quadrant at McBurney's point, elevated temperature, nausea, and vomiting

6. Diagnosis: increased WBC; anorexia, decreased or absent bowel sounds, and ultrasound

7. Treatment: surgical removal

8. Preoperative nursing care: NPO, routine preoperative orders, and antibiotics

9. Postoperative nursing care: early ambulation, fluids by mouth as soon as tolerated, and routine surgical wound care

C. Inflammatory bowel disease

1. Most commonly describes ulcerative colitis and Crohn's disease.

   a. Both diseases have a familial inherited trait.

   b. Both diseases have an immune reaction.

   c. Caused by environmental and lifestyle factors

   d. Incidence: age 10-30, then ages 50-60 years old

   e. Incidence is higher in whites than non-whites.

   f. Both diseases affect a greater number of women than men.

2. Disorders often associated with inflammatory bowel disease are irritable bowel syndrome (IBS), peripheral arthritis of the large joints with swelling and redness, stomatitis, and increased incidence of thromboembolic events.

3. Other associated factors; diet and smoking

4. **Ulcerative colitis** – inflammation of the colon and ulceration of the mucous membrane affecting the inner wall of the lower colon and rectum

    a. Cause: unknown; predisposing factors – acute infections, emotional stress, autoimmune disorders

    b. Diagnosis: clinical symptoms, sigmoidoscopy and colonoscopy showing inflamed bleeding mucosa, endoscopic biopsy, and barium enema; CBC showing decreased hemoglobin and hematocrit

    c. Signs and symptoms

       i. Diarrhea, including nighttime diarrhea; stool containing mucus, blood, and pus up to 30 to 40 times per day

       ii. Vomiting, nausea, and dehydration; malnutrition and weight loss; anemia

       iii. Fever, arthritis, stress, and skin lesions

    d. Treatment and nursing care

       i. Blood transfusion; TPN; high-calorie, high-vitamin diet

       ii. Rest, anxiety reduction

       iii. Correction of fluid and electrolyte imbalance

       iv. Pain management and psychological support

       v. Careful observation of number and characteristics of stool; perineal care and protective barrier

       vi. Surgery – removal of diseased area, usually ileostomy

    e. Drugs: antidiarrheal drugs, corticosteroids, antibiotics, immunomodulators, and biological response modifiers

5. **Regional enteritis (Crohn's disease)** – chronic inflammation affecting all layers of intestinal wall in the lower part of the ileum and ascending colon, characterized by loss of appetite, malabsorption, loss of electrolytes, and loss of protein

    a. Chronic inflammation leads to abscesses and fistulas, causes hypertrophy and fibrosis of the intestines, and can lead to obstruction.

    b. Cause: unknown; could be genetic, autoimmune, infection, excessive emotion, milk products, or fried foods

    c. Incidence is mostly in women 15 to 30 years old.

    d. Diagnosis: abdominal x-ray, colonoscopy, sigmoidoscopy, GI or barium enema, and fecal occult blood stool cultures, WBC and sedimentation rate (will be increased with reactive protein), ultrasound in women to rule out gynecological disorders

    e. Signs and symptoms

       i.   Slow progression with periods of remission and exacerbation

       ii. Pain in lower right quadrant

       iii. Abdominal cramping and spasms after meals

        iv. Nausea

        v. Diarrhea with blood, anorexia, and weight loss

        vi. Fluid and electrolyte loss

        vii. Inflammation that can lead to abscesses, fistulas, and perforation of intestines

    f. Treatment

        i. Two types of diet based on client needs, TPN to rest bowels

        ii. Antidiarrheal drugs, loperimide (Imodium), and Metamucil used carefully, antiemetics, corticosteroids, sulfonamide, iron, vitamins, immune modulators; avoid laxatives and aspirin because of hemorrhage risk.

        iii. Surgical intervention: bowel resection as a last resort because condition can recur after surgery.

  D. Diverticulitis

    1. **Diverticulum** is an outpouching of the intestinal mucosa and muscular layer; most common in the sigmoid colon

    2. **Diverticulitis** – inflammation of the diverticula with small herniations in colon wall; common in persons over 50 years, mostly in men

    3. Causes

        a. Diverticula form due to congenital weakness of large bowel.

        b. Low-fiber content in diet may also contribute.

        c. May result from normal slowing of intestinal tract in late years of life.

        d. Constipation and/or straining, stress

    4. Diagnosis

        a. Barium enema showing outpouching or colonoscopy if condition is not acute; barium enema with severe diverticula can cause rupture.

        b. CT scan with contrast, CBC, stool for occult blood

    5. Symptoms: change in bowel habits, constipation or diarrhea, dull steady pain in left lower abdominal quadrant, rectal bleeding, anorexia, low-grade fever

    6. Treatment

        a. Measures to allow colon to rest (i.e., NPO, IV fluids)

        b. Antibiotics as ordered

        c. High/low fiber diet still controversial; stool softener, drinking 6 glasses of water daily

        d. Surgical bowel resection if indicated

  E. **Peritonitis** – acute or chronic inflammation of peritoneum (membrane lining the abdominal cavity and covering viscera)

    1. Cause: results from bacterial invasion of the peritoneum – ruptured appendix, diverticulitis, perforated gastric/peptic ulcer, neoplasm, bowel strangulation, penetrating abdominal wound, ruptured ovarian cyst

    2. Signs and symptoms: severe abdominal pain, rigid abdomen with or without guarding or rebound, nausea and vomiting, paralytic ileus, tenderness, elevated temperature, tachycardia, leukocytosis

3. Treatment directed at eliminating the cause

    a. Position in Fowler's position to localize infection.

    b. Nasogastric tube to reduce distention

    c. IV fluid and electrolyte replacement

    d. Antibiotic therapy to combat spread of the infection

    e. Surgery to drain infected area

    f. Analgesics for pain relief

    g. Emotional support

F. **Irritable bowel syndrome (IBS)** – alteration in gastrointestinal motility characterized by periods of strong disorderly contractions and periods with no contractions

1. Bowel pattern changes from periods of severe diarrhea to constipation.

2. This is a group of symptoms rather than a disease.

3. Cause: inherited tendency towards disease occurring more in women and young adults to the middle years

4. In periods of emotional stress, flare-ups are common.

5. Infection can also aggravate the condition.

6. Diagnosis: clinical history, colonoscopy, sigmoidoscopy, barium enema, and GI series to determine other contributing disorders

7. Signs and symptoms: constipation, diarrhea, bloating, abdominal discomfort, and distention

8. Treatment

    a. Diet: high fiber; avoid foods that are gaseous.

    b. Eat small frequent meals; increase fluids; reduce stress.

    c. Drugs like Metamucil add bulk to stool and decrease diarrhea or constipation.

    d. Antispasmodics to decrease discomfort from spasms

    e. Antidepressants to improve emotional outlook

G. **Intestinal obstruction** – blockage of flow of intestinal contents – can be mechanical or from paralysis

1. Mechanical – occurs as a result of strangulated hernia or adhesions

2. Paralytic – occurs when there is decrease in or absence of peristalsis resulting from infection, abdominal surgeries, or trauma

3. Diagnostic tests: abdominal x-ray showing buildup of gas or fluid, CT scan, CBC with elevated WBC and electrolytes

4. Signs and symptoms: abdominal pain, vomiting (possibly fecal matter), absence of bowel movements; bowel sounds could be absent or high pitched.

5. Treatment: NPO, nasogastric tube to suction fluid, electrolyte replacement, pain control, prepare for surgery, prophylactic antibiotics

H. Ileostomy

1. Stoma formed by bringing ileum to outer abdominal wall following total **colectomy** (removal of the colon)

PEARSON

    a. Conventional: small stoma in RLQ requires pouch at all times because of continuous effluent.

    b. Continent (Kock pouch): lower portion of terminal ileum used to construct an internal reservoir with a nipple valve located near suprapubic area; a catheter inserted into the stoma every 3-4 days empties the reservoir.

  2. Colostomy can be formed and named based on portion of colon used. The type of stool varies depending on the location of the stoma (see Table 1).

Table 1. Ostomy Location and Type of Stool	
Location	*Characteristic of Stool*
Ascending colon	Liquid mush
Right transverse colon	Mush to semi-formed
Left transverse colon	Semi-formed soft
Descending or sigmoid colon	Soft to hard

  3. Types of stoma

    a. **End stoma:** formed with proximal bowel after abdominoperineal resection done following rectal cancer

    b. **Loop stoma:** a loop bowel (usually transverse colon) is pulled to outside wall of abdomen; a bridge under the loop usually holds it in place.

    c. **Double-barrel stoma:** often temporary; bowel is dissected and both ends of colon are brought out to the abdominal wall to form two stomas; the proximal stoma is the functioning part; the distal (mucus fistula) allows mucus to drain.

  4. Preoperative care

    a. The client visits with the nurse specialist to prepare emotionally and to help select a site for the stoma.

    b. This aids in having a properly fitted appliance.

    c. Bowel preparation: cleansing enemas until clear to reduce potential for infection

    d. Oral agent such as GoLyTely is given.

    e. Prophylactic antibiotics to sterilize the bowel

  5. Postoperative nursing care

    a. Inspect stoma every 8 hr; new stoma should be pink to red, moist, same as oral mucous membrane; bluish colon indicates poor blood supply; black colon indicates necrosis.

    b. Initially stoma is swollen, then size gradually decreases.

    c. Change appliance PRN; provide skin care.

    d. Support emotional concerns.

    e. Instruct client to avoid foods with odor and gas.

I. **Gastroesophageal reflux disease (GERD)** – regurgitation or reflux of stomach content into lower esophagus; leads to esophagitis, thickening, and narrowing

  1. Causes: alcohol, drugs, increased caffeine, and increased estrogen

  2. Signs and symptoms

    a. Heartburn in midsternal area, regurgitation

      b.   Pain radiating into back, neck, jaw, or both arms

      c.   Relieved within 3-5 minutes without liquid antacid

  3.   Diagnosis: barium swallow with esophagoscopy and x-ray

  4.   Treatment

      a.   Antacids with H_2 antagonist, proton pump inhibitors

      b.   Diet modification: avoid spicy, acidic, fatty foods with caffeine or gas. Take small frequent meals; sit erect up to 2 hours after eating.

      c.   Avoid tight clothing around abdomen.

      d.   Sleep with head of bed elevated 4 to 6 inches.

J. **Peptic ulcer disease** – a break in the mucous membrane lining in the stomach, duodenum, or esophagus from irritation or infection.

  1.   Erosion of the stomach can invade the musculature and lead to bleeding or perforation.

  2.   Cause: exact unknown; contributing factors:

      a.   Altered levels of gastric acid

      b.   Tobacco and alcohol use

      c.   Aspirin or other nonsteroidal drug use

      d.   Caffeine

      e.   Personality factors

      f.   *Helicobacter pylori*

  3.   Ulcers are named based on location in the stomach. Most common are gastric and duodenal.

  4.   Gastric ulcer

      a.   Signs and symptoms: burning, aching, or gnawing pain in upper epigastrium 30 minutes to 2 hours after meals, unrelieved by foods or antacids; epigastric tenderness; belching, nausea, and vomiting; bleeding: melena or hematemesis

  5.   Duodenal ulcer

  6.   Midepigastric pain 2-4 hours after meals, relieved by foods and antacids; melena and sometimes hematemesis; nausea, vomiting, anorexia

  7.   Diagnosis: upper GI series, endoscope test for *H. pylori*

  8.   Treatment

      a.   Aimed at lowering stress

      b.   Avoid caffeine, alcohol, and spicy foods; encourage client to eat small, frequent, bland foods.

      c.   Administer medications such as antacids, histamines (H_2 receptors), antagonists; cytoprotective proton pump inhibitor, antibiotics, bismuth.

      d.   Encourage lifestyle changes.

      e.   Prepare for surgery if necessary:

          i.   Pyloroplasty with vagotomy

          ii.   Subtotal gastrectomy (see under Gastric cancer below)

K. Gastric cancer

1. Malignancy of the stomach, mostly in males

2. Causes: *H pylori* infection, pernicious anemia, diet high in smoke or cured foods

3. Diagnosis: upper GI series, gastroendoscopy

4. Signs and symptoms:

   a. Nausea, vomiting, anorexia, indigestion, pain, discomfort

   b. Weight loss, anemia

5. Treatment:

   a. Subtotal **gastrectomy** or total gastrectomy used to treat cancer, involves partial or total removal of stomach

   b. Subtotal gastrectomy: two common surgeries – Billroth I and Billroth II

      i. Billroth I: 75% of the distal portion of the stomach is removed

      ii. Billroth II: 50% of distal portion of the stomach is removed

   c. **Vagotomy**: resection of vagus nerve to prevent vagal stimulation and to lower production of hydrochloric acid

6. Preoperative care as for any surgery:

   a. Build up nutritional state – may need TPN supplement, vitamins, and minerals

   b. Nasogastric tube may be inserted to remove fluid and gas and rest the stomach.

7. Postoperative care:

   a. Pain relief around the clock

   b. Vital signs, Fowler's position to facilitate drainage

   c. Provide comfort, relaxation, back rubs.

   d. Ensure patency of nasogastric tube.

   e. Monitor incision for infection and healing.

   f. Promote ambulation, monitor return of bowel sounds, begin progressive diet.

   g. Watch for complications, bleeding, distention, pernicious anemia, and dumping syndrome.

      i. Pernicious anemia – vitamin B$_{12}$ deficiency after gastrectomy; decrease or absence of intrinsic factor – vitamin B$_{12}$ is given PO, parenterally, or intranasally of each month for life.

      ii. Dumping syndrome

         (a) Develops post surgery once subtotal gastrectomy clients begin to take food

         (b) Sudden rapid entry of food into the jejunum

         (c) Not properly mixed with digestive enzymes

         (d) Signs and symptoms: weakness, dizziness, sweating, nausea, cramps, diarrhea, palpitations, hypotension, syncope; occurs 5-30 minutes after eating

         (e) Treatment:

            (1) Instruct to eat small frequent meals.

    (2) Meals should be high-protein and low-carbohydrate.

    (3) Fluids should not be given until 1 hour before or 2 hours after meals to slow gastric emptying.

    (4) Duration of symptoms: up to 6 months after surgery

L. Hernia

  1. **Hernia** – protrusion of a loop of tissue or organ through a weakened area in muscle wall

  2. Common hernias by location

    a. **Hiatal hernia:** protrusion of the lower part of the esophagus and part of stomach, slides through into lower portion of thorax

    b. **Umbilical hernia:** protrusion at umbilical region

    c. **Inguinal hernia:** protrusion containing intestines or spermatic cord at inguinal opening

    d. **Femoral hernia:** intestine protruding through femoral ring, mostly in females

  3. Types of hernias

    a. **Reducible hernia:** protruding tissue or organ can be replaced by pressure on the organ or manual manipulation back into abdominal cavity.

    b. Irreducible or **incarcerated hernia:** protrusion cannot be pushed back through the opening.

    c. **Strangulated hernia:** protrusion in which blood supply to the protruding part is cut off.

  4. Causes: congenital weakness, surgical incision, injury to the part where strangulation occurs

  5. Signs and symptoms: lump or local swelling at the site; pain, more pronounced on coughing. If hernia becomes strangulated, the client will have symptoms of an intestinal obstruction.

  6. Treatment: surgery (herniorrhaphy or hernioplasty)

  7. Preoperative: as for any surgery

    a. Discourage from coughing

  8. Postoperative: splint to cough or sneeze

    a. Avoid strenuous activity (pushing, pulling, and lifting) for 6-8 weeks.

M. Hemorrhoids

  1. Varicosities of veins in the rectum – either internal, external, or both

  2. Seen at age 20-50 years

  3. Cause: exact, unknown; contributing factors

    a. Increased abdominal pressure

    b. Standing/sitting

    c. Inherited tendency

    d. Constipation/straining

    e. Obesity/pregnancy

4. Signs and symptoms: bleeding with defecation or blood streaks; pain with defecating, sitting/walking; discomfort; itching

5. Diagnosis

   a. Clinical findings on examination and history

   b. Proctoscopy showing internal hemorrhoids, CBC may show decreased Hb and Hct

6. Treatment

   a. Conservative approach: diet with sufficient bulk food, stool softeners, fluids, exercise, warm compresses, sitz baths, topical anesthetics

   b. Surgical treatment: hemorrhoidectomy

7. Preoperative care: routine preoperative care

   a. Cleanse bowel with laxatives or enemas.

8. Postoperative care

   a. Assess for bleeding at operative site.

   b. Change rectal dressing every 2-3 hours PRN.

   c. Side lying to prone position

   d. Ambulation early, padded chair when sitting

   e. Pain control

   f. Stool softeners for elimination

   g. Analgesics for first bowel movement postoperatively

   h. Diet: high-fiber, increased fluids

   i. Sitz bath after each bowel movement for 2 weeks

   j. Report bleeding or exudates from rectum.

III. Diseases of the Accessory Organs of Digestion

   A. Special diagnostic tests and examinations

      1. X-ray examinations:

         a. The gallbladder and ducts that carry bile may be visualized by x-ray; if an opaque dye is used, the test can detect stones or tumor in the gallbladder or common bile duct.

         b. **Cholecystogram**, gallbladder studies, and cholangiogram are terms used to describe x-ray examination of the gallbladder using radiopaque dyes.

         c. Preparation of the client requires administration of cathartics and enemas until return is clear.

            i. Informed consent

            ii. Check allergy to iodine

            iii. Give 6 Telepaque tablets orally after evening meals q 5 minutes.

            iv. NPO after midnight

            v. High-fat meal can be given after test begins to stimulate gallbladder emptying.

            vi. Report any vomiting after drug is given.

PEARSON

2. Liver biopsy

    a. Aids in diagnosis of liver disease to identify cancer, cirrhosis, hepatitis

    b. Needle inserted via skin; small sample taken; client at risk for bleeding because organ is highly vascular.

    c. Before biopsy, informed consent, coagulation studies, NPO 6-8 hours

    d. During procedure, client should be positioned back or left side; tell client to hold still and hold his or her breath.

    e. Post-procedure: bed rest for 24 hours, lying on right side first 2 hours, small roll under biopsy site or sandbag to provide pressure for 4-6 hours; assess for bleeding until vital signs are stable.

3. Bilirubin test

    a. Bilirubin is a pigment normally found in the blood and removed by the liver; when the liver is diseased, bilirubin accumulates in the blood and produces jaundice.

4. Endoscopic retrograde cholangiopancreatography (ERCP)

    a. Provides visualization of the biliary system, pancreatic duct

    b. Test uses a fiberoptic scope inserted through mouth, esophagus, and stomach, into duodenum.

    c. Radiopaque dye is injected to provide visualization.

    d. Preparation:

        i.   NPO for eight hours prior

        ii. Informed consent

        iii. Instruct client to lie completely still.

    e. Post procedure

        i.   NPO until gag reflex returns

        ii. Monitor for signs of pancreatitis.

        iii. Nausea, vomiting, abdominal pain

        iv. Diminished or absent bowel sounds

        v.   Hypovolemic shock

B. **Jaundice** – name indicating that there are excessive amounts of bile pigment in the blood; refers to a group of symptoms rather than a disease

    1. Types of jaundice

        a. Obstructive jaundice – caused by plugging of the bile ducts

        b. Nonobstructive jaundice – associated with damage to the liver cells

        c. Hemolytic jaundice – hemolysis means destruction of the red blood cells; with large numbers of red blood cells destroyed, pigment is released into the blood, and jaundice develops.

    2. Nursing care

        a. Relief of itching of the skin – soothing baths, mild lotions, frequent changing of bed linens

        b. Indigestion due to blockage of the flow of bile into the intestinal tract – low-fat diet, relief of constipation

  c. Close observation of the color of the urine and stools: the urine may be dark due to excretion of the bile by the kidneys; stool may be light (clay colored) because of lack of bile

  d. Observe client for signs of bleeding, because the liver manufactures prothrombin, which plays an important role in blood clotting.

C. **Hepatitis** – inflammation of the liver from virus or chemical

 1. Types

  a. Viral hepatitis A (HAV) transmitted by contamination found in water, feces, saliva, and sexual contact; mostly children to young adults.

   i. Incubation period: 10-40 days; recovery: 4-6 weeks

   ii. Prevention: vaccine available

  b. Viral hepatitis B (HBV) transmitted by blood and body fluids

   i. Incubation: 28-160 days; places client at risk for cancer

   ii. Prevention: vaccine available

  c. Viral hepatitis C (HCV) transmitted by blood and body fluids

   i. Incubation: 2 weeks to 6 months; becomes chronic, leads to high risk of cirrhosis and cancer

   ii. May need liver transplant

  d. Viral hepatitis D (HDV) occurs with hepatitis B; transmitted by blood and body fluids

   i. Co-infection

   ii. Incubation: 1-10 weeks

   iii. Can progress to cirrhosis and chronic hepatitis

  e. Viral hepatitis E (HEV) transmitted by fecal-oral route or contaminated food and water

   i. Found in areas with poor sanitation

  f. Hepatitis G (HGV) transmitted by blood: IV users, prenatal, or tissue donation.

 2. Diagnostic tests

  a. Elevated bilirubin, alanine aminotransferase (ALT), and aspartate aminotransferase (AST)

  b. Lactic dehydrogenase (LDH), alkaline phosphatase, and gamma glutamyl transferase (GGT) are elevated.

  c. Elevated prothrombin time (PT) and international normalized ratio (INR)

 3. Signs and symptoms

  a. Early symptoms similar to those of an upper respiratory infection.

  b. Later there is local tenderness over the liver and the appearance of jaundice and pruritus, muscle pain, malaise, headache, nausea, vomiting, dyspepsia, diarrhea, fever, chills, photophobia, enlarged lymph nodes.

 4. Treatment and nursing care

  a. Reduce fatigue.

  b. Hydrate.

    c. Monitor electrolytes.

    d. Administer ordered vitamin K, fresh frozen plasma, and immunoglobulin.

    e. Decrease medication and avoid alcohol because liver cannot metabolize medications.

    f. Teach good personal hygiene to prevent spread of infection.

    g. Instruct clients that they will be unable to donate blood.

D. **Cirrhosis** of the liver – chronic disease characterized by degeneration of liver cells; cells are replaced by fibrous and scar tissue.

    1. Types of cirrhosis

        a. **Laennec's cirrhosis:** resulting from alcohol overuse and malnutrition – fat deposited in liver cells and leads to scarring

        b. **Postnecrotic cirrhosis**: result of viral hepatitis, causes inflammation and death of cells

        c. **Cardiac cirrhosis**: result of right-sided heart failure, when the liver becomes enlarged (hepatomegaly) and fibrous tissue infiltrates

        d. **Biliary cirrhosis**: result of obstruction of common bile duct and blocked bile excretion

    2. Diagnostic tests

        a. Elevated liver enzymes

        b. Prolonged prothrombin time and INR

        c. Obstruction of bile duct found on endoscopic retrograde cholangopancreatography (ERCP)

        d. Esophagoscopy showing varicose veins of the esophagus

        e. Ultrasound of liver

        f. Liver biopsy

        g. Paracentesis to withdraw fluid from abdominal cavity

    3. Cause: specific cause unknown; associated with vitamin deficiency

    4. Signs and symptoms

        a. Early symptoms are the same as those for acute hepatitis.

        b. Later, congestion of the blood vessels that drain the digestive organs and transport the blood to the liver (the portal circulation) leads to accumulation of fluid within the intestines and eventually into the abdominal cavity

        c. **Ascites** – excess fluid within the abdominal cavity; this condition is relieved by withdrawing the fluid from the cavity **(paracentesis)**

        d. Other symptoms include edema, jaundice, and small hemorrhages under the skin.

    5. Treatment and nursing care: no known cure for cirrhosis; treatment is symptomatic; drugs such as lactulose reduce ammonia levels.

        a. Bed rest – best position is with head and shoulders elevated if the client has ascites.

        b. Weigh client daily.

  c. Low-salt diet for edema relief

  d. Care of skin important

  e. Be alert for signs of internal bleeding.

  f. Dietary treatment consists of a high-protein, low-sodium, low-fat diet.

  g. Mental changes can be expected in the last stages: monitor for delirium, convulsions, or coma.

6. Complications: portal hypertension, ascites, esophageal varices, jaundice, and hepatic encephalopathy

7. **Esophageal varices** – varicose veins of the esophagus

  a. Cause: portal hypertension

  b. Tortuous veins can rupture and cause hemorrhage.

  c. Cause of rupture: coughing, sneezing

  d. Diagnosis: medical history, bleeding, endoscopy

  e. Signs and symptoms: hematemesis, melena, shock, enlarged liver and spleen, ascites, jaundice

  f. Treatment for nonbleeding varices

    i. Prophylactic beta blockers to decrease blood pressure and decrease risk of bleeding

  g. Treatment for ruptured varices

    i. Ensure patent airway; administer O_2 as ordered.

    ii. Keep NPO; IV fluids and electrolytes.

    iii. Monitor level of consciousness.

    iv. Blood transfusion

    v. Administer vasopressin IV or in superior vena cava to cause vasoconstriction of local blood vessels to decrease portal hypertension and bleeding.

    vi. Administer nitroglycerin IV to lower blood pressure and increase blood flow to heart.

    vii. Gastric lavage with iced saline to remove swallowed blood from stomach

    viii. Ice also causes local vasoconstriction.

    ix. Insert Blakemore-Sengstaken tube.

    x. Inflated balloon presses on wall of esophagus to prevent bleeding.

    xi. Client in bed, head elevated 30 to 45 degrees to prevent aspiration.

Additional Resources Found on MyNursingLab

- Digestive System animation
- Performing a Gastric Lavage video
- Drug Chart: Drugs Affecting the Gastrointestinal System

MODULE 3

Medical-Surgical Nursing

Submodule 3.12 Reproductive Disorders

Learning Objectives

3.12.1 Describe common diagnostic tests used to detect reproductive disorders.

3.12.2 Describe manifestations, treatment, and nursing care for clients with common female reproductive disorders.

3.12.3 Describe manifestations, treatment, and nursing care for clients with common male reproductive disorders.

3.12.4 Describe manifestations, treatment, and nursing care for clients with sexually transmitted infections.

Note: **Prior to beginning this unit, the student should review the anatomy and physiology of the female and male reproductive systems.**

    I.   **Female Reproductive Disorders**

        A. Assessment

            1. History

                a. Menstrual history, onset of menses **(menarche)**

                b. Pregnancy and delivery history

                c. Fertility issues

                d. Methods of contraception

                e. Related medical history

                f. Family history

            2. Physical examination

                a. Pelvic exam – explain procedure

                    i. Have client void before procedure.

                    ii. Lithotomy position

                    iii. Prepare equipment: light, gloves, speculum, and lubricant.

                    iv. Drape client.

                    v. Remain at client's side near head.

                    vi. Following exam, provide tissues for removing lubricant; assist as needed.

      b.   Breast examination based on inspection and palpation

      c.   **Papanicolaou (PAP)** smear – scraping of cervical tissue for analysis; useful in diagnosing cancer of cervix

      d.   Vaginal smears and cultures – diagnose infections

      e.   **Mammography** – x-ray of breasts; helps diagnose cancer of breast

      f.   Ultrasonography – of breast, to distinguish solid from cystic masses; of abdominal and pelvic region, to detect abnormalities

           i.   Pelvic exam: client drinks 1 quart of water 45 minutes to 1 hour prior to exam to distend bladder.

      g.   **Laparoscopy** – examines interior of abdomen using scope via abdominal incision

           i.   Local anesthesia and conscious sedation

           ii.   Informed consent needed

           iii.   Baseline vital signs, bladder empty before procedure

           iv.   Following procedure, monitor vital signs; report increase in temperature.

           v.   Observe for bleeding and monitor pain.

           vi.   Explain there may be shoulder and abdominal pain related to CO_2 insufflation.

           vii.   Provide discharge instructions.

      h.   **Colposcopy** – examines tissues of the vagina and cervix using a lighted microscope; may be accompanied by endoconical curettage for biopsy; done early in menstrual cycle

      i.   **Conization** – removal of a cone-shaped wedge of cervical tissue for biopsy

           i.   Monitor for bleeding; maintain packing for 12-24 hours.

           ii.   Refrain from sexual intercourse and douching until MD advises.

      j.   **Dilatation and curettage (D&C)** – stretching of the cervix and removal of tissue from the wall of the uterus; used as a diagnostic and therapeutic treatment

           i.   Light IV sedation; routine preoperative care

           ii.   Postprocedure care – routine postoperative care; check for voiding, monitor for bleeding; teach client to avoid sexual intercourse and douching until MD advises.

B.   Disorders of menstruation

   1.   **Amenorrhea** – absence of menses

      a.   Causes

           i.   Malnutrition

           ii.   Obesity

           iii.   Extreme stress

           iv.   Anemia

           v.   Oral contraceptives

           vi.   Pregnancy

vii. Diabetes

viii. Severe illness

ix. Endocrine tumors

b. Treatment – based on cause

c. Nursing care: Provide support and information to help decrease anxiety, and encourage compliance with treatment plan.

2. **Dysmenorrhea** – painful or difficult menstruation

a. Causes

i. Primary dysmenorrhea not pathologic, related to prostaglandins causing uterine contractions

ii. Secondary dysmenorrhea may be due to:

(a) Endometriosis

(b) Pelvic infection

(c) Fibroid tumors

(d) Other reproductive anomalies

b. Treatment

i. Drugs used to inhibit prostaglandin synthesis, aspirin, NSAIDs

ii. Hormone replacement therapy (HRT)

iii. Hormone adjustment

iv. Surgery for tumor removal

c. Nursing care

i. Combination of exercise and rest

ii. Warm baths

iii. Well-balanced diet, nonconstipating diet

3. **Menorrhagia** – excessive blood loss during menses

a. Causes

i. Uterine tumors

ii. Pelvic inflammatory disease (PID)

iii. Endocrine problems

b. Treatment – based on cause

c. Nursing care

i. Teach client to count pads.

ii. Balanced diet high in iron

iii. Encourage rest.

4. **Metrorrhagia** – bleeding between menstrual periods

a. Causes – similar to menorrhagia; may be early sign of cervical cancer

b. Treatment – based on cause

  c. Nursing care: Teach client to count pads.

C. **Menopause** – a natural part of the aging process; begins with premenopausal periods; gradual decline in hormone production leading to a permanent cessation of menses

 1. Signs and symptoms

  a. Premenopausal – erratic menses, hot flashes, night sweats

  b. Menopause – absence of menses

  c. Vaginal dryness

 2. Treatment

  a. Hormone replacement therapy (HRT) for some women

  b. Dietary changes including phytoestrogens (soy, tofu, flax seed, black cohash), adequate calcium intake

  c. Regular weight-bearing exercise

 3. Nursing care

  a. Education aimed at controlling symptoms

D. Uterine fibroid tumor – benign tumor

 1. Signs and symptoms

  a. Menstrual disturbances

  b. Urinary frequency

  c. Constipation

  d. Backache

  e. Uterine enlargement

 2. Treatment

  a. Excision of small tumors

  b. **Hysterectomy** (removal of uterus) for large tumors

 3. Nursing care

  a. Education and explanation of plan of care

  b. Routine preoperative and postoperative care same as for abdominal surgery

E. **Endometriosis** – excessive growth of endometrial tissue elsewhere in pelvic cavity

 1. Signs and symptoms

  a. Pelvic discomfort

  b. Dyspareunia

  c. Fatigue

  d. Infertility

 2. Treatment

  a. Hormone therapy to suppress ovulation

  b. Surgery hysterectomy, salpingectomy, and/or oophorectomy

 3. Nursing care

a. Emotional support

b. Education regarding treatment and medication plan

c. Routine preoperative and postoperative care

F. **Pelvic inflammatory disease (PID)** – an infection of the pelvis, outside the uterus; most organs involved are the fallopian tubes, ovaries, pelvic connective tissue, peritoneum, pelvic veins

1. Causes

   a. Organisms such as *Streptococcus, Gonococcus, Chlamydia, Trachoma, Mycoplasma,* and coliform bacteria

   b. Transmitted by sexual intercourse, abortion procedures, childbirth, intrauterine devices; postpartum

2. Signs and symptoms

   a. Abdominal fullness, pressure, pain, and cramps

   b. Chills, fever, nausea, vomiting, malaise

   c. Purulent vaginal discharge, spotting between menstrual cycles

   d. Elevated WBC, positive vaginal culture

3. Treatment

   a. Bed rest in mid-Fowler's position to facilitate drainage

   b. Analgesics for pain, and antibiotics for infection (penicillin)

4. Nursing care

   a. Monitor vital signs, WBC culture.

   b. Warm compresses or heating pad to abdomen for comfort and circulation

   c. Teach good perineal care, sexual abstinence during treatment.

5. Negative outcomes: stricture formation and obstruction of fallopian tubes leading to infertility

G. **Prolapse of uterus** – downward movement of uterus through vaginal opening

1. Causes

   a. Weakened supporting muscles from repeated pregnancies

   b. Congenital weakness

   c. Atrophy of supportive muscles and ligaments

2. Signs and symptoms

   a. Pain

   b. Lower abdominal pressure

   c. Stress incontinence

   d. Dyspareunia

   e. Backache

3. Treatment

   a. Use of pessary in vagina to support uterus

   b. Surgical repair of supporting muscles and ligaments

   c. Hysterectomy

H. Cystocele and rectocele

  1. **Cystocele** – herniation of bladder into vaginal wall

   a. Cause: weakened supporting muscles and ligaments

   b. Signs and symptoms

     i. Pelvic pressure

     ii. Stress incontinence

   c. Treatment

     i. Anterior colporrhaphy

   d. Nursing care

     i. Postoperative care: Foley care, I&O, analgesics for pain, pelvic exercises, no weight bearing or lifting, good perineal care, avoidance of sexual intercourse in immediate postoperative period

  2. **Rectocele** – abnormal protrusion of rectum into vaginal wall

   a. Causes: weakened supporting muscles and ligaments

   b. Signs and symptoms

     i. Constipation

     ii. Hemorrhoids

     iii. Backache

     iv. Lower abdominal pressure

   c. Treatment

     i. Antibiotic therapy

     ii. Analgesics for pain

   d. Nursing care

     i. Semi-Fowler's position to aid in pelvic drainage

     ii. Heat applications to increase circulation and comfort

     iii. Review safe sex principles with client.

I. Cancer of the female reproductive organs

  1. Cervical cancer

   a. Cause: abnormal cells in neck of uterus

   b. Signs and symptoms

     i. Asymptomatic in early stage

     ii. Menstrual disturbances

     iii. Postmenopausal bleeding

PEARSON

          iv.   Bleeding after intercourse

          v.   Abnormal Pap smear

    c. Treatment

          i.   Conization

          ii.   Radiation in advanced cases

          iii.   Chemotherapy

    d. Nursing care

          i.   Education and support

          ii.   Use of time, distance, and shielding with radium implant use

          iii.   High-protein, high-residue diet to avoid straining with bowel movements

          iv.   High fluid intake – 2000-3000 mL daily

          v.   Antiemetics as needed

          vi.   Routine postop care if surgery is performed

2. Uterine cancer

    a. Cause: abnormal cells in uterine lining

    b. Signs and symptoms

          i.   Postmenopausal bleeding

          ii.   Metrorrhagia

          iii.   Bleeding after intercourse

    c. Treatment

          i.   Surgery (hysterectomy)

          ii.   Chemotherapy

          iii.   Radiation

    d. Nursing care

          i.   Observe for vaginal hemorrhage, malodorous vaginal discharge.

          ii.   Observe for urinary retention.

          iii.   Change perineal pads every 3 to 4 hours and PRN.

          iv.   Listen for renewed bowel sounds.

          v.   Monitor for fever.

          vi.   Monitor I & O.

3. Ovarian cancer

    a. Malignant tumor – a cancerous growth found on the ovary

    b. Can be the primary site of the cancer or a secondary site caused by metastasis from the GI tract, breast, pancreas, or kidney

    c. Signs and symptoms

          i.   Pelvic pain

          ii.   Menstrual disturbances

   iii. Abdominal distention

   iv. Constipation

   v. Dyspareunia

   vi. Palpable mass

  d. Treatment

   i. Cyst may be observed for regression in size.

   ii. **Oophorectomy** (removal of ovaries)

   iii. Removal of all reproductive organs

   iv. Estrogen replacement therapy

   v. Chemotherapy

   vi. Radiation

4. Breast cancer

  a. Causes

   i. Heredity: cancer in first-degree relative

   ii. Advancing age

   iii. Obesity

   iv. Diet high in protein and fats

   v. Early menarche, late menopause

  b. Signs and symptoms

   i. Nonpainful nodule

   ii. Nipple retraction, discharge

   iii. Skin dimpling

  c. Treatment

   i. **Lumpectomy** – removal of lump

   ii. Simple **mastectomy** – removal of breast

   iii. Modified radical mastectomy – removal of breast, pectoralis minor muscle, and some adjacent lymph nodes

   iv. Radical mastectomy – breast removal, pectoralis muscles, fascia, and lymph nodes

   v. Radiation

   vi. Chemotherapy

   vii. Corticosteroids and possible hormone therapy

  d. Preoperative nursing care

   i. Offer emotional support.

   ii. Teach coughing, deep breathing, leg exercises, and use of incentive spirometer.

  e. Postoperative nursing care

   i. Elevate affected arm above level of heart to decrease edema.

        ii.   Report any numbness or swelling in affected arm – may indicate new circulatory impairment.

       iii.   Assist with postoperative exercises.

       iv.   Monitor for hemorrhage.

       v.   Avoid using affected arm for B/P or IV fluid administration.

       vi.   Monitor and empty Hemovac drainage.

       vii. Assist client getting out of bed (OOB); support the operative side.

       viii. Encourage arm exercises according to MD orders.

       ix.   Monitor for potential side effects if receiving chemotherapy and/or radiation.

       x.   Suggest meeting with Reach to Recovery or similar group for emotional support.

II. Male Reproductive Disorders

  A. Physical assessment

    1. History

    2. Physical examination

      a. Examination of penis, scrotum, testes, and breasts by observation and palpation

      b. Digital rectal examination (DRE) of prostate gland

      c. Ultrasound for male genitourinary problems

      d. Cystourethroscopy

      e. Blood tests

         i.   PSA prostate-specific antigen; normal is less than 4 ng/L.

         ii. PSA prostatic acid-phosphatase; normal is less than 3 ng/L.

      f. Infertility tests

      g. Urinalysis

  B. **Benign prostatic hypertrophy (BPH)** – benign condition appearing after age 50 in which growth of prostate tissue puts pressure on and constricts the urethra

    1. Signs and symptoms

      a. Urinary pattern changes – difficulty starting stream and/or diminished urinary force

      b. Leaking, dribbling, incontinence

      c. Urgency

      d. Dysuria

      e. Hematuria

      f. Nocturia

      g. Recurring infection

    2. Treatment

      a. Medical – medications to relax smooth muscles

b. Surgical

    i. **Transurethral resection of the prostate (TURP)** – scope inserted into urethra with removal of some of the obstructing prostatic tissue

    ii. **Prostatectomy** – surgical removal of the prostate gland through a suprapubic, retropubic, or perineal incision

3. Nursing care

    a. Maintain adequate bladder drainage via catheter.

    b. Continuous bladder irrigation (or triple lumen catheter) is used following transurethral resection.

        i. One lumen is used for inflating bag (usually 30-mL bag), one lumen for outflow of urine, and one for irrigating solution instillation.

        ii. Run solution in more rapidly with bright red drainage or clots; when drainage clears, decrease to about 40 drops/minute.

        iii. If clots cannot be rinsed out with irrigating solution, notify charge nurse and physician.

    c. Provide fluids to prevent dehydration (2 to 3 liters every 24 hours).

    d. Provide high-protein, high-vitamin diet.

    e. Observe for signs of hemorrhage and shock.

    f. Instruct client in perineal exercises to regain urinary control by squeezing perineal muscles by pressing buttocks together and holding for as long as possible. Repeat this process ten times every hour.

    g. Ambulate early as ordered.

    h. Observe for complications.

C. Prostate cancer

1. Exact cause unknown – contributing factors:

    a. Family history

    b. Advancing age

2. Signs and symptoms

    a. Initially asymptomatic

    b. Dysuria

    c. Hesitancy, frequency

    d. Nocturia

3. Treatment

    a. Medications to suppress testosterone

    b. Prostatectomy

        i. Simple **prostatectomy** – surgical removal of prostate gland

        ii. Radical prostatectomy – removal of prostate, seminal vesicles, and section of bladder neck

    c. Radiation and seed implantation may be used.

    d. **Cryosurgery** – freezing tissue

4. Nursing care

    a. Routine postoperative care: monitor vital signs, teach routine postoperative exercises.

    b. Maintain urinary catheter drainage.

    c. Maintain bladder irrigation.

    d. Observe for hemorrhage.

    e. Monitor intake and output.

    f. Administer pain medication as needed.

    g. Teach perineal exercises to help regain urinary control.

    h. Teach client to avoid Valsalva maneuver until healing is completed.

    i. Provide answers about sexual functioning.

D. **Prostatitis** – inflammation of the prostate gland

1. Causes: bacterial *(E. coli)* or nonbacterial

2. Signs and symptoms

    a. Fever, chills

    b. Frequency, urgency

    c. Nocturia

    d. Back pain

    e. Dysuria

3. Treatment

    a. Bacterial: antibiotics

    b. Nonbacterial: treated symptomatically with medications

E. Testicular cancer

1. Cause: unknown

2. Signs and symptoms – palpaple lump

3. Treatment

    a. Surgical removal of testes, epididymis, and spermatic cord

    b. Chemotherapy

    c. Radiation

III. **Sexually Transmitted Infections (STIs)**

A. Gonorrhea

1. A venereal disease caused by *Gonococcus*

2. Highly infectious disease, no immunity is established

3. Signs and symptoms

    a. About 90% of women with gonorrhea have no symptoms or very mild symptoms of a pelvic inflammatory disease.

4. Diagnosis – identification of the organism on a smear or culture

5. Treatment

    a. Large doses of penicillin or some other antibiotic

6. Nursing care

    a. Extreme care must be taken when caring for these clients; vaginal discharge is highly contagious.

B. Syphilis

    1. A venereal disease, but not restricted to the genital tract; it may involve any organs in the body.

    2. Cause: spirochete

    3. Signs and symptoms

        a. Primary stage – **chancres** (open sores) on the mouth or genital area which may subside without treatment, but the disease will still be present; secretions from chancre and client's blood both considered highly contagious

        b. Secondary and tertiary stages – may present symptoms of various serious diseases

    4. Treatment

        a. Use of antibiotics – most useful in the first stage

        b. After the disease has progressed to the third stage, little can be done for the client.

C. Genital herpes

    1. Signs and symptoms

        a. Incurable infection characterized by episodes of painful, reddened vesicles on the genitalia or rectum

        b. Primary sites: cervix in women and glans penis in men; accompanying lymph node enlargement

        c. Fever, malaise, dysuria, leukorrhea

    2. Treatment

        a. Antiviral agent – acyclovir

        b. Teach to keep lesions clean and dry; wear loose, absorbent underclothes.

        c. Sitz bath to enhance comfort

        d. No sexual intercourse while lesions are active

        e. Adequate nutrition; Pap smear follow-up

D. Chlamydia

        a. Most common STI in the United States; causes symptoms similar to gonorrheal infections

        b. Cause – *Chlamydia trachomatis*

    271

        c. Signs and symptoms

            i. Males

                (a) Urethritis, dysuria, frequency, watery mucoid discharge

                (b) Complications include epididymitis, prostatitis, infertility.

           ii. Females

                (a) Often asymptomatic but may have mucopurulent cervicitis, dysuria, frequency, local soreness

                (b) Complications include salpingitis, PID, ectopic pregnancy, and infertility.

        d. Treatment – antibiotic therapy (doxycycline, tetracycline, erythromycin)

E. **Condylomata** – genital or venereal warts

    1. Often seen with other STDs such as gonorrhea and trichomoniasis

    2. Highly contagious

    3. Cause: human papillomavirus (HPV)

    4. Signs and symptoms

        a. Small growths that grow into large cauliflower-like masses

        b. Profuse, foul-smelling vaginal discharge

        c. Bleeding; may progress to genital and cervical dysplasia and cancer

    5. Diagnostic tests: inspection of perineum, culture, biopsy

    6. Treatment

        a. Cryotherapy

        b. Laser therapy

        c. Acid treatments

        d. Surgery

        e. Chemotherapy (5FU)

F. Trichomoniasis/candidiasis – very common STI; symptoms frequently seen only in women

    1. Causes: *Trichomonas vaginalis and Candida albicans,* respectively

    2. Signs and symptoms

        a. Itching

        b. Discharge

    3. Diagnostic tests: culture and inspection of affected tissues

    4. Treatment

        a. Antifungals

        b. Antiprotozoal drugs (metronidazole, flagyl)

Additional Resources Found on MyNursingLab

- Female Pelvis animation
- Breast Self Exam video
- Male Pelvis animation
- Drug Chart: Drugs Affecting the Reproductive System

MODULE 3

Medical-Surgical Nursing

Submodule 3.13 Genitourinary System

Learning Objectives

3.13.1 Describe diagnostic tests and nursing care for common genitourinary disorders.

3.13.2 Describe treatment and nursing care for common genitourinary disorders.

Note: **Prior to beginning this unit, the student should review the anatomy and physiology of the genitourinary system.**

I. **Kidney Function Tests**

    A. Used to determine the kidney's ability to remove waste products from the blood, dilute the urine, or concentrate the urine.

    B. Various types of kidney function tests; nurse must be familiar with hospital policies and physicians' orders when preparing the client and assisting with these tests.

    C. Blood tests

        1. **Blood urea nitrogen (BUN)** – determines the amount of urea and waste accumulating in the blood; normal range 10 to 20 mg/dL.

        2. **Serum creatinine** – determines the amount of creatinine in the blood; creatinine is the end product of muscle and protein metabolism; normal levels for males are 0.6 to 1.2 mg/dL and for females are 0.5 to 1.1 mg/dL.

        3. **Prostate-specific antigen (PSA)** – a blood test; elevated levels are the result of prostate cancer, prostatitis, or benign prostatic hypertrophy (BPH); normal is 0 to 4 ng/mL.

    C. **Urinalysis** – one of the most common tests done to detect the presence of disease in the kidneys and bladder.

        1. Abnormal constituents include pus, bacteria, albumin, and glucose; each may indicate specific diseases.

        2. Routine urinalysis can be done as a random specimen or the first thing in the AM.

        3. Test can be done using diagnostic strip tests for pH balance, specific gravity, glucose, ketones, albumin, blood, and bilirubin.

        4. Collection of specimen

            a. Clean-voided specimen requires cleansing of external genitalia prior to client voiding.

            b. Sterile specimen is collected by catheterization.

            c. Specimens should be properly labeled and sent to the laboratory immediately.

        5. Normal findings: pH: 4.6 to 8; specific gravity: 1.010 to 1.025.

6. Findings of glucose, ketones, bacteria, albumin, or bilirubin are considered abnormal.

7. Microscopic examination of urine: finding of a few cast cells (epidermal cells) and of very few to no WBCs and RBC is still considered normal.

8. Normal color of urine is pale yellow to amber.

9. Normal odor should be mildly aromatic.

D. Urine culture: urine is examined for micro-organisms causing an infection in the urinary tract.

   1. Obtain **clean-catch** specimen:

      a. Cleanse perineal area around urethra.

      b. Instruct client to start void.

      c. Insert container to collect specimen.

      d. End voiding.

E. **24-Hour urine** – entire volume collected over 24 hours

   1. First voided specimen is discarded.

   2. Collect all urine thereafter.

   3. Last void at time test ends

   4. Done for creatinine and ketosteroid

F. **Urine specific gravity** – Measurement of kidney's ability to concentrate urine and of state of hydration

   1. Compared to density of distilled water

   2. Normal specific gravity is 1.010-1.025.

   3. Reduced in diabetes insipidus

   4. Increased in dehydration

G. X-ray examination of the urinary tract

   1. **KUB x-ray** – abdomen including kidneys, ureters, and bladder (KUB)
No preparation is needed.

   2. **Intravenous pyelogram** – dye is injected into the vein and excreted through the kidney. into the urine; films are taken as radiopaque dye passes through the kidneys, ureters, and bladder to outline their structures.

      a. Preparation – informed consent

         i. Check for allergy to iodine

         ii. Laxative night before

         iii. NPO for 8 to 10 hours before test

         iv. Inform client of a warm feeling experienced when dye is injected.

         v. Monitor vital signs during procedure.

      b. Postprocedure: increase fluids to increase excretion of dye.

   3. **Retrograde pyelogram** – dye is injected directly into the ureters by way of a catheter passed through the bladder; the test is done at the same time as a cystoscopy.

      a. Check allergy to iodine and seafood; NPO, laxative as prescribed.

      b. Low-residue diet the day before.

      c. Postprocedure: watch for bleeding at venipuncture site and in urine, also increase fluids.

  4. **Cystography** – visualization of the interior of the bladder through the use of a special instrument called a cystoscope

      a. Useful in diagnosing tumors or local infections.

      b. The physician can also remove small stones, obtain a biopsy from growths, and relieve strictures by using the cystoscope.

      c. If a biopsy is planned, NPO after midnight, enemas as ordered, and sedative.

      d. Postprocedure: analgesics, sitz bath, force fluids, check urine for bleeding and clots, and administer antimicrobial to destroy the specific microorganism causing the infection; rest and forcing fluids are important as long as the infection is present.

  5. **Angiography** – Renal arteriogram provides details of arterial blood supply to the kidneys; catheter inserted via femoral artery into aorta and to renal blood vessels

      a. Medium contrast injected via the catheter; allows series of x-rays to be taken.

      b. Instruct client of hot flushed feeling when dye is injected.

      c. Procedure lasts 30-90 minutes.

      d. Check allergy to iodine before the test.

      e. Check signed consent.

      f. NPO after midnight.

      g. Void before procedure

      h. Post procedure – pressure dressing to femoral artery for 4 to 5 hours

      i. Monitor vital signs and watch for bleeding.

      j. Neurovascular checks

H. **Renal biopsy** – Percutaneous insertion of needle into kidney to remove tissue sample

  1. Prior to procedure: assess vital signs, verify informed consent, coagulation studies

  2. NPO after midnight

  3. Postprocedure: vital signs, report hypotension or tachycardia; these changes indicate bleeding

  4. Pressure on puncture site for 30 minutes to prevent bleeding

  5. Bed rest, supine position for first 8 hours

  6. Increase fluids 1-2 L per day.

  7. Monitor urinary output and watch for bleeding.

  8. Monitor hemoglobin and hematocrit.

  9. No heavy lifting or strenuous exercise for 2 weeks.

I. Ultrasonography

  1. Can identify kidney's shape, size, location, collecting system, and tissue

J. CT scan and MRI of the abdomen can reveal pathology of kidneys.

II. **General Nursing Care of Clients with Urinary Disorders**

    A. Observation and accurate measurement of intake and output.

        1. Fluids are of primary importance in urological nursing.

        2. Output measures loss of body fluids.

            a. Total urinary output requires measurement of all urine excreted by the kidneys; may be obtained by having client void or from urethral catheter.

            b. Total output includes urine, emesis, watery stools, and an estimate of fluid lost through perspiration.

            c. Clients with edema are often weighed daily to estimate loss of body fluids; weigh at same time each day on same scales.

        3. Measurement of intake must include all fluids by mouth, administered into the vein, and through Levin tube or gastrostomy tube. Intake may be restricted in some cases.

        4. If catheter is irrigated and solution is allowed to drain into drainage bag, the amount of irrigating fluid must be subtracted from the total amount excreted to find the urinary output.

        5. Assess difficulty voiding and presence of urinary incontinence.

        6. Assess weight loss and weight gain.

        7. Check for presence of edema.

        8. Check characteristics of urine.

    B. Types of catheters

        1. Foley – held in place in the bladder by a balloon

        2. Coudé – tapered tip allowing easy insertion when client has BPH

        3. Urethral – passes into ureters

        4. Suprapubic – introduced through abdominal wall into bladder

        5. Texas or condom – connected to external male genitalia

    C. Care of the client using a retention catheter – retention catheter has a bulb on one end to hold it in place, and is left in bladder so that urine is constantly drained from bladder

        1. The drainage bag must always be kept below the level of the bladder to prevent reflux.

        2. Amount of drainage in bag is measured at least every 8 hours; observe color and content of drainage.

        3. Tubing and apparatus used for collecting urine must be sterile when connected to catheter to prevent introduction of microorganisms into the urinary tract.

    D. Urinary incontinence

        1. Involuntary voiding

        2. Types of incontinence

            a. Transient or temporary – caused by change in mental status, medication, increased fluid intake, immobility, and infection.

                i. Treatment – reversible if cause is corrected

    b. Total incontinence – continuous leakage of urine

       i. Cause: trauma to urethral sphincter

    c. **Neurogenic bladder** – caused by nerve damage, seen after prostate surgery or strokes

    d. **Stress incontinence** – leakage of urine from coughing, sneezing, laughing, or any straining; mainly affects women after multiple childbirths, loss of muscle tone, or aging; usually affects men, after prostate surgery; can be a few drops to a stream

    e. **Reflex/urge incontinence** – caused by bladder spasms and instability; leakage of urine is followed by urge to void; once leakage begins, no control in stopping; characteristic voiding pattern is frequent small amounts; decreased fluid intake causes urine to concentrate and increases spasms.

    f. **Incontinence with overflow** – results when bladder distends with urine and detrusor muscle does not contract.

       i. Causes: nerve injury in client with spinal cord injury, diabetes, blockage as in benign prostatic hypertrophy (BPH), cancer of prostate, postoperative urinary retention

       ii. Assessment: distended bladder, can have some leakage

       iii. Treatment: bladder training doing Kegel exercise, Credé maneuvers to empty bladder, or electrical stimulation, medications such as antispasmodic and tricyclic antidepressants.

III. Genitourinary Disorders

  A. Urinary tract infection

    1. Infection or inflammation of the urinary tract, including cystitis

    2. **Cystitis** – inflammation of the wall of the urinary bladder caused by gram-negative micro-organisms e.g., *E. coli;* more frequent in women because of proximity of bladder to urinary meatus

    3. Diagnosis: microscopic inspection of urine

    4. Symptoms: pain, burning on urination, frequency/urgency, hematuria, pyuria

    5. Treatment: increase fluids 2-3 liters to dilute urine, sitz bath for comfort, perineal care, diet, increase urinary acidity with cranberry juice; drugs as ordered (sulfonamides, urinary antiseptic, antispasmodics).

  B. **Glomerulonephritis** (Bright's disease)

    1. Inflammation of the glomerulus that can lead to its destruction

    2. Acute – seen 2-3 weeks after upper respiratory tract or urinary tract infection

      a. Causes: streptococcal infection and autoimmune processes

    3. Chronic – usually weeks after an acute episode

    4. Diagnosis

      a. Smoky color urine (coca cola color), hematuria.

      b. Increased BUN, creatinine, and specific gravity of urine

      c. Proteinuria, increased antistreptolysin O titers

5. Signs and symptoms

    a. Swollen, puffy face and feet

    b. Oliguria or anuria, fever, chills, fatigue, pallor, headache, and weakness

    c. Nausea, vomiting, anorexia, and flank pain

6. Treatment

    a. Monitor vital signs, daily weight, edema, intake and output.

    b. Watch for fluid overload and signs of congestive heart failure (CHF)

    c. Diet – increase calories, decrease protein

    d. Bed rest initially

7. Regulate fluid excess with diuretics.

    a. Regulate blood pressure with antihypertensive drugs.

    b. Treat infections with antibiotics.

C. Nephrotic syndrome

1. Caused by damage to glomeruli.

2. Signs and symptoms: proteinuria, hematuria, generalized edema, anemia, anorexia, malaise at times, irritability

3. Treatment

    a. Vital signs, bed rest, intake and output, assess edema, daily weights, abdominal girth

    b. Diet – low- to moderate-protein, low-sodium, high-carbohydrate

    c. Regulate blood pressure with antihypertensive drugs and diuretics

D. **Pyelonephritis** – inflammation of kidney leading to edema

1. Cause: *E. coli* organism

    a. Associated with diseases such as diabetes mellitus, urinary tract infection (UTI)

2. Outcome could be atrophy of kidney and nephrons

3. Diagnosis

    a. Urinalysis with bacteria and pus

    b. Urine culture to identify organism

    c. IVP to detect structural changes or obstruction

    d. Increased BUN and creatinine

4. Signs and symptoms: nausea, vomiting, diarrhea, hypertension, and signs of an infection

5. Treatment

    a. Rest and comfort

    b. Intake and output

    c. Promote fluid and nutrition

    d. Medication: antibiotics for infection; antispasmodics for discomfort

E. Renal calculi

   1. **Urolithiasis** – stones in the urinary tract

   2. **Nephrolithiasis** – stones in the kidney

   3. **Ureterolithiasis** – stones in the ureters

   4. **Cystolithiasis** – stones in the urinary bladder

   5. Composition of stones: calcium and uric acid

   6. Causes

       a. Diet with large amounts of calcium

       b. Uric acid

       c. Family history

       d. Sedentary lifestyle

       e. Urinary tract infections

       f. Hyperthyroidism

   7. Diagnosis: kidney-ureter-bladder (KUB) x-ray, intravenous pyelogram (IVP), cystoscopy, ultrasound to identify presence and location of stones

   8. Abnormal urinalysis

   9. Signs and symptoms:

       a. Renal colic, severe pain in flank radiating to groin and inner thigh

       b. Pain accompanied by nausea, vomiting, sweating, urinary urgency, frequency, and hematuria

   10. Treatment:

       a. Strain all voided urine for stones. Send to laboratory for analysis

       b. Increase fluids 2-3 L per day.

       c. Intake and output

       d. Analgesics for pain or heat application

       e. Antispasmodic agents to relieve spasms

       f. Diet – regulated based on cause of stones

           i.   Calcium stones: acid ash diet, decrease in dairy products and acidic foods

           ii. Uric acid stones: decreased purine intake, may need allopurinal to reduce uric acid

       g. Cystoscopy done to remove stones in bladder or ureters

       h. **Extracorporeal shock wave lithotripsy (ESWL)** – noninvasive method of breaking up stones in the kidney and aiding passage

           i.   Ultrasonic waves used under fluoroscopy to visualize break up of stones

           ii.   Stones passed within a few days are sent for analysis

           iii. Preparation before procedure: consent and NPO after midnight

    iv. Postoperative: watch for bleeding and passage of stones

        (a) Vital signs until stable

        (b) Intake and output

        (c) Treat pain.

        (d) Increase fluids

i. **Percutaneous lithotripsy** – invasive method used to break up stones in kidneys, ureters, and bladder

    i. Cystoscopy or nephroscopy incision to place tube in kidneys.

    ii. Ultrasonic wave applied under fluoroscopy

    iii. Nephrostomy tube or indwelling catheter inserted

    iv. Chemical irrigation may then be used to break down stones

    v. Clearing stones takes 1-5 days

    vi. Following procedure, increased fluid needed

    vii. Monitor client for bleeding or infection.

j. **Ureterolithotomy** – open incision to remove stone from ureters if lithotripsy fails

k. **Pyelolithotomy** – surgical incision in pelvis of kidney to remove stone

l. **Nephrolithotomy** – surgical incision into the kidney to remove stone

m. **Nephrostomy** – surgical incision into kidney for the purpose of providing for drainage from the kidney.

n. **Nephrectomy** – total or partial surgical removal of a kidney

    i. Postoperative care after nephrectomy

        (a) Client must be checked carefully for tubes and catheters that may have been inserted during surgery; these may be attached to various types of drainage or irrigation equipment

        (b) Hemorrhage is a common complication following surgery of the kidney.

        (c) Dressing may be tinged with bright pink drainage, but presence of blood should be reported.

        (d) Some drains have a sterile safety pin (Penrose) attached to the end; these must never be left open or attached to the bed linen or the client's clothing.

        (e) Adequate drainage from the unaffected kidney is of concern to the surgeon; the nurse is responsible for the accurate measuring and recording of urinary output from the bladder.

        (f) Fluids may be restricted during the immediate postoperative period in order to avoid overburdening the kidney.

        (g) Administer fluid as prescribed; packed red cells may be needed.

        (h) Urine output should be 30 to 50 mL per hour.

        (i) Daily weight and urine specific gravity.

        (j) Position semi-Fowler's to promote drainage.

        (k) Encourage deep breathing, coughing.

(l) Monitor for paralytic ileus.

(m) Antiembolic stocking to prevent embolism

(n) Pain control

(o) Irrigate tubes only if ordered

IV. Renal Failure

A. Acute renal failure

1. Rapid loss of kidney function

2. May be reversible or irreversible

3. Cause can be *perirenal* (outside of kidney)

   a. Causes: severe kidney infection, mercury poisoning

4. *Intrarenal* (inside the kidneys)

   a. Shock\transfusion, ischemic condition, e.g., tubular necrosis

   b. Cardiovascular conditions that decrease cardiac output

5. Phases

   a. **Oliguric phase** – characterized by inability to regulate electrolytes or excrete fluid and metabolic waste

      i. Seen in first 8-15 days

      ii. Urine output less than 400 mL\day

      iii. Fluid excess can lead to heart failure

      iv. Pulmonary edema and electrolyte imbalance

      v. Signs and symptoms

         (a) Uremia, nausea, vomiting, anorexia, pruritus

         (b) Drowsiness, disorientation, edema with electrolyte imbalance, sudden drop in urinary output, tingling, coma, Kussmaul respiration, cardiac arrhythmias

         (c) Tingling extremities, sudden drop in urine output, disorientation, drowsiness, coma

      vi. Treatment: Restrict fluid to 400-1000 mL\day. Give prescribed diuretic (Lasix) to promote diuresis.

   b. **Diuretic phase** – excessive urinary output 4-5 L/day

      i. Watch for dehydration, hypovolemia, hypotension, tachycardia, level of consciousness.

      ii. Treatment: give IV fluids and electrolytes as prescribed to maintain balance.

   c. **Recovery phase** – when urinary output returns to normal

      i. Takes 1 to 2 years

      ii. Treatment: monitor vital signs, neurologic status, intake and output; weigh daily; bed rest to conserve energy; diet – potassium, protein, and sodium restricted; protect against infection; chest physiotherapy; aseptic catheter care; prevent skin breakdown; monitor for presence of uremic frost; bowel care; stool softener

B. Chronic renal failure

1. Comes on gradually and leads to irreversible loss of kidney function

2. Two phases seen: uremic and end-stage renal function

3. Causes

   a. May be seen after acute renal failure

   b. Usually a complication of systemic disease (diabetes; hypertension [HTN], obstructive renal disease, infection, or autoimmune processes)

4. Outcome: dialysis for rest of life

5. Diagnosis: elevated BUN above 50 mg\dL

   a. Elevated creatinine levels above 5 mg\dL

   b. Electrolyte imbalance: hypocalemia, hyperkalemia, hypermagnesemia, hyperphophatemia, metabolic acidosis, and anemia

6. Signs and symptoms:

   a. Anorexia, nausea, confusion, lethargy, decreased strength of muscles causing joint pain; headache, diarrhea, or constipation

   b. **Uremic frost** (white powder on the skin), Kussmaul breathing, edema, hypertension, disorientation, convulsions, and coma; skin dusky yellow, tan, or grey.

   c. **Uremia** – accumulation of nitrogenous waste leading to decreased alertness, Kussmaul breathing, gradual loss of consciousness

7. Treatment

   a. Fluid restriction to prevent fluid overload; intake equal to excretion plus 300-600 mL for insensible loss

   b. Diet to control electrolyte imbalance; increased carbohydrates and fats, low protein, sodium, potassium and phosphorus to decrease buildup of nitrogenous waste

   c. Intake and output, daily weight to detect edema

   d. Treat anemia and prevent fatigue by providing rest periods; client may need blood products iron and epoeitin alfa (Epogen) to maintain hemoglobin and hematocrit.

   e. Monitor for gastrointestinal bleeding.

   f. Skin care: to decrease pruritus, cleanse and provide meticulous hygiene but avoid use of soap

   g. Antihistamine and antipruritics as prescribed

   h. Oral care to prevent infection and ulceration

   i. Psychological support: prepare for dialysis

   j. Hyperkalemia: monitor cardiac status, watch for arrhythmias, administer sodium polystyrene sulfonate (Kayexalate) to lower blood potassium levels

   k. Hypermagnesemia: monitor for cardiac arrhythmias and neuromuscular deficit resulting in loss of deep tendon reflexes; avoid medications and foods with magnesium

      l.   Hyperphosphatemia: administer calcium carbonate, calcium acetate to lower serum phosphorus levels

C. **Hemodialysis** – use of artificial kidney to remove waste and excess water from the blood

1. The blood flows from the client's body through tubes to the dialyzer; waste passes into dialysate solution; the cleansed blood is returned to the client's body via another tube.

2. Hemodialysis takes 3-4 hrs and is performed 3 to 4 times/week

3. Side effects: fatigue, hypotension, dizziness, nausea, cardiac dysrhythmias, angina, fluid and electrolyte loss

4. Anticoagulant, e.g. heparin, used to prevent clot.

5. Antihypertensive medications should not be given before dialysis because they can cause severe hypotension.

6. Water-soluble medications become ineffective as they are dialyzed out of the body.

7. Weigh client before and after dialysis to determine loss.

8. Post-dialysis: monitor vital signs, watch for bleeding, administer withheld medication

9. Hemodialysis requires placement of temporary or permanent venous access device in nondominant arm

    a.   Purpose is to access the bloodstream for removal and return of blood to the body during dialysis

    b.   Temporary venous access device can be inserted in subclavian or femoral vein

    c.   There are two types of permanent venous access devices:

        i.   **Vascular access graft** – placement of a synthetic tube used to link a vein with an artery.

           (a) The blood vessels are those of the arm, the basilic or cephalic vein and the radial or brachial artery.

           (b) Maturity of graft takes 2 weeks.

        ii.   **Arteriovenous (AV) fistula/shunt** – made by suturing a vein and artery together

           (a) Maturity takes 2-4 months.

10. Caring for venous access devices

    a.   After procedure, check for bleeding.

    b.   Assess neurovascular status of arm, report any compromise.

    c.   Check for patency by palpating for a thrill or ausculating for a **bruit** (swishing sound) at the site.

    d.   Diminished or absent bruit or thrill is reported to MD immediately.

    e.   Do not use the arm for blood pressure, placement of IV, drawing blood, or injections.

    f.   Instruct client not to lift heavy objects, bend arm, or rest head on arm during sleep.

    g.   Instruct client not to wear constricting clothing or use jewelry or handbags over site; these may cause dislodgement of device.

    h.   Watch for signs of infection and report.

11. Peritoneal dialysis provides ability for client or family to perform in home dialysis; the peritoneal membrane is used as a semipermeable membrane, across which waste and fluid are removed from the blood into a dialysate solution instilled in the peritoneal cavity via a peritoneal catheter. The exchange process consists of three steps: filling, dwell time, and drainage.

    a. Fill – 1500-2000 mL of sterile dialyzing solution

    b. Dwell – amount of time solution is left in abdominal cavity (several hours)

    c. Drain – time it takes to drain all solution

12. Types of peritoneal dialysis

    a. Continuous ambulatory peritoneal dialysis (CAPD) is most common, consists of 3 exchanges in the day and one at night

    b. Continuous cycle peritoneal dialysis (CCPD) can be done at home or hospital; uses an automated cycling machine programmed to deliver inflow, dwell time, and outflow

        i. Advantage: can dialyze during sleep and be dialysis-free in wake time

    c. Intermittent peritoneal dialysis (IPD) is done 3-5 times per week for 10-12 hours.

    d. Nursing concerns:

        i. Dialysate must be at body temperature to decrease discomfort.

        ii. Use aseptic technique at catheter site.

        iii. Weigh client before and after procedure.

    e. Complication: peritonitis due to sepsis; watch for fever, pain, and cloudy fluid

V. Renal Cancer of Kidney

  A. Cancer of the kidney

    1. Occurs more in men than women; cancers are aggressive and invasive, involving aorta or vena cava

    2. Diagnosis: x-ray, ultrasound, CT scan, renal arteriography

    3. Signs and symptoms: painless hematuria, mass palpable in flank, weight loss, fever, malaise

    4. Treatment: nephrectomy, chemotherapy, or radiation

    5. Kidney transplant

      a. Sources: human or cadaver

      b. Selection: tissue typing to find suitable match

      c. Donor must have two healthy functioning kidneys

      d. Matches most commonly occur with relatives

      e. Indication: provide recovery for client with renal failure

      f. Organ rejection – a result of the body's natural defense against invasion

      g. Treatment: drugs to suppress the immune system

  B. Cancer of the bladder

    1. Incidence higher in men 50 to 70 years.

2. Cause: cigarette smoking, exposure to carcinogens, caffeine intake, and use of artificial sweeteners

3. Diagnosis: x-ray, CT scan, cystoscopy and biopsy, cytology of urine

4. Treatment: depending on area of bladder involved

   a. Chemotherapy into bladder

   b. Transurethral bladder resection

   c. Laser therapy via urethra into bladder

   d. **Cystotomy:** excision and removal of part of bladder

   e. **Cystectomy:** removal of bladder with urinary diversion

   f. Radiation therapy

   g. Urinary diversion – performed when removal of the urinary bladder is required. There are two types of urinary diversion: cutaneous and continent.

      i. Cutaneous diversion

         (a) **Ileal conduit** – a section of ileum or colon is removed, attached to the ureter, and stoma is brought out of abdomen for use as a conduit to drain urine continuously; an appliance is worn continuously, and concern is skin integrity

         (b) **Cutaneous ureterostomy** – not as commonly performed; ureters are brought out of the abdomen and a stoma is created. Most common complication is stricture formation and obstruction.

      ii. Continent diversion

         (a) **Kock pouch** – the urine is directed into the middle section of the ileum and a pouch is created.

         (b) The ureters create a nipple-valve stoma.

         (c) The stoma is catheterized at intervals to empty the pouch.

Additional Resources Found on MyNursingLab

- Kidney animation

- Urinary System animation

- Drug Chart: Drugs Affecting the Urinary System

MODULE 4

Growth and Development/Nursing Care of Children

Submodule 4.1 Growth and Development

Learning Objectives

4.1.1 Define key terms and patterns of growth and development.

4.1.2 Describe the developmental milestones, safety, and play activities for infant through adolescent stages.

4.1.3 Describe health promotion and nutritional needs for each age group.

4.1.4 Describe the needs of children during hospitalization.

  I. Growth and Development

    A. Definition of terms

       1. **Growth**: increase in size

       2. **Development**: maturation of structures; development is dependent on growth

       3. **Cephalocaudal**: directional term describing growth from head to toe

       4. **Proximodistal**: directional term describing development from trunk towards the extremities

    B. Principles of growth and development

       1. Orderly and predictable

       2. Different rates for different individuals

       3. Proceeds from simple to complex and general to specific

       4. Occurs at different rates for different structures

    C. Patterns of growth and development

       1. Infancy: most rapid period, head proportionately large

       2. Toddler/preschool: slow steady growth, trunk increases in size

       3. School age: continued slow growth, arms and legs grow fast

       4. Adolescence: fast growth period, increased trunk growth, maturation of gonads

    D. Factors that influence growth and development

       1. Heredity, race, and culture

       2. Gender

       3. Family support

       4. Environment

       5. Birth order

E. Theories of child development

Theorist	Erik Erikson	Jean Piaget	Sigmund Freud
Infancy Birth – 1 yr	Trust *vs* Mistrust	Sensorimotor	Oral (Id dominated)
Toddler 1 – 3 yrs	Autonomy *vs* Shame & Doubt		Anal (Bowel & Bladder Training, Ego Develops)
Preschool 3- 6 yrs	Initiative *vs* Guilt	Preoperational	Phallic (Oedipal Complex)
School Age 6 – 12 yrs	Industry *vs* Inferiority Concrete Operations	Preoperational	Latent (Superego Develops)
Adolescent 11- 18 yrs	Identity *vs* Isolation	Formal Operational	

F. Prevention and health promotion

    1. Primary prevention: aimed at preventing health problems

        a. Immunizations

        b. Control of risk factors

        c. Education

        d. Regular medical and dental care

        e. Adequate nutrition

    2. Secondary prevention: begins with diagnosis of disease followed by treatment.

    3. Tertiary prevention: aimed at rehabilitation with the goal of having the individual reach the highest level of functioning possible.

II. **Stages of Growth and Development, Safety, and Play Activities**

A. Stages of growth and development

    1. Infancy: birth through age 1

        a. Neonatal (0 - 28 days)

            i. Head is ¼ of total body length.

            ii. Behavior is under reflex control.

            iii. Extremities are flexed.

            iv. Hearing and touch develop.

            v. Vision is immature; eyes focus on lights.

            vi. Responds to music, and to being held, cuddled, and rocked

            vii. Normal apical pulse: 110-160/minute

        viii. Respirations: range from 30-50/minute, irregular, abdominal, and through nose.

        ix. Blood pressure: use correct size cuff.

        x. Immature temperature regulating mechanism

        xi. Eyes track poorly at birth and are tearless for first 2 months.

        xii. Meconium is the 1st stool within 24-48 hours after birth, followed by transitional stools; then formula-fed stools are yellow-green, or breastfed are seedy yellow.

b. 1-4 Months

    i. Good head control

    ii. Posterior fontanel closes.

    iii. Binocular vision develops; eyes follow an object.

    iv. Poor hand to mouth coordination; purposeful reaching.

    v. Crying to express needs.

    vi. Smile is instinctive at 2 months, social at 3 months; laughs at 4 months.

    vii. Regards mother's voice.

    viii. Explores feet.

    ix. Solitary play

c. 5 - 6 Months

    i. Doubles birth weight

    ii. Begins teething

    iii. Rolls over

    iv. Crawls

    v. Grasps and releases

    vi. Transfers objects from hand to hand

    vii. Sits with support

    viii. Cries when mother leaves; habits begin: thumb-sucking, favorite blankets, etc.

d. 7 - 9 Months

    i. Sits alone

    ii. Creeps

    iii. Stands and holds on for support

    iv. Pincer grasp develops.

    v. Feeds self with bottle

    vi. Verbalizes sounds

    vii. Starts to understand simple words such as "no"

    viii. 1st deciduous tooth, usually lower central incisor

e. 10 - 12 Months

    i. Triples birth weight

    ii. Cruises (walking and holding on for support)

    iii. Speaks 4-6 words; understands much more

    iv. Claps hands; waves bye-bye; enjoys rhythm games, cloth books, and building toys; explores; weans from bottle and breast

f. Newborn reflexes

    i. Moro (startle)

    ii. Babinski

    iii. Stepping

    iv. Tonic neck

    v. Rooting

    vi. Sucking

    vii. Swallowing

    viii. Grasp

    ix. Sneezing

    x. Blink

2. Toddler (12 Months - 3 Years)

a. Characteristics

    i. Egocentric, negative, dawdles

    ii. Slow growth: 4 - 9 lb over 2 years.

    iii. Normal pulse is 100 (80-120).

    iv. Normal respiration is 20-30.

    v. BP is 99/64.

    vi. Vision is still immature: observe for amblyopia/lazy eye.

    vii. Separation anxiety is common.

    viii. Parallel play

    ix. Ritualistic behavior

    x. 20 deciduous teeth usually by 2½ years - introduce tooth brushing

    xi. Language development: 400 words at 2 years and comprehends more, increases by 3 years; easily frustrated.

    xii. Anterior fontanel closes by 18 months.

b. Toilet training

    i. Bladder training after bowel training; must walk well first.

    ii. Has temper tantrums, uses "no" excessively, is curious and easily frustrated, wants immediate gratification, needs limits set, needs consistency.

3. Preschool (3 - 5 years)

    a. Characteristics

        i. Slow growth

        ii. Nursery school starts.

        iii. Concerned about body integrity (wants band-aids, shows fear of doctors, hospitals, etc.

        iv. Conscience or superego develops.

        v. Sibling rivalry is common.

        vi. Imaginary playmates, magical thinking

        vii. Cooperative play (associative play)

        viii. Role playing, imaginative fantasy, day dreaming

        ix. Sexual curiosity and masturbation are common. Sexual questions should be answered honestly.

        x. Clay, finger paints, water play, sandbox

4. School-age child (6 - 12 years)

    a. Modest

    b. Abstract thinking begins: learns to read, write, or do basic math.

    c. Interested in board games; follows rules.

    d. Competitive play and sports begin.

    e. Growth continues.

    f. Deciduous teeth begin to fall out.

    g. Bones grow; have more fractures.

    h. Vision matures.

    i. Language skills improve.

    j. Peers are very important.

5. Adolescence (12 - 18 years)

    a. Rapid growth period; vital signs are near adult ranges.

    b. Attempts to cope with body image

    c. Daydreams

    d. Peer pressure increases.

    e. Interest in opposite sex

    f. Explores and attempts to identify values and beliefs

    g. Fears include acne, homosexuality, obesity, and social failure.

    h. Struggle for independence

    i. Development of secondary sex characteristics

B. Safety tips
    1. Infants
        a. Factors:
            i. Increased mobility
            ii. Exploration of environment
            iii. Oral stage
            iv. Poking fingers into openings
        b. Types:
            i. Falls
            ii. Aspiration
            iii. Ingestion
            iv. Poisoning
            v. Burns
            vi. Drowning
            vii. Motor vehicle crashes
        c. Preventive measures:
            i. Keep crib rails raised.
            ii. Never leave infant unattended on a high surface.
            iii. Support young infant's head and neck.
            iv. Keep small objects out of reach; never prop bottles.
            v. Never use plastic on mattress, etc.
            vi. Cover electrical outlets, remove dangling wires, lock medications, and gate staircases.
            vii. Check bathwater temperature and never leave child alone in or near water.
            viii. Use back-facing car safety seats in back seat of car.
    2. Toddlers
        a. Factors:
            i. Curiosity
            ii. Walking/independence
            iii. Climbing ability
            iv. Failure to recognize danger
            v. Tendency to put everything in mouth
            vi. Tendency to open drawers, closets, etc.
        b. Types:
            i. Falls, burns, drowning
            ii. Ingestion/poisons

             iii. Suffocation

             iv. Motor vehicle crashes

       c. Preventive measures:

             i. Supervise.

             ii. Bar windows; guard stairwells.

             iii. Turn in pot handles on stove; use safety seats.

             iv. Examine toys for sharp or small pieces.

             v. Lock poisons away.

             vi. Do not leave pails or tubs of water where toddlers can find them.

3. Preschool

       a. Factors:

             i. Runs, jumps, climbs

             ii. Rides tricycles

       b. Types:

             i. Falls

             ii. Drowning

             iii. Ingestion/poisoning

             iv. Burns

             v. Motor vehicle crashes

       c. Preventive measures:

             i. Use window/door locks.

             ii. Teach water safety.

             iii. Examine toys.

             iv. Supervise.

             v. Teach use of telephone: 911.

4. School age

       a. Factors:

             i. Fearlessness

             ii. Increased motor skills

             iii. More competitive play/sports

       b. Types:

             i. Falls

             ii. Sports injuries

             iii. Drownings

             iv. Burns

             v. Motor vehicle crashes

             vi. Bicycle

     c. Preventive measures:

        i. Teach safety measures.

        ii. Teach rules of sports and water safety.

        iii. Teach fire prevention.

5. Adolescent

    a. Factors:

        i. Driving

        ii. Increased interest in sports

        iii. Feeling of invincibility

        iv. Desire for peer approval

        v. Tempted by experimentation

    b. Types:

        i. Motor vehicle crashes

        ii. Drowning

        iii. Sports injuries

        iv. Suicide

        v. Drug abuse

    c. Preventive measures:

        i. Offer driver's education.

        ii. Teach sporting rules.

        iii. Be alert for signs of depression.

        iv. Educate about drug abuse.

        v. Know friends' whereabouts.

        vi. Keep communication lines open.

C. Play activities

1. Infant

    a. Solitary play: noninteractive

    b. Appropriate playthings

        i. Mobiles (colorful) stimulate

        ii. Rattles

        iii. Large blocks

        iv. Soft dolls/toys

        v. Large soft balls

        vi. Washable books

        vii. Take-apart toys with large pieces

2. Toddler

    a. Parallel/side-by-side; plays alongside rather than with another child.

    b. Short attention span

    c. Appropriate playthings

        i. Pull/push toys: enhance walking

        ii. Play dough

        ii. Blocks

        iv. Containers

        v. Telephones

        vi. Large puzzles

        vii. Books, crayons, paints

        viii. Musical instruments

        ix. Large riding toys

3. Preschool

    a. Cooperative play: begin sharing, taking turns

    b. Dramatic play: try on roles

    c. Appropriate playthings

        i. Dress-up clothes

        ii. Paints, paper, crayons, clay

        iii. Riding toys

        iv. Dolls

        v. Work tools

        vi. Puzzles

        vii. Musical instruments

4. School age

    a. Cooperative play: interactive

    b. Competitive play: follow fixed rules and regulations

    c. Team sports, clubs, gangs

    d. Appropriate playthings

        i. Arts and crafts

        ii. Simple science toys

        iii. Magic

        iv. Puzzles

        v. Collections

        vi. Board games

vii. Reading/books

viii. Bicycles

ix. Computer games

5. Adolescent

   a. Peer group dominates

   b. Appropriate activities

      i. Sports/teams

      ii. Clubs

      iii. Arts/crafts

      iv. Music

      v. Part-time job

      vi. Movies

      vii. Computers

III. Health Promotion and Nutritional Needs

A. Recommended immunizations

Recommended Age	Immunization	Comments
2 Months	DTP, HbCV, OPV	
4 Months	DTP, HbCV, OPV	
6 Months	DTP, HbCV	
15 Months	MMR, HbCV	
15-18 Months	DTP, OPV	
4-6 Years	DTP, OPV	Tuberculin testing at or before entry to school
11-12 Years	MMR	
14-16 Years	Td	Repeat every 10 years

1. Contraindications for immunization

   a. Acute febrile illness

   b. Administration of steroids, radiation, cancer chemotherapy

   c. Alterations in immune system

B. Dental care

1. Begin tooth brushing when teeth appear.

2. Begin dental examinations by age 2½ –3 years.

3. Do not give milk or juice bottles at naptime or bedtime.

4. Supplement fluoride if not added to drinking water.

C. Pediatric medications

    1 Oral medications

        a. Never administer to crying infant.

        b. Hold infant in a slightly reclining position.

        c. Place liquid into side of mouth by dropper or needleless syringe.

    2. Intramuscular injections

        a. Infants: use vastus lateralis or ventrogluteal.

        b. Children over 2: use posterior gluteal, ventrogluteal, or quadriceps femoris.

    3. Intravenous solutions

        a. Given by pump or microdrops: delivers drop factor of 60 microdrops per mL.

    4. Ear drops

        a. Under 3 years: pull pinna down and back.

        b. Older child: pull pinna up and back.

    5. Eye drops

        a. Place in middle of lower conjunctival sac.

    6. Fluid requirements (see Nutrition section for details)

        a. Infants: total body water constitutes 80% of body weight; therefore, more prone to dehydration.

        b. Early signs of dehydration: dry lips, mucous membranes; decreased urinary output, reduced weight, lethargy

        c. Moderate to advanced dehydration: depressed fontanels; sunken eyeballs; loss of turgor; oliguria; rapid, weak pulse; restlessness; convulsions

D. Nutrition

    1. Newborn

        a. Breast milk or formula: 6 - 8 feedings/day, 3-4 hours apart, not more than 32 oz/day

        b. Vitamin and mineral (iron) supplements offered after 4 months

        c. Water may be given between feedings.

    2. Infant

        a. Solids are introduced one new food at a time for several days sometime after first 4 - 6 months.

            i. Rice: first solid food followed by other cereals

            ii. Yellow and green vegetables

            iii. Noncitrus fruits; no citrus fruits, nuts, or shellfish until 1 year

            iv. Teething biscuits from 6 months on.

            v. Meats and egg yolks after age 6 months

      vi. Junior or mashed coarser foods at age 9 months

      vii. Finger foods by 10 months

  b. Cup between 3 - 6 months

  c. Never add milk or juice into night bottle; it leads to dental decay.

  d. Steady weight gain indicates adequate intake.

3. Toddler

  a. Full range of meats, vegetables, fruits, and cereals

  b. Offer small, colorful portions; vary textures and flavors.

  c. Avoid use of concentrated sweets.

  d. Ritualistic food habits and decreased appetites are common.

  e. Finger foods

4. Preschool

  a. Appetite wanes.

  b. Choose from basic food groups.

  c. Likes and dislikes develop.

5. School age

  a. Food habits are well established.

  b. Offer a nutritious breakfast.

  c. Seeks peer approval

  d. Influenced by media

6. Adolescent

  a. Patterns are well established and difficult to change.

  b. Usually very concerned about weight and fitness

  c. Food fads and dieting are common.

  d. Peer pressure is very influential.

IV. Needs of Children during Hospitalization

A. Infant

1. Hospitalization interferes with eating and sleeping habits.

2. Promote trust by following home routines.

3. Encourage visitation or rooming-in.

4. Provide pacifier for comfort.

5. Encourage visual, auditory, and tactile stimulation.

6. When taking vital signs, take least invasive first.

B. Toddler: suffers most from separation.

1. Stages of separation anxiety

  a. Protest: cries for mother; rejects attention from others

      b.   Despair: becomes apathetic and withdrawn

      c.   Denial: represses feeling for mother, responds to anyone, regresses to earlier stages

   2.   Encourage visiting.

   3.   Allow favorite items from home.

   4.   Provide opportunities for play.

   5.   Reassure child that parents will return.

   6.   Do not punish for regressive behavior.

   7.   Encourage independence and child's participation in activities.

   8.   Tell the child if something will hurt.

C. Preschooler

   1.   Explore child's understanding of illness/hospitalization; seen as a punishment.

   2.   Identify child's fears.

   3.   Provide play therapy.

   4.   Encourage verbalization.

   5.   Accept regressive behavior.

   6.   Reassure child that he/she is going home.

   7.   Allow choices where possible.

   8.   Maintain home routines when possible.

   9.   Explain simple procedure; use simple words.

   10. Provide information about 2 hours prior to procedure.

D. School age child

   1.   Minimize separation from peers and family.

   2.   Allow for privacy due to modesty.

   3.   Accept crying.

   4.   Encourage participation in self-care.

   5.   Provide choices.

   6.   Give praise when earned.

   7.   Maintain peer/family contact.

E. Adolescent

   1.   Explore their understanding of their illnesses.

   2.   Support positive self-esteem.

   3.   Explain all procedures.

   4.   Encourage peer visits.

   5.   Respect privacy and need for independence.

Additional Resources Found on MyNursingLab

- Newborn Reflexes: Stepping video
- Newborn Reflexes: Sucking video
- Infancy: A Major Life Transition video
- Communicating with Toddlers video
- Handling Temper Tantrums (video)
- Health Maintenance for School Aged Children video
- The Importance of Physical Activity video
- Teens: Mental and Spiritual Health
- Eating Disorders (video)

PEARSON

MODULE 4

Growth and Development/Nursing Care of Children

Submodule 4.2 Pediatric Disorders

Learning Objectives

4.2.1   Describe diagnostic tests, treatment, and nursing care for common respiratory disorders affecting infants and children.

4.2.2   Describe diagnostic tests, treatment, and nursing care for common gastrointestinal disorders affecting infants and children.

4.2.3   Describe the diagnostic tests, treatment, and nursing care for common hematological disorders in infants and children.

4.2.4   Describe the diagnostic tests, treatment, and nursing care for common cardiovascular disorders in infants and children.

4.2.5   Describe diagnostic tests, medical and surgical treatment, and nursing care for infants and children with endocrine disorders.

4.2.6   Describe diagnostic tests, medical and surgical treatment, and nursing care for infants and children with neurological disorders.

4.2.7   Compare diagnostic tests, symptoms, treatment, and nursing care for infants and children with common musculoskeletal disorders.

4.2.8   Compare diagnostic tests, symptoms, treatment, and nursing care for infants and children with common genitourinary disorders.

4.2.9   Describe diagnostic tests, treatment, and nursing care for common skin disorders affecting infants and children.

4.2.10 Discuss classification, estimation, treatment, and nursing care for infants and children with burn injuries.

4.2.11 Describe the diagnosis, treatment, and nursing care for common eye and ear disorders.

   I. **Respiratory System**

      A. Respiratory system diagnostic tests

         1. Character and quality of respirations

            a. Normal (*eupnea*)

            b. Rapid (*tachypnea:* > 60/min)

            c. *Hyperpnea:* deep respiration

            d. *Apnea:* cessation of respirations

         2. *Arterial blood gas (ABG):* assesses gas exchange

            a. Explain procedure to parents and child.

      b.   Apply firm pressure to puncture site after procedure.

      c.   Keep specimen on ice and transport to lab.

      d.   Assess for bleeding.

3.   *Pulmonary function test (PFT):* measures lung rate and volume

      a.   Explain procedure to parents and child.

4.   *Chest x-ray:* shows lung condition

      a.   Explain procedure to parents and child.

      b.   Hold child still during test.

5.   *Computerized axial tomography (CAT) scan:* scan provides multi-dimensional pictures.

      a.   Explain test to parents and child.

      b.   Obtain informed consent.

6.   *Magnetic resonance imaging (MRI):* helps identify obstruction and tissue perfusion.

      a.   Explain procedure to parents and child.

7.   *Sputum analysis:* detects abnormalities and allows for culture and sensitivity.

      a.   Explain procedure for collection into sterile container.

8.   *Bronchoscopy:* gives direct visualization of trachea and bronchi.

      a.   Permits collection of respiratory secretion

      b.   Explain procedure to parents and child.

      c.   Administer presedation.

      d.   Obtain informed consent.

B. Respiratory system disorders of the upper airway

   1.   **Croup:** viral infection producing spasms of larynx usually at night

      a.   Symptoms: onset usually at night and in cold weather, barking cough, hoarseness, low-grade fever, restlessness

      b.   Treatment and nursing care

          i.   Provide high humidity (run hot shower at home), oral fluids, and antipyretics (acetaminophen).

          ii.   Keep child calm to ease respirations.

          iii.   Use cool mist vaporizer in room.

          iv.   Encourage clear fluids when coughing subsides.

   2.   **Laryngotracheobronchitis** (LTB): viral or bacterial infection of larynx, trachea, and bronchi, producing inflammation, edema of a purulent exudate that obstructs the airways.

      a.   Symptoms: barking cough, hoarseness, respiratory stridor, retractions of chest wall, pallor or cyanosis, restlessness, irritability, and fever.

      b.   Treatment and nursing care: Observe respiratory effort, monitor vital signs, provide high humidity (croup tent), administer oxygen, administer IV fluids for adequate hydration, give prescribed medications (antibiotics), help reduce child's anxiety, be supportive.

3. **Epiglottitis:** acute inflammation of the epiglottis usually caused by bacterial H influenzae, pneumococci, or hemolytic beta streptococci; a prior history of a URI is very common; may lead to complete respiratory obstruction.

   a. Symptoms: sudden onset, high fever, orthopnea, excessive drooling, irritability, restlessness, wheezing, stridor, retractions of chest wall, tachycardia, and thready pulse.

   b. Treatment and nursing care: Transfer to hospital, do not examine, allow child to sit upright on parent's lap, observe closely, monitor IV fluids, reassure and support child and parents, administer antibiotics as prescribed, intubate or perform tracheostomy as necessary.

4. Acute **otitis media:** middle ear infection, which may be secondary to an upper respiratory infection, measles, or scarlet fever.

   a. Symptoms: fever, pulling ears, irritability, turning head side to side, vomiting or diarrhea, bulging eardrum that may rupture spontaneously with purulent drainage.

   b. Treatment and nursing care: Antibiotics, antipyretic therapy, analgesic, ear drops, antihistamines, decongestants, and myringotomy (surgical insertion of drainage tubes).

   c. Complications: chronic otitis media, impaired hearing or deafness

5. Upper respiratory infection or *nasopharyngitis* (common cold): causes include rhinovirus, respiratory syncytial virus (RSV), adenovirus, and influenza.

   a. Symptoms: fever, irritability, anorexia, mouth breathing, sneezing, coughing, aches, and nasal discharge.

   b. Treatment and nursing care: Antipyretics, decongestants, cough suppressants, fluids, rest, and good hygiene.

6. **Tonsillitis:** inflammation of tonsils; causes include beta-hemolytic streptococci, other bacterial infections, viruses, recurrent tonsillitis, peritonsillar abscess.

   a. Symptoms: enlarged cervical nodes, fever, hypertrophy of tonsils, and difficulty swallowing and breathing.

   b. Indications for tonsillectomy: recurrent tonsillitis, peritonsillar abscess, enlarged cervical nodes, hypertrophy of tonsils, and difficulty swallowing and breathing.

   c. Indications for adenoidectomy: chronic otitis media, impaired persistent rhinitis, voice alteration, hypertrophy of adenoids, persistent mouth breathing, and excessive snoring.

   d. Postoperative care: position semiprone with head turned to side until alert; observe for signs of hemorrhage; administer ice collar, cool liquids, mouth rinses, and analgesic (no aspirin); ensure rest for a few days.

C. Respiratory system disorders of the lower airway

1. **Bronchiolitis:** acute interstitial pneumonia caused by respiratory syncytial virus (RSV) and other viruses.

   a. Prevalence: caused by viral infection during first 6 months and up to 2 years of age during winter and spring months.

   b. Symptoms: coryza, tachypnea, intercostal and suprasternal retractions, dry cough, fever cyanosis, dehydration, restlessness, and irritability.

   c.   Treatment and nursing care: elevation of head and chest, high humidity with oxygen (croup), hydration with IV or oral fluids, antibiotic therapy to control secondary bacterial infection, maintenance of open nasal airway.

   d.   Complications: cardiac failure, respiratory failure, severe dehydration, and bacterial bronchopneumonia.

2.   Bacterial **pneumonia** (pneumonococcal is most common): infection in lungs

   a.   Prevalence: birth to 4 years in winter and spring.

   b.   Symptoms: mild upper respiratory infection with sudden refusal to eat, vomiting, diarrhea, respiratory distress, and high fever.

   c.   Treatment and nursing care: antibiotic therapy (penicillin G), fluids, antipyretics, high humidity with oxygen, respiratory therapy; position for comfort, and monitor vital signs and I and O.

3.   **Asthma:** an allergic response to allergens, causing smooth muscle of bronchi and bronchioles to go into spasm with mucosa, and an increase of mucus.

   a.   Prevalence: infants with infantile eczema may develop asthma later, 3 years or older, may disappear with puberty.

   b.   Symptoms: abrupt hacking cough, wheezing, difficulty breathing on exhalation, and coughing up thick mucus; attacks occur at night and may last for a short time or several days.

   c.   Treatment and nursing care: determine allergens with skin tests and eliminate them; advise to avoid emotional situations; administer antihistamines and corticosteroid bronchodilators during an attack, such as epinephrine, ephedrine, pseudoephedrine, or aminophylline; administer humidified oxygen, expectorant, and antibiotics for an infection; increase fluids; and teach breathing exercises.

4.   **Cystic fibrosis:** a disorder of the exocrine glands affecting many organs of the body.

   a.   Incidence: inherited as a recessive trait; occurs 1:2000 live births.

   b.   Symptoms: meconium ileus in newborns; cough; wheezing; recurrent bronchial infections; malnutrition; frequent, bulky, foul smelling stools; distended abdomen; flabby muscles, and a salty taste when skin is kissed.

   c.   Diagnosis: family history, elevated sodium chloride level in sweat, x-ray findings, absent pancreatic enzymes, lowered trypsin in stool, and a positive Dipstix test for increased protein content of meconium in a newborn.

   d.   Treatment and nursing care: increased protein, salt, and caloric intake with decreased fat intake; water soluble vitamins; pancreatic enzyme supplement given with meals and snacks: prevention and control of pulmonary infection; and cupping, clapping, and postural drainage with aerosol therapy.

   e.   Complications: respiratory infections, pancreatic fibrosis, biliary cirrhosis, sinusitis, heat and prostration.

5.   **Sudden infant death syndrome (SIDS** or crib death): sudden unexpected death of infant

   a.   Prevalence: under 6 months of age, during night, and mainly in winter months.

   b.   No known cause; many theories such as low maternal age, maternal cigarette smoking, or low birth weight; postmortem examination fails to show cause of death; offer bereavement counseling and emotional support.

II. Gastrointestinal System

A. Diagnostic tests

1. *Upper GI imaging:* barium swallow outlines stomach and small intestine.

   a. NPO after midnight.

   b. Explain procedure to parents and child.

   c. Help hold child still if needed.

   d. Monitor bowel movements after test.

   e. Shield genitals with lead apron.

2. *Barium enema* (lower GI series): allows visualization of the colon.

   a. Liquid diet 24 hours prior.

   b. Bowel prep before.

   c. Explain procedure to parents and child.

   d. Shield genitals with lead apron.

3. *Stool specimen:* tests for GI bleeding, infection parasites, and fat.

   a. Explain procedure to parents and child.

   b. Collect specimen in proper container and transport promptly to lab.

4. Scopes

   a. *Endoscopy* (visualization of esophagus, stomach, and duodenum)

   b. *Proctosigmoidoscopy* (inspection of the rectum and sigmoid colon)

   c. *Colonoscopy* (inspection of descending, transverse, and ascending colon)

   d. Obtain informed consent.

   e. Explain procedure to parents and child.

   f. Liquid diet 24 hours prior.

   g. NPO after midnight.

   h. Bowel prep before.

5. *Gastrointestinal intubation:* to decompress stomach before or after surgery, to administer feedings and or medications, and to diagnose and treat.

   a. Maintain careful I & O records.

   b. Monitor electrolytes.

   c. Measure and observe gastric drainage.

   d. Provide good oral care.

B. Gastrointestinal disorders

1. **Colic:** intermittent abdominal distress caused by immature GI tract.

   a. Prevalence: first 3 months in early evening and night.

   b. Symptoms: cries, draws legs up on abdomen, clenches fists, passes gas by mouth or rectum, and abdomen is tense and distended.

   c. Treatment and nursing care: anticolic bottles and nipples, formula change, antispasmodics, tranquilizers, and proper feeding and burping technique.

PEARSON

2. Vomiting and diarrhea

   a. Symptoms: may cause electrolyte imbalance and dehydration, and may be accompanied by fever.

   b. Treatment and nursing care: Record number, amount, and character of vomitus, stools, and urine; monitor temperature, skin condition, weight, and state of activity; fluid and electrolyte replacement; special mouth care; no rectal temperatures; isolation until cause of diarrhea determined.

3. Congenital hypertrophic **pyloric stenosis:** hypertrophy of pyloric sphincter muscle, causing partial or total obstruction of stomach exit.

   a. Symptoms: projectile vomiting when infant is 2 or 3 weeks of age, constant hunger, dehydration, failure to gain weight, constipation, decreased urinary output, palpable mass over pylorus, and visible left to right peristaltic waves.

   b. Treatment and nursing care: surgical enlargement of pyloric muscle (*pyloromyotomy*).

   c. Preoperative nursing care: intravenous fluids; small, frequent, thickened feedings; frequent burping; and upright positioning on right side.

   d. Postoperative nursing care: give small amounts of liquids first, position upright during feedings and upright right side after feeding, maintain I & O records, and keep incision clean and dry.

4. **Intussusception:** telescoping of portion of intestine into adjacent distal section of intestine.

   a. Prevalence: ages 4 months to 10 months; more frequent in boys

   b. Symptoms: sudden intermittent abdominal pain; "current jelly-like" stools with increasing absence of stools, vomiting, abdominal distention, symptoms of shock, dehydration, fever.

   c. Treatment and nursing care: emergency reduction of telescoped bowel by barium enema or surgical reduction, or gastric decompression. Prepare for barium enema; monitor I & O, vital signs, bowel sounds, and incision for signs of infection or inflammation.

5. **Hirschsprung's disease** (congenital megacolon): absence of parasympathetic ganglion nerve cells within wall of distal colon and rectum.

   a. Symptoms: no meconium stools, "currant jelly stools," bile stained emesis, abdominal distention, and constipation with overflow diarrhea,

   b. Treatment and nursing care: initially barium enema, if necessary a temporary colostomy and resection of involved colon, careful I & O, monitor vital signs and return of bowel signs, administer medications as ordered, and provide emotional support to parents and child.

6. **Meconium ileus:** obstruction of small intestine by exceptionally thick meconium, often indicative of cystic fibrosis or an imperforate anus.

   a. Symptoms: bile-stained emesis, abdominal distention, absence of meconium stool, and possible intestinal perforation.

   b. Treatment and nursing care: special enemas, intravenous replacement fluids, and oral administration of pancreatic enzyme; or surgical resection of intestine with temporary ileostomy.

7. **Cleft lip and palate:** failure of bone and tissue of upper lip and palate to fuse at midline; inherited and congenital; partial or complete, unilateral or bilateral; single disorder or both at same time.

    a. Symptoms: difficulty sucking and feeding; swallows a lot of air, causing distention; respiratory distress; choking episodes during feeding; and high risk for aspiration.

    b. Treatment and nursing care: lip repair

        i. Surgical repair at a few weeks of age (10 weeks or 10 lb).

        ii. Preoperative nursing care: feed in upright position, use special nipple, and offer emotional support to parents.

        iii. Postoperative nursing care: Logan bow, use of elbow restraints, no crying or sucking permitted, medicine dropper or syringe for feeding on unaffected side, side lying position in recovery room to prevent aspiration.

    c. Treatment and nursing care: palate repair at about 18 months of age.

        i. Preoperative nursing care: special feeders and nipples, use of an obturator.

        ii. Postoperative nursing care: prone or side lying position in recovery room to prevent aspiration, feeding with large spoon to prevent damage to repaired palate, elbow restraints, mouth care after feedings.

        iii. Potential problems: speech, hearing, tooth misalignment, and frequent otitis media

8. **Celiac disease:** inability to tolerate dietary wheat and rye gluten (gluten-induced enteropathy).

    a. Symptoms: chronic diarrhea with bulky, greasy, foul-smelling stools; progressive malnutrition; anorexia; irritability; frequent respiratory infections; distended abdomen; muscle wastage.

    b. Treatment and nursing care: gluten-free diet, supplemental vitamins and minerals, stool monitoring, emotional support for parents and child.

9. **Hernia:** protrusion of part of bowel through a weakened area in the abdominal wall.

    a. Types: inguinal and umbilical.

    b. Prevalence: more frequent in boys.

    c. Symptoms: palpable or visible lump in involved area

    d. Treatment and nursing care: may heal spontaneously, surgical hernia repair (herniorrhaphy), sterile dressing for 24 hours postoperatively for inguinal herniorrhaphy.

    e. Complications: incarceration or strangulation of bowel.

10. **Phenylketonuria** (PKU): faulty metabolism of phenylalanine, an amino acid found in protein foods; also caused by a missing hepatic enzyme, phenylalanine hydroxylase; failure to treat condition leads to brain damage and mental retardation.

    a. Symptoms: brain damage and mental retardation caused by high level of phenylalanine in blood and phenylpyruvic acid in urine between 2 and 6 weeks of age.

    b. Treatment and nursing care: Blood test done on third or fourth day of life; low phenylalanine diet with a special formula and synthetic protein foods.

III. Hematological System

A. Diagnostic tests

1. Blood typing: explain procedure to parents and child, handle sample carefully, and observe site for bleeding.

2. Coagulation studies: to analyze clotting bleeding times, platelet count, PT and PTT. Monitor lab and drug therapy, and observe for bleeding.

B. Hematological disorders

1. **Iron deficiency anemia:** red blood cells are smaller than normal and deficient in hemoglobin.

   a. Prevalence: children under 3 years and adolescent girls

   b. Symptoms: pallor, irritability, anorexia, listlessness, and low hemoglobin and hematocrit levels.

   c. Treatment and nursing care: iron fortified formula; oral administration of iron preparation; diet of iron rich foods, and IM injections of iron dextran complex in severe cases.

2. **Hemophilia:** a hereditary coagulation disorder characterized by a disturbance of blood clotting factors; appears in males, but is transmitted by females as a recessive sex-linked characteristic.

   a. Diagnosis: when child begins to crawl or walk, clotting time and partial thromboplastin time (PTT) are prolonged.

   b. Types of hemophilia and involved clotting factors: hemophilia A (classic) involves Factor VIII; hemophilia B (Christmas) involves Factor IX; hemophilia C (von Willebrand) involves Factor XI.

   b. Symptoms: prone to bruising and prolonged bleeding following injury; soft tissue hematomas, hematuria, anemia, and GI bleeding; bleeding into joints causes pain, swelling, and limited motion; and repeated hemorrhages cause deformity.

   d. Treatment and nursing care: for prevention, guard against injuries, pad toys and other objects, and administer deficient factors; for hemophilia C, fresh frozen plasma or whole blood for severe hemorrhage, direct pressure and cold compresses on bleeding areas, fibrin foam in wound, analgesics (no aspirin), bed cradle, ice packs, and joint immobilization for hemarthrosis with passive range of motion after bleeding subsides to prevent deformities, high protein diet, iron, and vitamin C with protein snacks; avoid injections.

3. **Idiopathic thrombocytopenic purpura** (ITP): caused by destruction of platelets in the spleen; an autoimmune disorder caused by a virus or by drugs

   a. Thrombocytopenic purpura is caused by failure of the bone marrow to produce platelets.

   b. Diagnosis: low platelet count, prolonged bleeding time, impaired clotting time, and positive capillary fragility test.

   c. Symptoms: petechiae and ecchymosis, anemia, internal and external bleeding, and enlarged spleen; remission and relapses are common.

   d. Treatment and nursing care: corticosteroids to reduce bleeding, whole blood and platelet transfusions, iron administration of anemia, splenectomy to elevate platelet level, chemotherapy for those who do not respond to corticosteroids or splenectomy; avoid trauma and aspirin; bed rest during active bleeding.

4. **Sickle cell anemia:** a hereditary form of hemolytic anemia occurring mainly in blacks.

   a. Low concentration of oxygen causes RBCs to become sickle-shaped and die quickly when the abnormal hemoglobin molecule hemoglobin S is present.

   b. Diagnosis: sickle cell prep, sickledex, hemoglobin, and electrophoresis.

   c. Symptoms: anemia; sickle cells block blood vessels causing severe pain in organs and bones; sickle cell crisis occurs when oxygen need is increased by cold, emotional stress, or infection.

   d. Treatment and nursing care (no cure): avoid factors that increase need for oxygen; advise genetic counseling for prevention and detection, bed rest, increased fluids, analgesics, oxygen, steroid therapy, good skin care, and blood transfusions during crisis, general health maintenance, and stress avoidance.

5. **Leukemia:** neoplastic disease of blood-forming tissues with an increase in immature leukocytes and a decrease in erythrocytes, hemoglobin, and platelets, resulting in anemia and bleeding; peak age 2-5 years.

   a. Exact cause unknown, causative factors believed to be radiation, certain chemicals, certain viruses, and familial tendency.

   b. Classified according to:

      i. Maturity of cells - acute and chronic

      ii. Type of WBC - lymphocytic, granulocytic, and monocytic.

   c. Diagnosis: CBC, bone marrow biopsy and lymph node biopsy, chest and skull x-rays.

   d. Acute lymphocytic leukemia (ALL): a rapidly progressive disease affecting mainly children and young adults involving immature cells (blasts).

   e. Symptoms: sudden onset coinciding with acute upper respiratory infection; bleeding tendency involving nose, mouth, stomach, rectum, urinary tract, petechiae, and purpura; dyspnea; fatigue; tachycardia; weight loss; malaise; fever; sweating; heat intolerance; pallor; joint and bone pain; anemia; uric acid stone; prone to infections; and enlarged lymph nodes and spleen.

   f. Treatment and nursing care: supportive measures aimed at limiting complications; chemotherapy to induce remission; radiation and immunotherapy; transfusions of platelets, packed RBC s and WBCs; antibiotics to control infection; special mouth care; soft diet; force fluids; hypothermia measures; analgesics; tranquilizers; antiemetics; bone marrow transplants; observe for signs of infection and side effects of chemotherapy and radiation; offer emotional support; teach and practice good hygiene; handle with care to limit painful episodes.

IV. **Cardiovascular System**

   A. Diagnostic tests

   1. *Electrocardiography* (ECG): detects injury, conduction delays, arrhythmias, ischemia and necrosis. Explain procedure to parents and child.

   2. *Chest x-ray:* provides size and shape of heart, and pulmonary circulation. Explain procedure to parents and child.

   3. Echocardiography: evaluates cardiac structures and functions. Explain procedure to parents and child.

4. *Cardiac catheterization:* evaluates functions, heart pressure, and oxygen saturation. Explain procedure to parents and child; monitor vital signs and I & O; observe for bleeding from site after test.

B. Cardiovascular disorders

1. Acyanotic heart defects

   a. **Patent ductus arteriosus** (PDA): opening between aorta and pulmonary artery remains after birth.

      i. Symptoms: pale skin, slow weight gain, feeding problems, frequent respiratory infections.

      ii. Treatment and nursing care: pharmacological treatment with diuretics; use of Indomethacin to help close defect or surgery to ligate defect. Explain plan of care to parents, monitor vital signs, pulse oximetry, I & O and daily weights, provide rest to reduce cardiac demands, and keep head of bed elevated to ease breathing efforts.

   b. **Pulmonary stenosis:** obstruction of blood flow from the right ventricle at the pulmonary valve

      i. Symptoms: usually asymptomatic, but may have decreased exercise tolerance, dyspnea, or precordial pain.

      ii. Treatment and nursing care: surgical valvulotomy. Explain all procedures and treatment to parents; monitor vital signs, pulse oximetry, I & O, and daily weights; provide rest to reduce cardiac demands; and keep head of bed elevated to ease breathing efforts.

   c. **Aortic stenosis:** obstruction of blood flow from the left ventricle at the aortic valve.

      i. Symptoms: chest pain, systolic murmur, syncope dyspnea, fatigue, narrow pulse pressure, weak pulse or CHF, poor feeding.

      ii. Treatment and nursing care: aortic valvulotomy or valve replacement, digoxin and diuretics for signs of heart failure, anticoagulant therapy to prevent clot formation, prophylactic use of antibiotics to prevent bacterial endocarditis. Explain all procedures and treatment to parents; monitor vital signs, pulse oximetry, I & O, and daily weights; provide rest to reduce cardiac demands; and keep head of bed elevated to ease breathing efforts.

2. Cyanotic defects

   a. **Tetralogy of Fallot** is four defects: pulmonary stenosis, ventricular septal defect, hypertrophy of right ventricle, overriding aorta (aorta straddles the ventricular septal defect).

      i. Symptoms: cyanosis, feeding problems, poor weight gain, slow growth and development, dyspnea, fatigability, clubbing of fingers and toes, squatting, and anemia.

      ii. Treatment and nursing care: palliative with Blalock-Taussig shunt, total correction between 3 and 5 years of age, digoxin and diuretics for signs of heart failure, anticoagulant therapy to prevent clot formation, prophylactic use of antibiotics to prevent bacterial endocarditis. Explain all procedures and treatment to parents; monitor vital signs, pulse oximetry, I & O, and daily weights; rest to reduce cardiac demands and keep head of bed elevated to ease breathing efforts.

PEARSON

3. Acute **rheumatic fever**: a systemic disease affecting connective tissue and endothelial tissue; sequela to group A beta-hemolytic streptococcal infection.

    a. Prevalence: peak between ages 5 and 15; high family incidence; more common in winter and spring.

    b. Symptoms: range from mild to severe, affecting different body organs

        i. **Polyarthritis** (migratory, hot, swollen, tender enlarged joints)

        ii. **Carditis** (murmurs, rapid and irregular pulse, pericarditis, cardiac enlargement, or CHF)

        iii. **Chorea** (purposeless, involuntary, rapid movements associated with muscle weakness)

        iv. **Erythema marginatum** (irregular red rash on trunk and extremities)

        v. Painless subcutaneous nodules over joints of knees, elbows, wrists, occiput, knuckles, and spine; fever; fatigue; abdominal pain; epistaxis; and anemia

    c. Diagnosis: Jones criteria: fever, arthralgia, ECG changes, elevated sedimentation rate, and c-reactive protein.

    d. Treatment and nursing care: penicillin, erythromycin, or sulfonamides; aspirin to control joint pain and lower fever; steroid therapy to prevent permanent heart damage; bed rest for 4 to 12 weeks; careful positioning; good skin care; protect from infections; emotional support; passive diversions; and prophylactic antimicrobial therapy indefinitely.

V. Endocrine System

  A. Diagnostic tests

    1. Endocrine function studies: measures hormone levels and their effectiveness

    2. Radioimmunoassay: measures minute amounts of hormones

  B. Endocrine disorders

    1. Type I diabetes mellitus

      a. Juvenile diabetes

        i. Chronic systemic disorder

        ii. Always insulin dependent

        iii. Rapid onset, usually low weight

        iv. No insulin produced: cells unable to utilize glucose, glucose spills into urine.

        v. Signs of **polyuria** (excess urination), **polydipsia** (excessive thirst), and **polyphagia** (excessive hunger)

        vi. Usually 7-13 years at onset

        vii. Observe for weakness, fatigue, headache, nausea/vomiting, and abdominal cramps.

        viii. Urine testing taught 6-7 years of age: use dipstick Clinitest, (Accu-Chek, Accu Test Strips, or other).

        ix. Insulin self-administration taught usually after 7 years of age.

        x. Normal blood glucose 80-120.

b. Signs of **hyperglycemia** (high blood glucose): dry, flushed skin; general malaise; nausea/vomiting; abdominal pain; apple breath; red lips; dehydration; and sunken eyes.

c. Causes of hyperglycemia: infection, overeating, stress, or insulin overdose.

d. Treatment and nursing care: regular insulin and fluid and electrolyte replacement; provide client/family teaching.

e. **Hypoglycemia** (low blood glucose) causes: excessive exercising, eating too little or too late, vomiting, insulin under-dosage.

   i. Signs: fatigue, weakness; personality changes; hunger; pale, clammy skin; diaphoresis; lethargy; tremors; convulsions; loss of consciousness; and death.

   ii. Treatments

     (a) Conscious client: oral carbohydrate (CHO), orange juice, and sugar

     (b) Unconscious client: IM or SQ glucagon, or IV glucose.

f. Insulins:

   i. Regular (clear, short-acting): onset 30 minutes, peaks 2-4 hours

   ii. NPH (cloudy, intermediate-acting)

     (a) May mix both above, but draw up clear (regular) first.

     (b) Do not shake vials.

     (c) Rotate injection site to prevent lipodystrophy.

     (d) Remind child to eat before peak time.

2. **Tay-Sachs disorder:** an inherited abnormal gene causes the lack of an enzyme that breaks down fatty material in the brain.

a. Symptoms: between 3-6 months muscle weakness appears progressing to paralysis.

b. Treatment and nursing care: supportive and palliative care for infant and family.

3. Hypothyroidism may be congenital, causing a lack of thyroid hormone.

a. Symptoms: appear after few months, include lethargy, jaundice, feeding problems, and hypotonia.

b. Treatment and nursing care: thyroid hormone replacement and client/family teaching

VI. Neurological System

A. Diagnostic tests

1. Computerized tomography (CT) scan: produces a multidimensional image with or without contrast. Explain procedure to parents and child, obtain informed consent, assist child to remain still during test, and check for allergies to contrast medium.

2. Magnetic resonance imaging (MRI): allows for great detail of images. Explain procedure to parents and child, obtain informed consent, assist child to remain still during test, and alert radiology if child has any metal objects or implants (i.e. pins, screws).

3. *Electroencephalography* (EEG): shows electrical brain activity, test is noninvasive. Explain procedure to parents and child, and assist child to remain still during test.

4. *Ultrasonography:* uses sound waves to detect abnormalities in blood flow, and/or lesions. Explain procedure to parents and child, and assist child to remain still during test.

5. *Lumbar puncture:* cerebral spinal fluid is aspirated from the sub-arachnoid space in the lumbar region for analysis. CSF pressure can be measured. Obtain informed consent prior to test, hold child still in side-lying or knee-chest position. Explain procedure to parents and child.

6. *ICP monitoring:* directly measures intracranial pressure. Obtain informed consent prior to test and explain procedure to parents and child.

7. *Cerebral angiography:* Using the femoral artery, radiopaque dye is injected, allowing for visualization of the cerebral vessels. Explain procedure to parents and child, obtain informed consent prior to test, check for allergies to dye, assist child to remain still during test, monitor pulses, and monitor for bleeding after test.

8. *Electromyography:* detects neuromuscular disorders, nerve damage, and motor neuron defects. Explain procedure to parents and child, obtain informed consent prior to test, assist child to remain still during test, and monitor for bleeding after test.

9. Eye examinations: allow for visualization of the internal structures and detect certain disorders. Explain procedure to parents and child.

10. Ear examinations: allow for visualization of the internal structures, and may determine hearing acuity. Otoscope is used. In small child (under 3), pinna is pulled down and back; in an older child, pinna is pulled up to straighten ear canal. Explain procedure to parents and child.

B. Neurological disorders

1. **Hydrocephalus:** increased cerebrospinal fluid in ventricles of brain, resulting in enlargement of the head and pressure changes in the brain; may be communicating or noncommunicating.

   a. Symptoms: enlargement of head, symptoms of increased intracranial pressure, strabismus, "sunset eyes," delayed closure of anterior fontanel, poor muscle tone of extremities, prominent forehead, shiny scalp with prominent scalp veins, helplessness, and lethargy.

   b. Treatment and nursing care: measure head circumference daily; give small, frequent feedings; support head and turn frequently; surgical insertion of ventriculoperitoneal or ventriculoatrial shunt; observe for increased intracranial pressure, dehydration, and infection; teach care to parents and offer emotional support.

2. **Spina bifida:** imperfect closure of spinal vertebrae

   a. *Spina bifida occulta:* imperfect closure of spinal canal without involvement of spinal cord and meninges; discovered by x-ray; no treatment needed.

   b. **Meningocele:** meninges protrude through opening in spinal canal forming a sac filled with cerebrospinal fluid.

   c. *Meningomyelocele (myelomeningocele):* protrusion of meninges and spinal cord through opening in spinal canal; causes incontinence, partial or complete lower extremity paralysis and sensory disturbance; frequently accompanied by hydrocephalus.

   d. Preoperative treatment and nursing care: prevent sac from injury and infection, position on side or abdomen, use care in lifting, good skin care, adequate nutrition; observe sac, measure head frequently; surgical correction within first 24 hours of life; offer emotional support to parents.

    e.   Postoperative treatment and nursing care: position on abdomen until incision is healed; rehabilitation includes ambulation, bladder and bowel management, emotional support, and encouragement for family.

3. **Cerebral palsy:** nonprogressive disorder of motor centers and nerve pathways.

    a.   Incidence: 1-3:1000 persons; caused by prenatal infections or anoxia before or during birth, by trauma, or by infections of central nervous system.

    b.   Types: may be mild, moderate, or severe.

        i.   *Spastic CP:* increased muscle stiffness, stretch reflex, jerky motions and contractures, and scissors gait.

        ii.   *Athetoid CP:* involuntary, uncoordinated, purposeless movements.

        iii.   *Ataxic CP:* loss of sense of balance and difficulty with spatial relationships.

        iv   Mixed types: one type usually predominates.

    c.   Symptoms: involuntary muscle movements may include seizures, possible mental retardation, behavior problems, special sensory defects, and speech and eating difficulties.

    d.   Treatment and nursing care: aimed at limiting disability and making the most of remaining abilities. Drug therapy includes muscle relaxants and anticonvulsants; physical, speech and occupational therapy; orthopedic surgery; special braces, appliances, and feeding aids; and special education classes. Offer high-calorie diet to help meet demands. Teach ROM exercises to limit contractures. Provide activities that stimulate growth and development. Provide a safe environment, and help family establish realistic goals.

4. Seizure disorders

    a.   *Epilepsy*: chronic, recurrent, idiopathic, convulsive disorder

        i.   Incidence: 1% of population has seizure disorders.

            (a) Grand mal: 50% of seizure disorders

            (b) Petit mal: 10% of disorders

            (c) Mixed: 20% of disorders

        ii.   Unknown cause, possibly genetic defects; onset between 4 and 8 years of age.

        iii.   Classifications and symptoms:

            (a) *Grand mal epilepsy:* may be preceded by aura and loss of consciousness; involuntary movements of eyeball; generalized tonic and clonic movements; may bite tongue, be incontinent, and drool; duration varies; clonic movements followed by relaxation, then drowsiness or stupor.

            (b) *Petit mal epilepsy:* lasts less than 30 seconds and can include loss of consciousness, staring gaze; may have rolling eyes or slight body tremors, no recollection of seizure; frequency of one or two each month to several hundred daily; may disappear at puberty or develop into grand mal attacks.

            (c) *Focal (Jacksonian) seizure:* may be motor or sensory, of brief duration, involuntary unilateral movements in one area progressing to adjacent areas, possible disturbance of consciousness, may lead to grand mal.

> (d) *Psychomotor seizures:* coordinated and repetitive but inappropriate movements, seizure of brief duration, possible disturbance of consciousness, possible confusion or drowsiness afterward.
>
> (e) *Akinetic seizures:* brief loss of consciousness and muscle tone, but no tonic or clonic movements; possible drowsiness after attack.
>
> (f) *Status epilepticus:* series of grand mal seizures without regaining consciousness; may result in brain damage; treated as a medical emergency.

iv. Diagnosis: history and EEG

v. Observe and record seizure:

> (a) Onset time and behavior before seizure
>
> (b) Site where seizure began and ended
>
> (c) Areas of body involved, progression, eye position, and types of movement
>
> (d) Incontinence, amount of perspiration, respiratory changes, color, drooling, and degree of consciousness
>
> (e) Length of seizure and behavior after seizure

vi. Treatment and nursing care: anticonvulsant drug therapy depending on seizure type. Phenobarbital (Luminal), phenytoin (Dilantin), ethosuximide (Zarontin), and diazepam (Valium); caregiver must know side effects for the above drugs.

b. *Febrile convulsions:* generalized seizures occurring early in the course of fever.

i. Symptoms: body stiffness, loss of consciousness, clonic movements, irregular breathing, and inability to swallow saliva.

ii. Treatment and nursing care: Reduce fever, turn head to side to prevent aspiration during seizure, suction mouth, and pad crib sides to prevent injury.

5. Head injuries

a. Type: may be concussion or skull fracture.

b. Symptoms: headache, drowsiness, anorexia, blurred vision, vomiting, or unconsciousness

c. Treatment and nursing care: observe for signs of increased intracranial pressure; observe head size and tension of fontanels; assess reflexes; offer teaching and emotional support.

6. *Down syndrome (mongolism):* congenital defect of embryo caused by chromosomal abnormality.

a. Symptoms: small head; low ears; upward-outward slanted eyes; short, flattened bridge of nose; thick, fissured, and protruding tongue; short hands with incurved fifth finger and single palmar crease; wide space between first and second toes; lax muscle tone and loose joints; coarse, dry hair; slow development; mental retardation with mean IQ of 50; poor resistance to infection; and other congenital anomalies.

b. Treatment and nursing care: maintain adequate nutrition, provide safe environment, observe for signs of physical complications, provide stimulation to help development of potential, encourage parental acceptance, and offer teaching and emotional support.

VII. Musculoskeletal System

A. Diagnostic tests

1. Computerized tomography (CT) scan: produces a multidimensional image with or without contrast. Explain procedure to parents and child, obtain informed consent, assist child to remain still during test, and check for allergies to contrast medium.

2. Magnetic resonance imaging (MRI): allows for great detail of images. Explain procedure to parents and child, obtain informed consent, assist child to remain still during test, and alert radiology if child has any metal objects or implants (i.e. pins, screws).

3. *Myelography:* invasive procedure in which dye is injected to detect spinal cord abnormalities. Explain procedure to parents and child, obtain informed consent, assist child to remain still during test, and check for allergies to contrast medium. Child may feel a warm, burning sensation during test. After test, instruct to lie still with head elevated, encourage fluids, and check for voiding.

4. *Arthroscopy:* visually examines internal joint cavity. Explain procedure to parents and child, obtain written consent, note allergies, possible NPO after midnight.

5. X-rays: detect fractures, bone deformities, calcifications, density and joint problems. Explain procedure to family and child, provide lead apron for genital area, help hold child still if necessary.

B. Musculoskeletal disorders

1. **Clubfoot** (talipes equinovarus): unilateral or bilateral turning of the foot inward and downward with heel drawn up.

   a. Treatment and nursing care: manipulation by stretching exercises for flexible type. Adhesive strapping and manipulation exercises: Denis Browne splint, abduction bar, and foot plates. Manipulation and casting: cast changes frequently until deformity corrected, then cast in overcorrected position; surgical correction of tendons and bones followed by casts, special shoes, and exercises. Assess for pulses and circulation; movement, color, and temperature in distal areas. Provide good skin care. Help parents and child adjust to immobility.

2. Congenital dislocation of hip (*hip dysplasia*): partial or complete displacement of head of femur from hip socket (acetabulum).

   a. Symptoms: asymmetry of gluteal skin fold with deeper creases on affected side, limited abduction of affected hip, shortened extremity, delayed walking, and limp.

   b. Treatment and nursing care: Splint brace or harness worn continuously in some cases, Bryant traction used in some, placing both legs in traction for babies under 3 years or 35 lbs; others have closed reduction under general anesthesia, followed by the use of a hip spica cast with an abduction bar. Assess for pulses, circulation, movement, color, and temperature in distal areas. Provide good skin care. Help parents and child adjust to immobility.

3. *Juvenile rheumatoid arthritis* (JRA) or Still's disease

   a. Prevalence: onset between 1 and 6 years of age, females more often affected, aggravated by emotional stress and fatigue.

   b. Symptoms: painful joint movement; subcutaneous nodules; growth retardation; intermittent fever (high in evening, normal in morning); irritability; rash; enlargement of liver, spleen, and lymph nodes; anemia; anorexia; and pallor.

c. Treatment and nursing care: Heat therapy, warm compresses, splints used to prevent contractures, aspirin to relieve pain and reduce swelling, joint exercise to prevent ankylosis, steroid therapy for severe systemic disease; provide limited activities followed by rest periods. Help parents and child adjust to limitations.

4. *Duchenne's muscular dystrophy*: inherited group of diseases that cause muscle degeneration and wasting

   a. Incidence: onset within first three years of life; affects 1:10,000 males; hereditary, sex-linked, recessive condition; life expectancy limited to teenage period.

   b. Symptoms: difficulty in walking, owing to muscle weakness; Gower's sign (self-climbing procedure when rising from seated to standing position); cardiac and or pulmonary failure.

   c. Treatment and nursing care: keep child ambulatory as long as possible; ROM exercises to maintain mobility; orthopedic appliances such as splints, braces, high top sneakers, or the use of a foot board to prevent foot drop; supportive treatment; offer family counseling and support.

5. Structural *scoliosis*: lateral curvature of spine, which may be congenital, postural, or idiopathic

   a. Incidence: 80% of cases are idiopathic; more common in girls.

   b. Symptoms: poor posture, uneven shoulder height, one hip more prominent, crooked neck, lump on back, waistline and hemline uneven, back pain, one breast appears larger, and fatigue

   c. Treatment and nursing care: Milwaukee brace worn 16 to 23 hours a day plus exercises; casts; Cotrel or halo traction; surgical Harrington instrumentation and posterior spinal fusion with plaster of Paris jacket for 6 weeks to 1 year, or surgical Dwyer instrumentation and anterior spinal fusion with plaster of Paris jacket for 3 to 4 months; log-roll turning postoperatively to prevent injury and damage; monitor vital signs; maintain correct body alignment; teach stretching exercises when capable; check for skin breakdown; promote positive self-esteem.

6. *Legg-Calve-Perthes disease:* a self-limiting form of necrosis to the femoral head. Eventually necrotic tissue is reabsorbed and replaced with healthy granulation tissue.

   a. Symptoms: hip pain, which worsens with activity, leading to decreased mobility and muscle wasting.

   b. Treatment and nursing care: Aimed at reducing the pain and discomfort. Braces are used to limit mobility. Caregivers are to be taught how to apply braces and to monitor for skin breakdown. Offer family counseling and support.

7. Cast care (review fractures in the Musculoskeletal System portion of the Medical Surgical module)

   a. Chemical changes in cast while drying causes discomfort to child.

   b. Expose wet cast to air to hasten drying.

   c. Turn and change positions frequently using palms rather than fingers to hold cast.

   d. Assess skin circulation: note color, temperature, edema, capillary refill, and mobility.

   e. Note any drainage or odor from cast.

   f. Prevent objects from being inserted into cast.

      g.   Do not use powder on skin near cast.

      h.   Petal edges of cast to keep cast dry.

      i.   Hip spica cast: a body cast extending from mid-chest to legs; legs are abducted with a bar between them.

         i.   Never lift or turn child with abduction bar.

         ii.   Perform cast care as listed above, but with additional measures: check respirations.

         iii.   Line the back of the cast with plastic or other waterproof material.

         iv.   Keep cast level, but on a slant, with the head of bed raised so that urine and stool will drain downward.

         v.   Use mattress firm enough to support cast, and pillows to support parts of cast if needed.

         vi.   Reposition child frequently to avoid pressure on skin and bony prominences; check for pressure as child grows.

    8.   Traction: general information

      a.   Traction decreases muscles spasms, and realigns and positions bone ends.

      b.   Traction pulls on the distal end of bones.

      c.   The two main types of traction are skin and skeletal: skin traction pulls indirectly on the skeleton by pulling on the skin via adhesive, moleskin, and/or an elastic bandage; skeletal traction pulls directly on the skeleton via pins or tongs.

      d.   Keeping the child in alignment can be difficult, because of increased mobility and lack of understanding of the treatment.

      e.   Weights must hang free; nurse should check for skin irritation, infection at pin sites, and neurovascular response of extremity.

      f.   Prevent constipation by increasing fluids and fiber.

      g.   Prevent respiratory congestion by promoting pulmonary hygiene using blowing games.

      h.   Provide pain reliever.

      i.   Provide developmental stimulation.

      j.   Bryant's traction

         i.   The only skin traction designed specifically for the lower extremities of children under age 2; the child is his or her own countertraction.

         ii.   Legs are kept straight and extended 90 degrees toward ceiling from the trunk; both legs are suspended even if only one is affected.

         iii.   Buttocks are kept slightly off the bed to ensure sufficient and continuous traction on the legs.

         iv.   Traction is usually followed by application of a hip spica cast.

VIII.Genitourinary System

    A.   Diagnostic tests

      1.   Urinalysis: determines characteristics, pH, specific gravity, properties, and presence of abnormal findings such as blood, bacteria, casts, and WBCs.

      2.   Blood tests: determine blood urea nitrogen (BUN), creatinine, and uric acid levels.

3. X-ray of kidneys, ureters, and bladder (*KUB*): detects size, shape, position, and condition.

4. *Cystourethrogram:* provides information about bladder and related structures during voiding. Explain procedure to parents and child, obtain informed consent, insert urinary catheter as ordered prior to start of test, and encourage fluids after catheter removal.

B. Genitourinary disorders

1. *Nephrotic syndrome:* chronic, intermittent, renal condition characterized by generalized edema (anasarca).

    a. Prevalence: between 2 and 6 years of age; more common in boys.

    b. Symptoms: edema first around eyes (periorbital edema); then involving arms, legs, abdomen, and scrotum; dyspnea; diarrhea; anorexia; irritability; fatigue; and susceptibility to infections.

    c. Treatment and nursing care: corticosteroid therapy, broad spectrum antibiotic, daily urine for protein, provide good skin care, elevate HOB to ease breathing efforts, turn and position frequently, take daily weights, carefully monitor I and O, restrict salt intake, and protect from others with infections.

2. *Acute glomerulonephritis:* inflammation of kidneys caused by allergic reaction to an infection elsewhere in the body; most frequent causative agent is group A beta hemolytic streptococci.

    a. Incidence: more common in 5 to 10 year old males in winter and spring; onset 1 to 3 weeks after initiating infection.

    b. Symptoms: decreased urine output, bloody or brown urine, periorbital edema, fever, malaise, headache, anorexia, vomiting and diarrhea, and hypertension.

    c. Treatment and nursing care: bed rest until hematuria subsides, antibiotic therapy, and hypotensive drugs; protect from fatigue and contact with persons with infections; maintain accurate intake and output and daily weight; provide liquid diet to soft to full as tolerated; read B.P. frequently; and restrict salt and protein in severe cases.

    d. Complications: hypertensive headache, drowsiness, convulsions, vomiting, CHF, uremia, and anemia.

3. *Wilms' tumor:* adenosarcoma in kidney that develops from abnormal embryonic tissue.

    a. Incidence: 10% of cancer in children; diagnosed before 3 years of age.

    b. Symptoms: mass in region of kidney, constipation, vomiting, abdominal distention, dyspnea, weight loss, pallor, and anemia.

    c. Pre operative treatment and nursing care: avoid palpating abdomen. Surgical procedure: radical nephrectomy; radiation therapy and chemotherapy to follow.

4. Acute *pyelonephritis:* urinary tract infection.

    a. Prevalence: between 2 months and 2 years of age; more frequent in girls.

    b. Symptoms: abrupt onset with fever, vomiting, diarrhea, irritability, and pus in urine.

    c. Treatment and nursing care: urine culture, and antibiotic therapy (sulfasoxazole, ampicillin, or nitrofurantoin); force fluids; encourage frequent bladder emptying; avoid bubble baths; and teach proper hygiene.

5. Undescended testicle (*cryptorchidism*)

    a. Incidence: affects 1% of male population; usually unilateral.

    b. Symptoms: tenderness in inguinal canal, possible torsion, spontaneous descent usually complete by first year.

    c. Treatment and nursing care: injections of human chorionic gonadotropin to lengthen spermatic cord, or surgical orchiopexy if medical treatment is unsuccessful; offer teaching and emotional support.

6. *Hydrocele:* accumulation of fluid within scrotum around testicle.

    a. Incidence: may accompany inguinal hernia.

    b. Symptoms: enlargement of scrotum.

    c. Treatment and nursing care: may correct itself, or surgical hydrocelectomy for chronic hydrocele.

IX. Skin (Integumentary System)

A. Diagnostic tests

    1. Microscopic examination: detects lesions and other abnormalities. Explain procedure to parents and child.

    2. *Gram stains and cultures:* identify causative organisms in underlying infections. Explain procedure to parents and child.

    3. *Patch tests:* identify allergens. Explain procedure to parents and child.

    4. *Skin biopsies:* diagnose disease. Explain procedure to parents and child, obtain informed consent, and follow prescribed treatment for biopsy site after test.

B. Skin disorders

    1. Infantile *eczema* (atopic dermatitis)

        a. Prevalence: from 2 months to 2 years; caused by allergens.

        b. Symptoms: reddened skin followed by papules and vesicles that break and weep serum that forms crusts and scales; appears first on head, neck, and extensor surfaces of arms and legs; causes intense itching and irritability.

        c. Treatment and nursing care: eliminate allergens, provide hypoallergenic diet, relief of itching and irritability, no small-pox vaccination, protection from infection, use elbow restraints to prevent scratching, and offer teaching and emotional support.

    2. *Diaper rash:* local skin irritation

        a. Causes: irritants, urine exposure, friction, and lack of air.

        b. Symptoms: erythema, maculopapular rash in diaper region, pain, and irritability.

        c. Treatment and nursing care: Keep area clean and dry, expose to air, use barrier type ointments such as zinc oxide, petroleum jelly, A and D ointment, or topical antibiotics if secondary infection occurs.

    3. Head lice (*pediculosis capitis*): caused by a parasite; commonly seen in children 3-10 years old.

        a. Symptoms: intense itching, nits may be seen attached to the hair shaft.

b. Treatment and nursing care: Shampoo with a pediculicide, followed by combing with a fine tooth comb to remove eggs (nits).

c. All bed linen, clothing, and furniture must be cleaned to prevent spread or re-infestation.

4. *Impetigo:* a superficial, highly contagious skin infection caused by streptococci or staphylococci.

   a. Symptoms: vesicles, pustules, erythema, and edema around lesion.

   b. Treatment and nursing care: Soak with medicated soap, topical anti-bacterial ointment, or systemic antibiotics for unresponsive cases; teach caregivers proper hygiene, such as to wash and separate linens.

5. *Acne vulgaris:* a common skin condition affecting adolescents.

   a. Symptoms: Hair follicles become blocked with sebum causing comedones to form. Papules, pustules and nodules may develop on face, chest, shoulders and back.

   b. Treatment and nursing care: Topical medication or systemic antibiotics may be used. Support and education on proper skin care should be offered. Teach clients to avoid picking lesions; hands should be kept away from the face.

C. Burns

1. Destruction of tissue by exposure to extreme heat, hot liquids, electrical agents, strong chemicals, or radiation

2. Burn injury is classified based on degree of tissue loss and surface area of body affected.

3. Classification

   a. Superficial partial thickness (1st degree): involves the epidermal layer.

   b. Dermal partial thickness (2nd degree): involves the epidermal and dermal layers.

   c. Full thickness (3rd degree): involves epidermal, dermal, subcutaneous layer, and nerve endings.

   d. *First degree* (superficial): erythema, edema, pain, and blanching.

   e. *Second degree* (partial): pain, oozing fluid, filled vesicles, shiny and wet appearance.

   f. *Third degree* (full): eschar, edema, but no significant pain because nerves have been destroyed

   g. Percentage of burned area based on surface area ("rule of nines")

4. Burn care stages

   a. *Emergent phase:* Objective is to stop the burning; phase lasts from first 24 hours after burn up to 3 days.

      i. Stopping different types of burns

         (a) Thermal: remove person and extinguish.

         (b) Flame: lower and log roll.

      (c) Electrical: note entry and exit sites of current.

      (d) Chemical: remove clothing, wash area profusely for 10-15 minutes, apply cold to decrease pain and create hypnotic effect, wrap in a cool moist towel or sheet, maintain airway, prevent sepsis, and transport to hospital.

  ii. Admission assessment

      (a) Assess the degree of burn.

      (b) Obtain a history: time of burn, how injury occurred, and cause.

      (c) Determine degree of burn: minor burns, less than 10% not involving face.

      (d) Assess for singed nasal hairs; soot around and in nostrils; red, swollen mouth; and dark mucous membranes.

  iii. Treatment and nursing care

      (a) Fluid loss: sudden shift of fluid from intravascular to interstitial spaces

      (b) Correct fluid loss: start IV and administer colloids

      (c) Prevent shock, which occurs in first 48 hours.

      (d) Monitor for dehydration, decreased blood pressure, or elevated pulse rate; thirst: or decreased urinary output.

      (e) Electrolyte imbalance, hyponatremia, hyperkalemia, low blood protein levels, and metabolic acidosis

      (f) Respiratory status: check for singing and soot in nasal passageways.

        (1) Maintain patent airway; intubate if needed. Suction to keep airway free.

        (2) Pulse oximetry and arterial blood gases

        (3) Oxygen administration as prescribed

        (4) Use of incentive spirometer

      (g) Pain management

      (h) Administration of tetanus toxoid prophylaxis

      (i) Wound care: cleanse and debride.

      (j) Insert Foley for hourly output; maintain minimum hourly output 30-50 mL; NPO; NG tube to suction.

      (k) To prevent paralytic ileus: antacid prophylactically. Prevent infection, which usually occurs 3 days after initial injury.

      (l) Record intake and output: physician uses this information to determine need for additional fluids.

      (m) Baseline weight and daily weight

b. *Acute phase* - Fluid shifts from interstitial back to intravascular spaces, resulting in diuresis and possible fluid overload, decreased cardiac output, and hypoproteinemia.

  i. Fluid remobilization - Maintain strict intake and output, weigh diapers.

  ii. Prevent infection: protective isolation and prophylactic antibiotic therapy maybe ordered.

PEARSON

          iii. Burn care: open or closed method

             (a) Debride wound to remove eschar.

             (b) Cover with biologic or biosynthetic skin.

          iv. Provide adequate nutrition diet.

             (a) Offer twice the amount of calories per day: high protein, high carbohydrate, and Vitamin C and additional nutritional supplements to provide healing.

          v. Prevent contracture.

             (a) Perform ROM exercise.

             (b) Mobilize once vital signs are stable and medical condition permits.

  c. *Rehabilitation phase*: Skin grafting allows wound closure; rehabilitation promotes optimal level of functioning.

          i. Promote psychological well being.

5. Complications of burns

  a. Infection of wound or respiratory tract.

  b. Contractures: may be prevented by proper positioning and adequate exercise.

  c. Loss of fluid through burn area causing shock for first 48 hours.

  d. Pulmonary changes from inhalation injury: look for singed nasal hair and soot around mouth and nostrils.

  e. Renal changes: decreased urinary output and frequent UTIs.

  f. Gastrointestinal changes: distention and paralytic ileus.

6. Methods of treating burn wounds

  a. Antimicrobials for burns: used to prevent or treat infection with either open or closed method.

  b. *Open method:* wound is thoroughly cleansed and left uncovered and exposed to air

  c. *Closed method:* wound is covered with nonadherent, absorbent dressings.

          i. Nursing precautions: guard against infection; use sterile sheets

          ii. Special unit is desirable.

  d. *Surgical method:* wound is debrided naturally, mechanically, surgically, or enzymatically.

7. *Skin graft:* Replacement of damaged skin with healthy skin to protect underlying structures

  a. Types

          i. *Split thickness graft:* half the epidermis removed by a dermatone.

          ii. *Full thickness graft:* removal of the outer epidermis.

          iii. *Pinch/insert graft:* small piece of skin removed with a needle.

  b. Sources of graft

          i. *Autograft:* uses client's own skin.

      ii.   *Allograft/homograft:* human skin, usually from a cadaver.

      iii. ***Heterograft/xenograft:*** obtained from animals such as pigs

  c. Preoperative care as usual except donor site prepared by cleansing.

  d. Postoperative care routine

      i.   Avoid weight bearing on extremity with graft site.

      ii. Elevate and immobilize graft site.

      iii. Assess site for infection, hematoma; antibiotic as prescribed.

      iv. Keep donor site clean and open to air.

      v. Prevent damage or pressure.

      vi. Protect from direct sunlight.

X. Special Senses

A. Eye

1. Eye examinations: for infant, not startling to loud noises, not responding to voices are possible indications; for child 3 or older, tonometry or pure tone audiometry test allow for visualization of the internal structures and detect certain disorders. Explain procedure to parents and child.

2. *Myopia:* nearsightedness: common in children, and treated with corrective glasses.

3. *Hyperopia:* farsightedness; treated with corrective glasses.

4. **Amblyopia:** use of one eye and not the other; unused eye fails to develop proper vision; treated with exercises and corrective glasses.

5. *Strabismus:* inability of eyes to coordinate function.

  a. Incidence: 1 to 2 percent of all children; occurs after infancy.

  b. Symptoms: deviation of eye, squinting, closing one eye to see, tilting head, clumsiness, and double vision

  c. Treatment and nursing care: patching unaffected eye, eye exercises, corrective glasses, surgical lengthening or shortening of muscle controlling eyeball position; offer teaching and emotional support.

6. *Cataract:* opacity of crystalline lens.

  a. Cause: may be hereditary, result from maternal infection during pregnancy, or metabolic disorders.

  b. Symptoms: diminished vision, strabismus.

  c. Treatment and nursing care: dilation of pupil with mydriatic eye drops, surgical iridectomy or lens fragmentation, corrective glasses; surgery results in average vision of 20/70; offer teaching and emotional support.

7. *Blindness:* legal blindness is considered vision of 20/200; treat as much like sighted child as possible; special classes to learn Braille; tape-recorded instruction: offer teaching and emotional support.

B. Ear

1. Ear examination: for infant, lack of response to loud noises and voices is possible indications; for child 3 or older, tonometry or pure tone audiometry test

2. Erythromycin prophylactically at birth to prevent ophthalmia neonatorum.

3. Acute *otitis media* (inflammatory disorder of the middle ear)

    a. May be bacterial or viral

    b. Infants and young child prone due to straight and wide ear canal

    c. Symptoms: fever, pain, crying and pulling at ear, upper respiratory symptoms

    d. Treatment and nursing care

        i. Administer antibiotics for 10 days and follow-up with ear checkup.

        ii. Use measures to reduce fever: acetaminophen, tepid sponge baths.

        iii. Use comfort measures.

        iv. Monitor for hearing loss.

4. Chronic otitis media with effusion: middle ear infection with persistent fluid

    a. May lead to hearing loss, scarring, or perforation

    b. *Myringotomy*: surgical insertion of ventilating tubes

5. Otitis externa: swimmer's ear; be sure ears are dried thoroughly after water immersion. Can instill hydrogen peroxide in intact ear canal for 5-10 seconds, then drain ear to aid water removal.

Additional Resources Found on MyNursingLab

- Normal Lung Sounds; 4 years old lung sounds

- SIDS video

- Congenital Heart Defects animation

MODULE 5.1

Maternal-Newborn Care

Learning Objectives

5.1.1. **Describe a normal pregnancy and prenatal period and possible complications.**

5.1.2. **Describe normal labor and delivery, possible complications, and the role of the practical nurse.**

5.1.3. **Discuss the postpartum period, common complications, and nursing care.**

5.1.4. **Describe the characteristics and nursing care of the normal newborn.**

5.1.5. **Discuss common disorders affecting the newborn.**

    I. Obstetrics

        A. Principles of obstetrical nursing

            1. Introduction

                a. Goal of health care is to reduce maternal and infant mortality associated with childbirth.

                b. Despite many advances in modern medicine, both women and children still die at childbirth.

                c. Four causes account for most infant deaths.

                    i. Low birth weight

                    ii. Congenital abnormalities

                    iii. SIDS

                    iv. Respiratory distress syndrome

            2. Obstetrical care

                a. Hospital main setting for childbirth.

                b. Some choose birthing centers.

            3. Public education

                a. Today, emphasis is placed on adequate prenatal care.

                b. Federal, state, and city governments have sponsored many maternal and child care programs.

                    i. School health programs

                    ii. Hospital-run prenatal clinics and well baby clinics

                    iii. Visiting nurse services

                    iv. Immunization programs

    4. Responsibilities of practical nurse

        a. Must have knowledge of:

            i. Normal functioning of reproductive organs

            ii. Normal processes of gestation and delivery

            iii. Physical and emotional demands of mother and child before, during, and after birth

B. Normal pregnancy

    1. Length approximately 280 days, which is equivalent to 10 lunar months, 9 calendar months, or 40 weeks.

    2. Physiological changes associated with pregnancy

        a. Circulatory

            i. Cardiac output increases 20-40%.

            ii. Blood pressure and pulse remain normal overall; in second trimester, there may be a slight decrease in BP.

            iii. Tissues retain excess fluid (about 3 quarts).

        b. Breasts

            i. May become painful or more sensitive

            ii. Become enlarged

            iii. Have increased pigmentation of areolae

            iv. Formation of colostrum

        c. Uterus

            i. Organ where implantation of fertilized ovum takes place

            ii. Enlarged to almost five times it normal size

            iii. Softer between cervix and its body (Hegar's sign)

        d. Vagina - changes to bluish color (Chadwick's sign)

        e. Cervix

            i. Contains mucus plug to protect fetus from bacteria

            ii. Softens during pregnancy (Goodell's sign, a probably sign of pregnancy); cervix softens more ("ripens") right before birth to permit delivery of child

            iii. Becomes bluish in color (Chadwick's sign)

        f. Abdomen

            i. Becomes enlarged

            ii. Appearance of striae gravidarum (stretch marks)

        g. Digestive tract - slowing of peristaltic action leads to nausea and constipation

        h. Urinary tract

            i. Frequency of urination due to pressure of uterus on bladder early and late in pregnancy

            ii. Kidneys work harder

    i.   Respiration - rate of respiration increases during last trimester to supply needed oxygen

    j.   Weight gain - total of approximately 25-35 pounds is considered normal.

    k.   Skin

        i.   **Striae gravidarum** - stretch marks

            (a) Caused by stretching and rupture of internal tissue

            (b) Occur on breasts, thighs, and abdomen

            (c) Usually lighten after delivery

    l.   Metabolism is accelerated

3.   Signs of pregnancy

    a.   Presumptive signs

        i.   Morning sickness - nausea and vomiting

        ii.   Absence of menstruation - amenorrhea

        iii.   Breast changes - enlargement, somewhat painful and tender

        iv.   Frequent urination common during early months

        v.   Quickening - feeling of fetal movement

        vi.   Fatigue

    b.   Probable signs

        i.   **Chadwick's sign** - cervix or vaginal walls turn bluish

        ii.   **Ballottement** - rebounding that occurs when doctor taps floating fetus within uterus

        iii.   Pigmentation - increasing deposits in skin of breasts, face, and abdomen

        iv.   **Goodell's sign** - softening of cervix

        v.   Contour of abdomen - change in contour due to changes occurring in uterus

        vi.   **Uterine soufflé** - a muffled swishing pulse heard over pregnant uterus; sound is in unison with the mother's heart beat and is due to rush of blood through large uterine vessels (same sound can be heard over large vascular tumors)

        vii.   Positive pregnancy tests

    c.   Positive signs

        i.   Palpation of fetal parts - head and back of child and often small parts may be felt about sixth or seventh month

        ii.   Fetal movements - felt by examiner

        iii.   Funic soufflé and fetal heart tone

            (a) **Funic soufflé** - fetal blood rushing through umbilical vessels

            (b) **Fetal heart tone** - heart sounds obtained through fetoscope

        iv.   Ultrasound, x-ray rarely done

4. Laboratory tests to determine pregnancy

    a. Immunologic laboratory - test on firstst voided urine specimen, 1-2 weeks after last missed period, 95-98% accuracy

    b. Home test - test on first voided urine specimen, 2 weeks after last missed period, 97% accuracy

    c. Radioimmunoassay (RIA) - test on serum 6-9 days after ovulation, almost 100% accuracy

    d. ELISA - enzyme-linked immunosorbent assay - done on woman's urine 7-8 days after ovulation

II. Prenatal Care

A. Medical supervision

    1. First visit to doctor or prenatal clinic should be made as soon as pregnancy is suspected.

    2. Physical examination

        a. Physical examination performed to determine overall health of mother-to-be; examination includes abdominal and vaginal examinations and taking of pelvic measurements

B. Important aspects of examination

    1. Medical history

        a. Previous diseases

        b. Previous surgeries

        c. Past pregnancies

            i. Number of pregnancies

            ii. Duration of pregnancies

            iii. Number of abortions and or stillbirths

            iv. Labor - prolonged, complications, etc.

            v. Delivery - spontaneous, breech, cesarean section, etc.

            vi. Health of living children

        d. Menstrual history

        e. Present pregnancy

    2. Family history

    3. Client's attitude

    4. Complete physical examination

        a. Skin and hair

        b. Eyes, ears, nose, and throat (including mouth and teeth)

        c. Thyroid

        d. Cardiovascular system

        e. Abdomen

        f. Pelvic exam

g. Extremities

h. Vital signs

5. Laboratory tests

a. CBC

b. Serologic test for syphilis

c. Urinalysis

    i. Examine for protein and sugar

    ii. Done at every prenatal visit

d. Rh factor and blood typing

e. AB0 compatibility

f. Papanicolaou smear

6. Approximate date of delivery (EDD) - **Naegele's rule** - determined by counting back three months from the first day of last menstrual period and adding one year and seven days.

7. Subsequent visits - usually scheduled every four weeks until eighth month of pregnancy, then every two weeks until ninth month, and then every week until delivery

8. Danger signals to report to doctor

a. Frequent headache

b. Edema of face, hands, or legs

c. Persistent vomiting and nausea

d. Constipation

e. Vaginal bleeding

f. Shortness of breath

g. Severe pain in lower abdomen or lumbar regions

h. Nervousness, sleeplessness, and apprehension

I. Escape of fluid from vagina

j. Chills and fever over 100 degrees F (37.8 degrees C)

k. Any infection or illness

l. Absence of fetal movements

m. Visual disturbances

C. Maternal hygiene during pregnancy

1. Clothing - comfortable; shoes with low, solid heels for balance

2. Breasts - bra for support because of breast enlargement and tenderness

3. Posture - good posture to lessen strain on muscles of back and thighs

4. Abdominal support

5. Douches - permitted only if advised by physician

6. Personal hygiene - daily baths or showers

7. Dental checkup as needed

8. Sleep and rest - necessary to avoid fatigue; irritability; rest periods should be taken periodically

9. Exercise according to prepregnant habits.

10. Elimination - increased urinary output, tendency toward constipation

11. Diet

    a. Regulate weight gain

    b, Meet nutritional needs of mother and child

    c. Adequate fluid to aid in elimination and fluid

D. Discomforts of pregnancy

1. Constipation - controlled by adding bulk and fluid to diet, exercising daily

2. Nausea and vomiting after first trimester

3. Pruritus - frequent bathing; use of lotion

4. Varicose veins - eliminate constricting clothes; rest with elevation of hips and legs; regular bowel movements; avoid crossing legs

5. Backache - wear well-fitting, low-heeled shoes

6. Hemorrhoids - dilated blood vessels in anal region

    a. Caused by interference with venous circulation due to pressure; condition aggravated by constipation

    b. Relief may be obtained by:

        i. Relieving constipation

        ii. Cold applications

        iii. Ointments or suppositories

7. Leg cramps

    a. Caused by:

        i. Pressure on nerves by uterus

        ii. Fatigue, tense posture

        iii. Low calcium intake

    b. Relief obtained by:

        i. Drinking adequate amount of milk daily

        ii. Not crossing legs

        iii. Avoiding restrictive clothing

        iv. Avoiding fatigue

        v. Wearing proper shoes

8. Flatulence

    a. Gas in digestive tract and a feeling of distension caused by:

        i. Bacteria in intestinal tract

        ii. Pressure exerted by growing uterus

       b. Relief obtained by:

          i.   Avoiding gas-forming foods

          ii. Chewing foods well

          iii. Daily regulation of elimination

9. Heartburn

       a. Caused by:

          i.   Worry, fatigue, nervous tension, emotional trauma

          ii. Improper diet

          iii. Enlarging uterus pressing on the stomach

       b. Relief obtained by:

          i.   Frequently eating small meals

          ii. Omitting fried, highly seasoned, or indigestible foods

10. Vaginal discharges

       a. May be caused by:

          i.   Yeast infection

          ii. Gonorrhea

          iii. Increased glandular activity of reproductive tract

       b. Treated by:

          i.   Good hygienic practices

          ii. If discharges are caused by venereal disease, the disease must be treated.

          iii. Medications as ordered by the physician

11. Insomnia

       a. Caused by shortness of breath due to pressure of uterus on the diaphragm

       b. Relieved by:

          i.   Abdominal breathing

          ii. Relaxation exercises

          iii. Warm drink at bedtime

E. Pregnancy teaching

1. Avoid alcohol completely during pregnancy.

2. Avoid tobacco - causes low birth weight

3. Medications only as prescribed by physician

4. Sexual relations - may continue throughout pregnancy unless complications

5. Review employment concerns.

6. Discuss travel plans.

7. Encourage attending childbirth education.

8. Encourage father's role.

III. Fetal Development

A. First month

1. Early development of eyes, ears, and nose

2. Length of embryo is approximately ½ inch

3. Embryo - from 1-8 weeks; fetus after 8th week

B. Second month

1. Formation of head and body

2. Development of extremities

3. Embryo approximately three inches

C. Third month

1. Appearance of downy hair **(lanugo)** on back and shoulders

2. Nail growth on fingers and toes

3. Sex differentiation obvious

4. Fetus approximately six inches

D. Fourth month

1. Detectable fetal heartbeat

2. Hair development on head

3. Fetus approximately 10 inches, 10 ounces

E. Fifth month

1. Appearance of eyebrows and eyelashes

2. Wrinkled, transparent skin

3. Cheesy material (vernix caseosa) covering body

4. Fetus approximately 12 inches, 1.2 lb

F. Sixth month   24 wks

1. Wrinkled, reddish skin, covered with vernix caseosa

2. Fetus approximately 14 inches, 2 lb

G. Seventh month   28 wks

1. Fetal movements evident

2. Fetus approximately 16 inches, 3-4 lb.

3. **Viability** - ability to live outside the uterus

4. May be viable at 24 weeks or weighing more than 400 gm

H. Eighth month

1. Fetus doubles weight

2. Fetus approximately 18 inches

3. Fetus has good chance of surviving if born at this stage

I. Ninth month

1. Skin unwrinkled

2. Disappearance of fine body hair

3. Fully developed baby

4. Weight is approximately seven pounds

IV. Disorders and Complications Occurring in Pregnancy

A. **Ectopic pregnancy** - fertilized ovum implanted outside of uterus within fallopian tube, abdomen, ovary, or cervix

    1. Symptoms similar to those of early pregnancy

    2. Intense pain may be felt on affected side.

    3. Vaginal bleeding or concealed bleeding may occur.

    4. Signs of hemorrhage and shock may occur.

    5. Early diagnosis and treatment crucial

    6. Surgical repair necessary

    7. Nursing care

        a. Keep client warm and quiet.

        b. Prepare for surgery.

        c. Observe and record vital signs.

        d. Prepare for blood transfusions.

        e. Give treatment for shock.

        f. Offer emotional support.

B. **Placenta previa** - placenta attached to lower uterine segment near or covering internal os.

    1. Most characteristic symptom is painless hemorrhage during last trimester.

    2. Treatment depends on status of cervix, parity, degree of previa, presence or absence of labor, and amount of bleeding.

        a. Blood replacement

        b. Prevention of shock

        c. Nursing care

            i. Keep client absolutely quiet.

            ii. Check vital signs and report and record.

            iii. Elevate foot of bed.

            iv. Intravenous fluids as ordered

            v. Continuous fetal monitoring

            vi. Observe amount of blood loss; report and record.

C. **Abruptio placentae** - premature separation of normally implanted placenta

    1. Primary cause unknown

    2. Symptoms

        a. Intense abdominal pain occurring in last trimester

        b. Vaginal bleeding - visible or concealed

      c.   Boardlike consistency in uterus; boardlike abdomen

      d.   Absence of fetal heart sounds

      e.   Symptoms of shock

   3.   Treatment

      a.   Blood replacement therapy

      b.   Uterus emptied either by vaginal delivery or cesarean section

      c.   Hysterectomy if uterus fails to contract

   4.   Nursing care

      a.   Monitor, report, and record vital signs.

      b.   Assist in preparation of client for immediate delivery, either vaginal or cesarean section

D. **Spontaneous abortion** or **habitual abortion** - expulsion of fetus before viability (24 weeks or 400 grams); no death certificate is required.

   1.   May be caused by ovular defects (50-60%), maternal factors (15%), abnormal fetal formation, immunologic factors, implantation abnormalities, infections, and hormonal problems.

   2.   Treatment

      a.   Absolute bed rest for threatened abortion

      b.   Sedatives to quiet uterus

      c.   Endocrine therapy

      d.   If abortion incomplete, dilatation and curettage may be necessary.

      e.   Blood replacement therapy may be necessary.

   3.   Nursing care is that of any clean surgical case.

   4.   Postpartum care if abortion is complete.

E. **Hydatidiform mole** - abnormal increase of chorionic tissue forming sacs (vesicles) resembling drops of water; associated with choriocarcinoma

   1.   Occurs early in pregnancy, causing death of embryo.

   2.   Symptoms include uterus enlarged beyond normal size for stage of pregnancy, brownish vaginal discharge, absence of fetus on x-ray, possible hemorrhage.

   3.   Treatment - immediate emptying of uterus

   4.   Emotional support and grief counseling

F. **Hyperemesis gravidarum** - excessive nausea and vomiting after first trimester

   1.   Symptoms

      a.   Persistent vomiting

      b.   Acetone and diacetic acid in urine

      c.   Weight loss

      d.   Dehydration

      e.   Low-grade fever

    f. Rapid pulse

    g. Scanty urine

2. Treatment

    a. Combat dehydration - parenteral fluids

    b. Relieve starvation - intravenous glucose, vitamins, and possibly tube feedings of high-vitamin, high-calorie diet

    c. Emotional support

    d. Therapeutic abortion if following:

        i. Jaundice

        ii. Delirium

        iii. Fever above 101 degrees F in spite of fluid intake

        iv. Steadily rising pulse rates above 130

        v. Retinal hemorrhages

G. Pregnancy-induced hypertension (PIH); also called gestational hypertension

1. Characteristics

    a. Hypertension

    b. Generalized edema and proteinuria

    c. Occurs after 7th month

2. **Preeclampsia** - early stages of PIH

    a. Occurs in latter half of pregnancy, during labor or puerperium

    b. Symptoms

        i. Nausea and vomiting

        ii. Edema and weight gain (caused by fluid retention)

        iii. Hypertension

        iv. Albuminuria

        v. Visual disturbances

        vi. Apprehension and depression

    c. Occurs in mild or severe form

    d. Treatment

        i. Preventive care early

        ii. Low-sodium, high-protein, 1500-calorie diet

        iii. Bed rest

        iv. Sedation

    e. Nursing care

        i. Accurate fluid intake and output record

        ii. Monitor fetal heart rate

        iii. Blood pressure every 4-6 hours

    iv. Daily urinalysis

    v. Sedatives for rest and to lower blood pressure (phenobarbital)

    vi. Vital signs checked as ordered and recorded

    vii. Quiet room, soft lights

    viii. Medication as ordered

    ix. Antihypertension medication

    x. Daily weight (same time each day)

3. **Eclampsia** - late, severe form of PIH; once called toxemia

  a. Symptoms appear in last trimester

    i. Seizures, convulsions, and coma

    ii. Edema

    iii. Albuminuria

    iv. Elevated blood pressure

  b. Treatment

    i. Prevention

      (a) Vigilant prenatal care

      (b) Early diagnosis and treatment of pre-eclampsia

      (c) Reporting of any symptom immediately

    ii. Sedation

    iii. Protect client from self-injury

      (a) Client never left alone

      (b) Padded side rails, suction and airway available

    iv. Protect client from external stimuli.

    v. Turn client's head to side to prevent aspiration of mucus and/or vomitus.

    vi. Intravenous administration to promote urination

    vii. Close observation and recording of signs to protect against complications (cerebral hemorrhage, congestive heart failure, respiratory paralysis, etc.)

    viii. Oxygen administered as needed

    ix. Condition improves when pregnancy ends.

4. Chronic hypertensive vascular disease

  a. Hypertension predates pregnancy.

  b. Occurs generally in obese multiparas

  c. Health of fetus may be compromised.

  d. Symptoms

    i. Hypertension

    ii. Headache

e. Treatment

    i. Hypotensive drugs

    ii. Rest

    iii. Low-sodium diet

    iv. Observe for signs of toxemia

    v. Interruption of pregnancy if symptoms become very severe

V. Disorders and Conditions Affected by Pregnancy

A. Heart disease

  1. Mainly rheumatic

  2. Regarded as fourth major cause of maternal death

  3. Treatment

    a. Adequate rest

    b. Avoidance of infection

    c. Observing for early signs of heart failure (edema, shortness of breath, etc)

    d. Digitalis

    e. May need complete bed rest in hospital

B. Diabetes mellitus

  1. Difficult to control in pregnant woman

    a. Changes in glucose tolerance

    b. Increased tendency to ketosis

  2. Complications

    a. Excessively large fetuses

    b. Slightly increased abortion rate

    c. Increased incidence of PIH

    d. Increased incidence of fetal death in utero

    e. Congenital defects

    f. Inhibition of lactation

    g. Neonatal complications

      i. Anoxia

      ii. Immaturity

      ii. Pulmonary problems

      iv. Hypoglycemia

  3. Treatment

    a. Strict medical supervision

    b. Termination of pregnancy before term if clinical course complicated

    c. Avoidance of infection

      d. Proper rest regimen

      e. May need several hospital admissions for supervision before term

C. Infectious diseases

  1. Syphilis

    a. Routine serology during pregnancy now legislated

    b. Intensive treatment for those diagnosed as positive

    c. Untreated cases result in fetal deformity, prematurity, and fetal death depending upon time of infection.

  2. Rubella (German measles)

    a. Exposure in first trimester causes severe malformation in fetus

    b. Infection after first trimester not dangerous

    c. Live vaccine, not given in first trimester; not safe anytime in pregnancy

    d. Generally therapeutic abortion is indicated in proven cases.

  3. Gonorrhea

    a. Can cause blindness in fetus (disease contracted by fetus during birth)

    b. Erythromycin ointment in baby's eyes immediately postpartum as prophylactic treatment.

VI. Labor and Delivery

A. Labor

  1. **Labor** - process by which fetus, placenta, and membranes are expelled from a woman's body

  2. Exact cause of labor is believed to be due to action of hormones and other factors.

  3. Fetus, placenta, and membranes expelled from pregnant woman's body after 38 to 40 weeks or 266 to 280 days of gestation

  4. In case of premature labor, management of delivery and labor is same as in full-term labor; however, premature infant is susceptible to respiratory problems and other complications.

B. Preliminary signs of labor

  1. **Lightening**

    a. Infant descends into pelvis

    b. May occur two weeks before labor

    c. Relieves pressure on diaphragm, so sense of being "lighter"

  2. **Braxton-Hicks contractions**

    a. False contractions which are irregular and intermittent

    b. May occur 2 weeks before labor in primiparas and immediately before labor in multiparas

  3. **Show** or **bloody show** - release of mucus plug (has pink tinge) from cervix

    4. **Rupture of membranes** (bag of waters)

        a. Gush of liquid from vaginal tract

        b. May occur days or weeks prior to labor

    5. Regular contractions

        a. Increase in frequency

        b. Stronger

        c. Result in cervical dilation

C. Stages of labor

    1. **First stage**

        a. Dilatation of cervix - early or latent phase, active phase, transition phase

        b. Usually lasts 12-18 hours for mother's first baby

        c. Contractions occur every 10-15 minutes.

        d. Membranes may rupture.

        e. Contractions begin to lengthen.

    2. **Second stage**

        a. From full dilation of cervix to delivery of baby

        b. Passage of fetus through birth canal

        c. Duration is 1-2 hours for first baby.

        d. Mother should be encouraged to relax between contractions.

    3. **Third stage**

        a. From birth of baby to separation and expulsion of placenta and membranes

        b. Duration is a few minutes.

        c. Contraction of uterus controls bleeding.

    4. **Fourth stage**

        a. From end of third stage to 1st hour after stabilization of vital signs of mother

        b. May experience chills

        c. Fundus and blood loss monitored

D. Pain relief

    1. Regional blocks

        a. Pudendal: into pudendal nerve in area of episiotomy

        b. Epidural: into epidural space in lumbar region

    2. Local infiltration

    3. General anesthesia - not used for vaginal deliveries; may be used for emergency C-section

E. Admission of woman in labor

    1. Client usually speaks with doctor before going to hospital.

    2. Physical preparation of client varies with hospital.

PEARSON

3. Practical nurse assists client in undressing and getting into bed.

4. Obtain necessary information concerning onset and duration of pain, whether membranes have ruptured, and previous labors if multipara.

5. Follow doctor's orders.

6. Keep accurate record of pains and duration.

7. Keep client in bed after rupture of membranes.

8. Provide comfort measures.

9. Observe client closely.

10. Provide emotional support.

F. The role of the practical nurse

    1. Nursing care

        a. Take vital signs and record; report all unusual symptoms to RN immediately.

        b. Apply external fetal monitor.

        c. Observe for rupture of membranes.

        d. Note contractions - duration and frequency.

        e. Observe client for any unusual symptoms and record:

            i. Change in vital signs

            ii. Excessive bleeding

            iii. Meconium in vaginal discharge

            iv. Prolapsed cord

            v. Shock

            vi. Exhaustion

            vii. Dehydration

            viii. Long, painful contractions

            ix. Change in fetal heart rate

        f. Encourage side-lying position.

        g. Encourage voiding.

G. Complications of labor and delivery

    1. Difficult labor **(dystocia)**

        a. May be caused by insufficiently strong contracting force

        b. May be caused by abnormal position of fetus in uterus

        c. May be caused by baby's being too large for birth canal

        d. May be necessary to deliver by cesarean section

    2. Abnormal presentation

    3. Prolapsed umbilical cord (cord flushed out of uterus when membranes rupture)

        a. Causes distress for baby - take FHR immediately.

      b.   Immediately elevate client's hips or place client in Trendelenburg position to relieve pressure on cord.

      c.   Requires emergency C-section

  4. Postpartum hemorrhage

      a.   May be caused by improper uterine involution

      b.   May be caused by lacerations of cervix, vagina, or perineum

      c.   May be caused by retained fragments of placenta

      d.   Lacerations are classified as first, second, or third degree.

  5. Multiple pregnancy

      a.   Condition in which two or more embryos develop at same time in uterus

      b.   Types of twins

         i.   **Fraternal** - develop from two fertilized eggs; each embryo has its own placenta, amnion, and umbilical cord

        ii.   **Identical** - develop from a single fertilized egg; one placenta exists, but there are two amnions and two umbilical cords

  6. **Abruptio placentae**

      a.   Premature separation of normally implanted placenta

      b.   Separation is complete or incomplete.

      c.   Occurs in late months of pregnancy or at onset of labor

      d.   Cause is unknown

      e.   Visible or concealed bleeding occurs.

      f.   Sudden intense uterine pain

  7. **Puerperal sepsis** - takes several days for symptoms to appear, including fever of 100.4 degrees F or higher

  8. **Placenta previa**

      a.   Implantation of placenta lower than normal

      b.   Painless vaginal bleeding in last half of pregnancy

H. Surgery and procedures

  1. Episiotomy and repairs

      a.   **Episiotomy** - cutting perineum in order to permit delivery of baby without lacerations

      b.   Episiotomy is sutured following delivery.

  2. Forceps delivery or vacuum extraction

      a.   Doctor assists baby through birth canal using obstetrical forceps or suction cup.

      b.   Forceps (and episiotomy) are often used for new mothers in their first births.

      c.   Forceps may be harmful to baby if applied incorrectly.

  3. Surgery

      a.   **Cesarean section** - opening of abdomen and uterus in order to deliver baby.

        b.   Following removal of the placenta, the uterus and abdomen are sutured.

        c.   Delivery by cesarean section requires special care of baby.

   4. **Version**

        a.   Turning baby in uterus from undesirable to desirable position

        b.   Types - external and internal

I.   Important factors of obstetrical nursing

   1. Primary objectives of nursing care

        a.   Safety of mother and baby

        b.   Overall wellness of mother

   2. Secondary objectives

        a.   Maintain asepsis.

            i.   Perineal care

           ii.   Comfort

        b.   Check and record vital signs at regular intervals.

        c.   Encourage frequent voiding.

        d.   Encourage rest and relaxation to help avoid fatigue.

        e.   Offer fluids (unless contraindicated) to prevent dehydration.

        f.   Check fetal heart rate every half-hour during first stage of labor; check fetal heart rate after every contraction during second stage; check fetal heart rate immediately after rupture of membranes.

        g.   Time contractions and record client's progress.

            i.   Duration of contractions

           ii.   Interval between contractions

          iii.   Rapid, irregular, slow, or absent fetal heart rate

          iv.   Meconium-stained vaginal leakage

           v.   Hyperactivity

        h.   Watch for and report signs of maternal danger.

        i.   Record all important data pertaining to mother's care throughout labor.

J.   Delivery

   1. Practical nurse may assist doctor or RN in delivery room with a routine delivery.

   2. Procedure:

        a.   Client is placed in modified lithotomy position; sterile strict asepsis is adhered to.

            i.   Preparation of pudendum

           ii.   Sterile draping of client exposing only introitus

        b.   Client is urged to push with contractions.

        c.   Episiotomy may be performed as head crowns.

        d.   Baby's mouth and nose are suctioned after delivery of head in order to remove mucus.

PEARSON

  e. After respiration is established, delivery is completed.

  f. Baby is placed on mother's abdomen.

  g. Cord is clamped and cut.

  h. Baby is wrapped in warmed garment and placed in warmer.

  i. Physician expresses placenta as it begins to separate from uterus.

  j. Physician examines placenta to determine if it is intact.

  k. Injection of oxytoxin may be given to mother to stimulate a firm, contracted uterus.

  l. Nurse should examine fundus to note size, position, and consistency.

  m. If episiotomy has been performed, it is repaired.

  n. Nurse cleans vulva and perineal area; a sterilized perineal pad is applied.

  o. Mother is sent to recovery until stable.

  p. Following birth

    i. Immediate care of mother

      (a) Allow rest.

      (b) Check blood pressure, pulse, and respirations often until they are stable.

      (c) Check fundus for firmness and level.

      (d) Encourage mother to void; check for bladder distention; maintain intake and output for 24 hours.

      (e) Offer fluids; if client complains of hunger, a light diet may be given.

      (f) Reassure mother that she and her baby are in good condition; encourage family visitation.

      (g) Report any change in client's condition.

      (h) Record vital signs and all other pertinent information concerning client.

    ii. Immediate care of newborn

      (a) Identification of new baby (methods used depend on hospital).

      (b) Care of baby's eyes - erythromycin drops instilled into each eye to prevent blindness caused by gonorrhea (ophthalmia neonatorum)

      (c) Umbilical cord checked for bleeding

      (d) Appraisal of newborn 1 minute after delivery and again at 5 minutes - Apgar score

      (e) Place infant in supine position with head slightly lowered.

      (f) Administer vitamin K as ordered.

      (g) Aspirate mucus from nose and throat as needed.

      (h) Dry and maintain body warmth.

      (i) Infant is transferred to nursery.

 E. Pain relief during labor

  1. Butorphanol tartrate (Stadol) - an opioid analgesic

  2. Meperidine HCl (Demerol) - an opioid analgesic

3. Naloxone (Narcan) - narcotic antagonist

4. Drugs may cause respiratory depression; monitoring is crucial.

VII. **Postpartum Care**

   A. **Puerperium** - time from end of labor to return of genital organs to normal; ranges from 6-8 weeks

   B. Normal puerperium

      1. Breasts

         a. Secrete **colostrum** (thin, protein-rich liquid) during first few days following delivery

         b. Lactation begins between second and fourth day.

         c. Medication can be given to dry up breasts if mother cannot or does not wish to nurse.

      2. Uterus

         a. **Involution** - process by which uterus returns to its normal state

         b. Uterus decreases in size and returns to its normal state in approximately 6 weeks.

         c. Involution entails:

            i. Firming of uterus

            ii. Descent of uterus into pelvis

            iii. Normal lochia

      3. Lochia

         a. Discharge from uterus

         b. Character

            i. **Lochia rubra** - bright red because of blood from placental site, mucus, and decidua

            ii. **Lochia serosa** - lighter, pinkish or brownish red because of serum from healing surfaces

            iii. **Lochia alba** - yellowish white

      4. Afterpains

         a. Caused by contraction and relaxation of uterus

         b. Occur more frequently in multiparas

         c. Occur frequently in mothers who are breastfeeding

         d. Treatment

            i. Administering analgesics

            ii. Explaining cause of pains to mother and reassuring her

      5. Return of menstruation

         a. Occurs in six to eight weeks if mother is not nursing child

         b. Occurs eight weeks after lactation ceases

6. Abdomen

    a. **Striae** (stretch marks) on abdominal walls do not usually remain

    b. Abdominal muscles regain tone with exercise.

C. Nursing care postpartum

  1. Daily observation of:

    a. Breasts - check for any signs of engorgement or any abnormality

    b. Uterus - check for height, consistency, and uterine size.

    c. Lochia - check for amount, color, and consistency.

    d. Perineum - observe to monitor healing process and to detect infection.

    d. Breasts for signs of engorgement or any abnormality

    e. Mother's emotional attitude

  2. Perineal care

    a. Given to keep mother clean and to prevent infection

    b. Procedure is determined by hospital.

  3. Bladder care

    a. Client is encouraged to void regularly.

    b. Catheterization is used only if client is unable to void.

    c. Urine output is greater than normal.

  4. Elimination

    a. Constipation is likely to occur.

    b. Regulation by diet, fluid intake, and regular pattern of elimination

  5. Activity

    a. Bed activity is encouraged.

    b. Activities out of bed are regulated by physician.

  6. Education of mother

    a. Taught to care for herself and her baby

    b. Emphasis placed on:

      i. Cleanliness

        (a) Daily shower taken for comfort

        (b) Tub baths permissible after a few weeks' time

        (c) Daily perineal care should be administered.

        (d) Shampoo the hair as needed.

        (e) All aspects for personal hygiene, including care of the hands and feet

      ii. Diet

        (a) Client is advised on proper diet.

        (b) Well-balanced diet essential to promote healing and ensure good health.

    (c) Green, leafy vegetables, lean meats, citrus fruits

    (d) Vitamin and mineral supplements may be prescribed by physician.

   iii. Rest and exercise

    (a) Quiet room and clean dry bed are essential.

    (b) Rest periods during day are necessary.

    (c) Adequate sleep; at least eight hours are recommended.

    (d) Daily exercise in form of walking is recommended.

    (e) Special exercises to promote muscle tone of abdomen are prescribed by doctor.

   iv. Elimination

    (a) Cleansing enema may be ordered on third day following delivery.

    (b) Client encouraged to void to prevent overdistended bladder

   v. Breast care

    (a) Breasts are bathed when bath is given (breasts are first part of body washed).

    (b) Special ointment may be ordered for nipples by doctor (if indicated).

    (c) Wearing a good, well-fitted brassiere will give necessary support and prevent muscle stretching.

    (d) Postpartum examination - scheduled by doctor usually 6 weeks after delivery.

 D. Complications postpartum

  1. Infection - **puerperal** fever

   a. Caused by bacteria, generally located in lower genital tract and rectum.

   b. Puerperal infection often caused by Staphylococcus and Streptococcus.

   c. Hospital personnel in maternity wards must be free from infections.

  2. **Mastitis** - infection of breasts

   a. Caused by entry of bacteria through cracks or tissues in nipples.

   b. Occurs most frequently during third to fourth week following delivery

   c. Symptoms

    i. Temperature is elevated.

    ii. Breasts become red and hard.

   d. Treatment

    i. Nursing may be discontinued if mastitis is severe.

    ii. Application of ice packs

    iii. Antibiotics

  3. Thrombophlebitis

   a. Usually occurs in legs.

   b. Affected area turns white, becomes swollen and painful.

    c. Affected part should not be rubbed or massaged.

    d. Treatment according to doctor's orders

  4. Postpartum depression

    a. If mother is insecure about ability to care for child, report concerns to RN.

    b. Reassure the mother.

  5. Postpartum hemorrhage

    a. Proper monitoring of fundus during hours immediately following delivery will provide early symptoms which should be reported immediately.

      i. Report 2 or more saturated pads per hour.

      ii. Report passing of heavy clots in post delivery period.

    b. Uterine and vaginal packing may be necessary.

  6. Puerperal sepsis

    a. Aseptic techniques during labor and throughout puerperium will prevent puerperal infections.

    b. Antibiotics and sulfonamide therapy may be necessary, depending upon type of organism causing infection.

    c. Prevention is the best defense against puerperal infection.

    d. Warm sitz baths may be ordered if episiotomy or lower genital tract is involved.

    e. Symptoms (must be reported immediately)

      i. Fever (temperature over 100.4°F or 38°C)

      ii. Local tenderness or pain

      iii. Green or yellow lochia

      iv. Unusual foul odor

VIII. Care of the Newborn

  A. Introduction

    1. Critical period for newborn is immediately after birth.

    2. Marked changes from life *in utero* to life outside uterus.

  B. Immediate care

    1. Directed toward assisting newborn in meeting basic needs

      a. Cord - inspected for presence of 2 arteries and 1 vein (3 vessels);observed frequently for bleeding

      b. Eyes - erythromycin drops instilled

      c. Airway - nose and mouth suctioned to remove accumulated mucus and amniotic fluid as needed

      d. Inspection

        i. Weight - average at birth about 7 lb

        ii. Length - average at birth 19"-21"

        iii. Temperature - rectal 98°-99°F

        iv. Recording of Apgar score (See Table 1. Apgar Score of Newborn Infant)

e. Birth registration - mandatory in all hospitals, hand prints or footprints are made and name bracelets according to policy

2. Baby is transferred to nursery.

3. Rooming-in

    a. Process whereby mother is able to care for her newborn baby at her bedside

    b. Newborn infant receives specialized, individualized attention from parents.

    c. Parents are given instructions on baby care from hospital staff through rooming-in.

Table 1. Apgar Score of Newborn Infant

		0	1	2
A	Appearance (color)	Blue, pale	Body pink, extremities blue	Completely pink
P	Pulse (heart rate)	Absent	Below 100	Over 100
G	Grimace (reflex irritability in response to stimulation of sole of foot)	No response	Grimace	Cry
A	Activity (muscle tone)	Limp	Some flexion of extremities	Active motion
R	Respiration (respiratory effort)	Absent	Slow, irregular	Strong cry

IX. General Characteristics of the Newborn

A. Weight

1. Range - 6.2-9.2 lb (2,900-4,000 grams)

2. 10% of this weight is lost in a few days, regained in next ten days (normal physiologic weight loss)

B. Length - 18"-22" (45-55 cm)

C. Temperature - 98°-99°F

D. Skin

1. Body covered by vernix caseosa.

2. Parts of body covered with lanugo.

3. Thinness of skin may result in peeling on the trunk and the extremities

E. Body color

1. Prominence of superficial veins

2. Mottled look

3. Ruddy complexion

4. Poor circulation in extremities making them appear bluish (acrocyanosis)

    F. Head

        1. Circumference of head - 12.2"-14" cm

        2. Accounts for 33-35.5 cm of total body length

        3. Two soft spots due to the skull bones not having united yet - anterior and posterior fontanel

            a. Anterior fontanel closes within 12-18 months.

            b. Posterior fontanel closes by end of 4th month.

    G. Face

        1. Expressionless eyes; closed most of the time

        2. Eyes may seem to be crossed due to weak muscles.

        3. Eyes are blue-gray in color.

        4. Nose is flat.

        5. Lower jaw appears to be receding.

        6. Tongue extends only as far as gums.

    H. Neck

        1. Short

        2. Has weak muscles which cannot support head

    I. Chest

        1. Round shape

        2. Breasts may be engorged due to hormones transmitted from mother via placenta.

    J. Abdomen

        1. Round shape

        2. Protrudes due to size of enclosed organs

        3. Rises and falls when baby breathes

    K. Extremities

        1. Arms and legs in fetal position (flexed)

        2. Hands semi-closed

        3. Bowed legs

        4. Continuous, purposeless movements when baby is awake

    L. Bones soft

X. Newborn's Responses to Internal and External Stimuli

    A. Sight

        1. Turns eyes to light

        2. Cannot focus until after 3 months

        3. Tears absent until 2 months

    B. Pressure: soothing effect produced by stroking and patting

    C. Hearing: delayed for several days

    D. Taste: aware of strong tastes (bitter, sweet)

    E. Thirst: present from beginning, demand for satisfaction

    F. Hunger: not always present at birth, but soon experienced

    G. Temperature: sensitive to cold and warmth

    F. Head

        1. Circumference of head - 12.2"-14" cm

        2. Accounts for 33-35.5cm of total body length

    H. Comfort: warm and fed

    I. Discomfort: cold and hungry

XI. Newborn's Growth Responses to External Stimuli

    A. Sleep: Newborn sleeps 20 hours of 24 hours in short periods.

    B. Development

        1. Builds new movements and perfects those he or she already has

        2. Finds more meaning in world around him or her

        3. Makes connection between what he or she sees and does

        4. Later modifies actions by intentional responses

XII. Physiological Changes

    A. Reflexes

        1. Has sucking reflex

        2. Can cough, sneeze, cry, and yawn

        3. Babinski, tonic neck, Moro, rooting, grasping, stepping, swallowing, and blinking

    B. Elimination

        1. Void and pass stools

        2. First stools are dark green called **meconium,** progress to yellow pasty (formula-fed infants) or yellow seedy (breastfed infants)

    C. Respirations

        1. 30-60 per minute

        2. Irregular

    D. Pulse

        1. 100-150 per minute

        2. Irregular

    E. Body temperature

        1. Baby's unit must be kept at constant temperature in order to maintain body heat.

    F. Body movements

        1. Disorganized

        2. Good muscle tone

        3. Constant, aimless moving

XIII. Daily Newborn Care

  A. Daily bath

      1. Clean skin and stimulate circulation.

      2. Routine varies according to hospital.

         a. Wash head.

         b. Use only water to cleanse eyelids - wipe from inner canthus outward.

         c. Observe cord - report unusual characteristics.

      3. Sponge bath given until cord heals.

      4. Safety precautions:

         a. Prepare all equipment beforehand; protect baby from drafts.

         b. Room temperature should be 75°- 80°F.

         c. Check water temperature with thermometer; should be 90° - 100°F.

         d. Support baby's head.

         e. Use soft towel and washcloth.

         f. Rinse and dry completely.

         g. In males, area around foreskin should be cleansed; if male infant has been circumcised, follow hospital procedure.

         h. Observe carefully for skin irritation or skin abnormalities; any such observations should be reported immediately.

  B. Weight

      1. Baby is weighed daily while in hospital.

      2. 10% of birth weight is usually lost by end of 3-4 days; regained by end of second week.

      3. Report and record weight daily.

  C. Elimination

      1. Urine usually pale yellow; baby usually voids twelve to fifteen times daily.

      2. Stool (meconium) passed four to five times daily.

  D. Feedings

      1. Baby taken to mother for nursing unless contraindicated.

      2. Breastfeeding

         a. Easiest, simplest, and most inexpensive way to feed baby

         b. Mother's milk and colostrum provide substances that protect baby from disease.

         c. Emotionally satisfying experience for mother and child

         d. Putting baby to breast stimulates milk secretion.

         e. Mother must be comfortable during nursing.

         f. Instruct mother in care of breast.

   3. Bottle-feeding

      a. Formula prescribed by doctor.

      b. Baby should be held during bottle feeding just as if he were being breastfed.

E. Record all observations.

   1. Respirations - rate and rhythm

   2. Stools - color and consistency, number of movements

   3. Voiding - frequency and color

   4. Alignment of body

   5. Sound of cry

   6. Reactions to noises and movements

   7. Weight loss and/or weight gain

   8. Color of body, extremities, face

XIV. Disorders of the Newborn

A. **Atelectasis** - incomplete expansion of lungs

   1. Causes

      a. Obstruction of bronchi

      b. Aspiration of mucus or amniotic fluid

   2. Symptoms

      a. Shallow, rapid respirations

      b. Mostly abdominal respirations

      c. Cyanosis

      d. Respiratory grunting, nasal flaring

   3. Nursing care - follow treatment ordered by physician.

B. **Asphyxia neonatorum**

   1. Obstruction of air passages by mucus or amniotic fluid

   2. May be mild or severe

   3. Symptoms

      a. Congested appearance

      b. Cyanosis

      c. Slow pulse

      d. Symptoms of asphyxia - blue lips; pale appearance; weak, rapid heart beat

   4. Treatment

      a. Stimulate respiration.

      b. Apply principles of resuscitation.

   5. Nursing care - follow treatment ordered by physician.

C. Caput succedaneum

    a. **Caput succedaneum** - a generalized edema of the scalp; resolves without treatment.

D. **Cephalhematoma** - hemorrhage between the periosteum and the skull bones

    1. Causes

        a. Birth injury

        b. Injury from forceps delivery

    2. Symptoms - swelling of scalp

    3. Treatment - no specific treatment since swelling usually disappears in 6-8 weeks

    4. Nursing care - close observation of infant

E. Hemorrhagic disease of the newborn

    1. Either internal or external bleeding

    2. Symptoms

        a. Increased bleeding and clotting time

        b. Decreased number of platelets

        c. Vomitus with blood stains

        d. Bleeding from cord stump or skin

        e. In severe cases - fever, anemia, cyanosis, and convulsions

    3. Baby usually responds quickly to blood transfusions and dosage of vitamin K.

F. Hemorrhaging from cord

    1. Caused by slipping of cord tie or clamp

    2. Treat by applying new ligature or clamp

G. **Ophthalmia neonatorum** - any conjunctivitis in newborn

    1. Causes

        a. Chemical conjunctivitis due to antibiotic ointment

        b. Infectious conjunctivitis due to staphylococci, pneumococci, or gonococci (appears during 2nd-5th day postpartum)

    2. Symptoms

        a. Inflammation of eyes

        b. Redness or swelling of lids

        c. Discharge

    3. Isolation precautions are taken and appropriate treatment given if bacterial.

H. **Icterus neonatorum** - physiologic jaundice

    1. Caused by immature liver functions and increased destruction of red blood cells during first 2 weeks of life

    2. Symptom - jaundice appearing on 2nd or 3rd to the 5th day of life

    3. Condition usually lasts only a few days

I. Erythema

   1. Newborn rash

   2. Cause unknown

   3. Symptom - blotchy rash appearing on back, shoulders, or buttocks

   4. Usually lasts only a few days, self-limiting

J. **Thrush** - *Candida* infection

   1. Transmitted by nipples, vagina, or by poor hygienic procedures

   2. Diagnosed by laboratory test

   3. Preventive measures

      a. Adequate cleaning of mother's nipples (or bottle nipples) prior to feeding

      b. Wash hands before handling baby.

   4. Treatment

      a. Daily observation and inspections of baby's mouth

      b. Take adequate precautions when using feeding apparatus or touching baby.

      c. Medications ordered by physician

K. **Erythroblastosis fetalis** - hemolytic disease of newborn; excessive destruction of red blood cells

   1. Due to incompatibility between mother's blood and fetus' blood

      a. Rh negative mother who:

         i. Has had more than one previous pregnancy resulting in an Rh positive child

         ii. Has been transfused previously with Rh positive blood

      b. Rh positive fetus

   2. Becomes apparent late in fetal life or soon after birth

   3. Prevention

      a. Typing of mother's blood

      b. Administration of anti-Rh gamma globulins (Rho-GAM) to mother 72 hours postpartum to protect future Rh positive children

   4. Symptoms

      a. Pathological jaundice - evident within 24 hours

      b. Anemia

      c. Enlarged liver and spleen if untreated

      d. Extensive edema if untreated

   5. Treatment

      a. Intrauterine transfusion (prevention)

      b. Exchange transfusions administered by physician

      c. Repeated small transfusions at later time

      d. Antibiotics to prevent infection

6. Nursing care

    a. Observe newborn's color, vital signs, urine, skin; report all changes immediately.

    b. Report any evidence of jaundice during first and second day.

    c. Apply sterile, wet compresses to umbilicus.

L. **Phenylketonuria (PKU)** - metabolic defect due to lack of development of hepatic enzyme phenylalanine

  1. Symptoms

    a. Progressive mental retardation if untreated

    b. Neurological disturbances

  2. Diagnostic tests

    a. Newborn blood sample to determine phenylalanine levels

    b. Special paper used to test urine to determine phenylalanine level

  3. Treatment

    a. Special diet soon after birth - low in phenylalanine and prepared commercially

    b. Monitor blood levels of phenylalanine

XV. Care of the Premature Infant

A. Prematurity

  1. Physical characteristics

    a. Depends upon age in weeks

    b. Lanugo may cover entire body; vernix caseosa is absent

    c. Poor control of body temperature

    d. Organs immature

    e. Body system not functioning to capacity

    f. Impaired respiration

    g. Weak sucking and swallowing

    h. Kidneys not functioning to capacity

    i. Thin, transparent skin

    j. Thin and delicate skin and mucous membranes

    k. More susceptible to infection

    l. Cry is a weak whine

B. Nursing care

  1. General principles

    a. Practical nurse assists in care of premature infants.

    b. Include all observations on nurse's notes.

    c. Supervised by RN with special training.

    d. Handle infant as little as possible.

    e. Maintain body temperature in range of 97°- 99°F

f. Maintain constant temperature 80°-90° and humidity 40%-60% in the incubator.

g. Record temperature of incubator each time temperature of baby is taken.

h. Give oxygen only when ordered by doctor and give prescribed concentration.

i. Feeding must be careful and unhurried; unusually by gavage method.

j. Formula and method of feeding ordered on individual basis.

k. Throat may need gentle suctioning of mucus between feedings.

l. Check carefully after feeding to see that no formula, which might be aspirated, is left in mouth or throat.

Additional Resources Found on MyNursingLab

- Conception (video)
- Preeclampsia (video)
- Delivery of Infant (video)
- Postpartum Assessment (video
- Circumcision (video)
- Cord Care to a Newborn's Cord Stump (video)
- Applying a Mummy Wrap (video)

MODULE 6.1

Older Adult Nursing Care

Learning Objectives

6.1.1   Describe demographics, myths, and common theories about aging.

6.1.2   Describe the normal physical changes of aging.

6.1.3   Describe the common psychosocial changes affecting older adults.

6.1.4   Discuss the nursing needs of older clients with common health problems.

I.   **The Older Person**

    A.   One in every eight Americans is 65 years of age or older.

    B.   More than 12.6% percent of the United States population is 65 years of age or older.

    C.   Life expectancy is approximately 80 years.

    D.   The elderly are most often affected by chronic illness.

    E.   Each person is unique.

    F.   Three major causes of death in the elderly are heart disease, cancer, and stroke.

    G.   Many myths and beliefs associated with aging exist today:

        1.   Cognition and learning ability decrease with age.

        2.   Old and infirm are the same thing.

        3.   The majority of older people are unable to adapt to change.

        4.   Most elderly live in nursing homes.

        5.   It is impossible for an older person to learn something new.

II.   **The Aging Process**

    A.   Aging process begins at conception and affects every body system.

    B.   Genes, state of health, diet, life experiences, environment, activity, and stress affect the rate of aging.

    C.   Aging is a universal biological phenomenon.

    D.   The biological and psychosocial processes of aging are interrelated and interdependent.

    E.   Not all body systems age at the same rate.

    F.   Theories of aging - no one theory completely explains the aging process.

        1.   Biological theories

            a.   Programmed aging - . People inherit a specific genetic program which then determines the rate of aging.

            b.   Error - Genetic mutations may be responsible for errors in cells, causing a decline in organ functioning.

   c. Autoimmune - Aging occurs as a result of the immune system becoming less efficient or less able to distinguish between foreign and host cells.

   d. Free radical - Free radicals produced as a result of metabolism cause chemical damage to cells, which interferes with normal body functioning.

   e. Wear and tear - Cells of the body wear out from prolonged use, causing the body to function less efficiently.

  2. Psychosocial theories- theories explore thoughts, feelings and behaviors affecting individuals as they age

   a. Disengagement theory - Aging is the process in which the elderly and society gradually withdraw or disengage. This is mutually satisfying as it allows older individuals to concentrate on their needs while society can prepare for the transfer of power.

   b. Activity theory

    i. This theory suggests that the older individual should remain active and involved for as long as possible.

    ii. Society should embrace the older person's continued involvement.

   c. Continuity - developmental theory

    i. This theory suggests that behavior patterns and basic personality traits remain the same throughout the life cycle.

    ii. Active individuals will likely remain active, while sedentary ones will remain inactive.

III. Characteristics of an Elderly Person

 A. Physical changes

  1. Number of cells is gradually reduced, with slower healing process.

  2. Recovery time from illness lengthens with more complications.

  3. Lean body mass decreases.

  4. Loss of subcutaneous tissue increases their sensitivity to cold.

  5. Height decreases due to loss of cartilage and thinning of vertebral disks.

  6. Cardiovascular system changes

   a. Vessels lose elasticity and lumen narrows, causing an increase in BP.

   b. More time is needed for the heart to return to resting stage.

   c. Heart muscle loses the ability to contract efficiently, decreasing cardiac output.

   d. Response to inflammation and healing slows.

   e. Heart valves become thicker and rigid from sclerosis, leading to arrhythmias.

   f. Blood pressure increases to make up for peripheral resistance and decreased cardiac output.

  7. Respiratory system changes

   a. Decreased ciliary action and cough reflex

   b. Lungs appear larger due to loss of elasticity.

   c. Calcification of the costal cartilage makes the rib cage more rigid.

   d. Decreased arterial blood O_2 level (pO_2)

    e.   Diameter of the anterior posterior chest increases.

    f.   Respiratory muscles weaken, therefore less lung expansion

    g.   Increase in residual lung volume

    h.   Less efficient gas exchange - all these changes put the older person at greater risk for respiratory infections.

8. Gastrointestinal system changes are less serious but bothersome.

    a.   Loss of teeth due to periodontal disease and poor dental care

    b.   Decreased taste sensation

    c.   Decreased salivary secretion

    d.   Slowed swallowing time

    e.   Decreased esophageal motility; greater risk for aspiration

    f.   Decreased stomach motility and capacity

    g.   Decreased hunger contractions and emptying time

    h.   Decreased peristalsis in the colon leading to constipation

    i.   Impulses to defecate slower and less noticeable

    j.   Decreased sphincter tone

    k.   Decrease in gastric and enzyme secretions; less absorption of nutrients

9. Genitourinary system changes

    a.   Fewer cells in kidney, causing a decrease in renal function

    b.   Bladder muscles weaken, less elasticity and capacity; urinary frequency, urgency, and nocturia are common.

    c.   Urethra has less muscle tone, and urine is more concentrated.

    d.   In the male, benign prostatic hypertrophy (BPH)

    e.   In the female, atrophy of the vulva

    f.   Ovaries become thicker and smaller; fallopian tubes atrophy and shorten.

    g.   Uterus and cervix become smaller, with atrophy of endometrium

    h.   Ovaries and testes cease to function; conception not possible

    i.   Drier, less elastic, and more alkaline vaginal canal

    j.   Decreased distribution of pubic hair and size of external genitalia

    k.   Sexual response time is slowed, but arousal period is lengthened.

10. Musculoskeletal system changes

    a.   Kyphosis occurs.

    b.   Joints enlarge; tendons and ligaments are less elastic; muscle spasms are common.

    c.   Muscles weaken.

    d.   Height decreases due to thinning vertebral disks.

    e.   Muscle mass and strength decreases. Exercise minimizes these losses.

f. Bone and mineral mass decreases, making bones more porous and brittle and more likely to fracture.

g. Varying degrees of flexion at wrists, hips, and knees with less joint mobility; endurance and agility diminish.

11. Nervous system changes

a. Decreased number of cells; altered equilibrium, proprioception and motor coordination

b. Decreased blood flow to and from brain; decreased pain perception

c. Delay in response and reaction time

d. Decreased need for sleep, but need for more rest

e. Memory of recent events diminished

f. Slowed reflexes

12. Endocrine system changes

a. Decrease in thyroid gland activity and metabolism

b. Hormone production decreases and endocrine glands are smaller

c. Regulation of electrolytes changes

d. Changes in endocrine system affect every other body system

13. Integumentary system changes

a. Fewer skin cells; increased skin pigmentation; less elastic and more delicate skin

b. Lines and wrinkles appear, and body temperature is difficult to maintain due to less subcutaneous fat.

c. Decreased secretions of perspiration and sebum

d. Thinning, graying, and dry scalp hair; nails become hard and brittle.

14. Sensory organs change.

a. All five senses become less efficient.

b. Vision changes

i Vision declines (presbyopia); peripheral vision decreases.

ii. Eyes adjust more slowly to light changes.

iii. Lenses become more opaque; cataracts and glaucoma may occur.

c. Hearing changes

i. Perception of high frequency impaired, followed by impaired perception of low notes

ii. Tympanic membrane experiences sclerosis and atrophies

iii. Increased cerumen in external ear

d. Senses of taste, smell, and touch diminish.

i. Reduced number of taste buds; sense of sweet and salty flavors lost before bitter and sour

ii. Decrease in ability to detect pressure and temperature changes in objects touching skin; pain sensation decreases.

iii. These sensory changes make the older client more at risk for falls and injury.

B. Psychosocial adjustments

1. Family changes

   a. Children becoming independent

   b. Changing roles

   c. Grandparenting

2. Widowhood or loss of life mate

   a. Facing new responsibilities

   b. Adjustments in lifestyle

   c. Loss of companionship

3. Retirement

   a. Preparedness for retirement

   b. Changes in roles, status, and identity

   c. Changes in leisure time

   d. May go through phases of retirement

      i. "Honeymoon" period - characterized by euphoria

      ii. Disenchantment - the reality of retirement sets in

      iii. Stability - person achieves understanding of retirement role

      iv. Termination period - person becomes ill or goes back to work

4. Awareness of mortality

   a. Reality of one's own mortality

   b. Life review

   c. Set goals to achieve

   d. Reminiscing is therapeutic and gives depth and meaning to life.

   e. Religious beliefs and family ties may be strengthened.

   f. Need to leave a legacy to be remembered

5. Living facility changes

   a. Present facility may be too large or too expensive or unsafe.

   b. Change in climate may be desired.

   c. Possible relocation to retirement community.

   d. Living with children may not be desired.

6. Shrinking social contacts

   a. Children grown and gone from home

   b. Rural area can be difficult to get around; urban area may cause fear.

   c. Hearing and speech deficits increase loneliness.

   d. Death of friends, relatives, peers or spouse, may cause depression and withdrawal.

IV. Common Disorders Found in the Elderly

A. Cardiovascular diseases

1. Congestive heart failure, myocardial infarction

2. Coronary artery disease, hypertension, arteriosclerosis

3. Arrhythmias, pulmonary emboli, varicose veins

4. Rheumatic heart disease, bacterial endocarditis

B. Cancer

C. Cerebrovascular accident (CVA), stroke (apoplexy), cerebrovascular disease (CVD), and transient ischemic attack (TIA)

D. Delirium

1. **Delirium** - an acute condition; if underlying causes are treated promptly it may be reversible.

2. It has an acute onset. If individual exhibits difficulty concentrating, decline in ability to perform ADL, disorganized thinking, or changes in LOC, suspect delirium as a response to a disruption in homeostasis due to:

   a. Infection

   b. Drug toxicity

   c. Alcohol intoxication or withdrawal

   d. Electrolyte imbalance

   e. Head trauma

   f. Sleep deprivation

   g. Changes in chronic illness

   h. New disease processes

3. Treatment is based on recognizing and treating the underlying causes.

E. Dementia

1. **Dementia** is cognitive impairment characterized by gradual, progressive onset.

2. It causes an alteration in cognitive functioning. It is irreversible.

3. Symptoms include impaired:

   a. Judgment

   b. Memory

   c. Abstract thinking

   d. Social behavior

4. Seen in:

   a. Alzheimer's disease

   b. Multi-infarct

   c. Huntington's chorea

   d. Parkinson's disease

   e. Multiple sclerosis

        f.   Brain tumors

        g. Korsakoff's syndrome

        h. Creutzfeldt-Jakob disease

    5. Treatment is aimed at reducing symptoms and undesired behaviors.

    6. Nursing care for delirium and dementia

        a. Provide a safe environment.

        b. Use a consistent approach to care.

        c. Assist client with ADL.

        d. Reorient as needed.

        e. Use short, simple directions and instructions.

        f.   Provide support to family and encourage caregiver support.

  F. **Depression** - extreme sadness or pathological grief reaction

  G. Respiratory diseases such as emphysema, pneumonia, asthma, and chronic bronchitis

  H. Degenerative arthritis (osteoarthritis), osteoporosis, fractures

  I. Parkinsonism, senile dementia

  J. Nutritional deficiencies, diabetes

  K. Chronic constipation and fecal impaction

  L. Incontinence, urinary and fecal; benign prostatic hypertrophy

V. Nursing Care of the Older Client

  A. Nursing observations and charting must be complete and accurate

  B. Nursing interventions

    1. Clients should be encouraged to participate in their ADL.

    2. Provide a safe environment

        a. Warm and stable temperature

        b. Nonslip floors, proper footwear, well lighted areas

        c. Prevention of burns

        d. Belongings within reach

        e. Hand rails and grips, assistive devices for ambulation

    3. Allow adequate time for activities of daily living

    4. Hygiene

        a. Fewer baths needed, lotions or creams to reduce skin dryness; special attention to pressure areas

        b. Special care trimming nails

        c. Provide good oral care

    5. Provide a nutritious diet

        a. Provide less quantity and higher quality of food with more protein and fewer carbohydrates and fats.

        b. Suspect dehydration if suddenly disorientation occurs.

    c. Caloric intake for older adults -1600 for females, 2200 calories for males

    d. 2500-3000 mL per day fluid intake

    e. Four or five small feedings instead of three large ones, with more flavoring in food

6. Adequate exercise

    a. Prolonged immobility can lead to complications.

    b. Normal range of motion in all joints

    c. Avoid fatigue.

7. Medications

    a. The older person's body's ability to absorb, metabolize, detoxify, and eliminate drugs is decreased.

    b. Certain drugs can accumulate and cause toxic effects.

    c. Intravenous fluids can cause circulatory overload.

    d. Avoid self-medication with home remedies and over-the-counter drugs.

    e. Cathartics should be given with care. Mineral oil depletes the body's stores of vitamin A. Saline cathartics cause dehydration.

    f. Medication problems of the elderly

       i. Inability to read instructions and pour liquids because of poor vision and tremors

       ii. Inability to open bottles with safety caps

       iii. May forget to take medication (or take them twice) because of poor memory

       iv. May not be aware of side effects of drugs

       v. **Polypharmacy** –taking many medications increases the risk of toxicity or interactions. See Table 1 for Medications Commonly Used by the Elderly.

TABLE 1.   COMMON GROUPS OF DRUGS USED BY THE ELDERLY

DRUG GROUP	NURSING IMPLICATIONS
Antacids	Observe for signs and symptoms of diarrhea, constipation. Teach elders to check sodium and sugar content on the label. Encourage elders to take antacid 1 hour after meals and not with other medications. Caution clients with history of cardiac or renal conditions.
Antibiotics	Observe for confusion, changes in hearing. Encourage fluid intake. Monitor weight, intake and output, specific gravity of urine. Observe for GI disturbances, diarrhea. Observe for secondary yeast or fungal infections of mouth or vagina.
Antidepressants/ Antipsychotics	Observe for tremor, spasms. Teach techniques to use with dizziness when changing positions, and methods to counteract dry mouth. Cautious use in clients with glaucoma, prostate, or cardiac conditions Observe for urinary retention.
Antihistamines	Observe for changes in blood pressure. Observe for anticholinergic effects: restlessness, delirium. Cautious use in clients with glaucoma, prostate, or cardiac conditions
Antihypertensives	Observe for depression, anxiety, disorientation. Monitor for bradycardia, angina, and hypotension.
Anti-inflammatory Agents	Teach importance of taking with food. Avoid if there is a history of peptic ulcer. Observe for nausea, vomiting, GI bleeding. Observe for psychological disturbances.
Cardiovascular Agents	Explain importance of keeping appointments for laboratory examination. Monitor heart rate and rhythm. Observe for orthostatic hypotension. Observe for adverse reactions: confusion, depression, vertigo, lethargy.
Diuretics	Observe for orthostatic hypotension, delirium, changes in mental function. Should be taken in the morning
Narcotics	Observe for hypotension, observe for adverse or idiosyncratic reactions (hallucinations, agitation, confusion). Monitor respiratory function.
Oral Anticoagulants	Monitor prothrombin times. Observe for bleeding. Explain importance of keeping appointments for lab work. Avoid aspirin-containing products. Institute safety measures to prevent injury.

Oral Hypoglycemic Agents, Tranquilizers, Sedatives	Observe for signs of hypoglycemia: weakness, headache, malaise. Monitor blood glucose levels. Observe for signs of oversedation: lethargy, confusion, agitation. Explain the need to avoid other depressants and alcohol. Observe for adverse and idiosyncratic reactions: delirium, orthostatic hypotension, cardiac dysrhythmias.

8. Incontinence

   a. Related to changes in muscular tone of bladder or bowel, disease, disorientation, or lack of proper signal

   b. Damages skin, lowers self-esteem, increases chances of infection

   c. Fecal impaction often mistaken for diarrhea or incontinence

9. Be alert to possible causes of confusion: drug reaction, dehydration, fever, or first sign of some disorder. Orient confused persons to time, place, and person whenever necessary; do not endorse senile behavior.

10. Arrange for a health worker to visit those living alone.

11. Make use of special services for the elderly

   a. Foster grandparents program

   b. Day care centers

   c. Continuing education

   d. "Meals on Wheels"

   e. Homemaker services

   f. Extended care facilities

   g. Senior citizen groups

C. Nursing interventions for the confused client

  1. Care of clients who wander

   a. Make environment safe and secure and allow person freedom to roam within it.

   b. Keep current photograph of individual on hand; have ID secured on person.

   c. Take individual for walk or provide some activity daily.

   d. Use distraction to decrease wandering.

   e. Help orient to present (reality orientation).

  2. Keys to solving problem behaviors

   a. Sudden changes in behavior need to be evaluated medically.

   b. Note any triggers to unwanted behavior.

   c. Check for any physical discomfort.

   d. Reduce environmental stimuli.

   e. Allow for choices whenever possible.

3. Suggestions for nighttime restlessness/sundowning syndrome

   a. Use night light.

   b. Reduce intake of stimulants.

   c. Follow bedtime routines.

   d. Provide short naps during day.

   e. Provide comfort items for sleep: teddy, doll, special pillow, or blanket.

4. Suggestions for reducing agitation

   a. Evaluate medical regimen and medications used.

   b. Try music to soothe.

   c. Reduce environmental stimuli.

   d. Simplify tasks.

   e. Provide nonstressful tasks that the person can accomplish e.g., folding linen, setting mats on table.

Additional Resources Found on MyNursingLab

- Nursing Issues and the Elderly (video)
- Pharmacology and the Elderly (video)

MODULE 7.1

Mental Health Nursing Care

Learning Objectives

7.1.1 **Distinguish between characteristics of mental health and mental illness.**

7.1.2 **Describe elements of a therapeutic relationship in mental health nursing.**

7.1.3 **Describe common theories of personality development.**

7.1.4 **Describe nursing care and treatment modalities for major mental disorders.**

    I. Mental Health and Mental Illness

        A. Mental health

            1. The individual develops mature coping mechanisms for everyday problems.

            2. The person accepts reality and acts appropriately.

            3. The person adjusts to the environment in a socially acceptable manner and maintains a certain degree of continuity and consistency.

            4. The person sets future goals and moves toward them.

            5. Mental health fluctuates day to day. No one characteristic is evidence of mental health, nor is lack of any one characteristic evidence of mental illness.

            6. Characteristics of mentally healthy behavior

                a. Independent personality

                b. Ability to adjust to change

                c. Tolerance of stress and frustrations

                d. Acceptance and knowledge of self

                e. Sincere concern for others

                f. Ability to love others

                g. Ability to be directed by inner values

                h. Ability to find outlets for basic needs

                i. Ability to appraise reality

        B. Mental illness

            1. Definition is usually based on what people think of as socially accepted behavior.

            2. Mental illness describes the state of an individual who is unable to cope effectively, establish satisfying relationships, or acknowledge reality, and who lacks a healthy self-concept.

            3. Mentally ill behavior is often considered bizarre and not in keeping with reality.

            4. Personal and social relationships are compromised.

PEARSON

C. Psychiatry

    1. The branch of medicine dealing with mental health and mental illness.

    2. It focuses on how and why people act the way they do, how to prevent mental illness, and how to deal with client's behavior.

D. Care of the mentally ill, past and present

    1. Social attitudes and viewpoints have influenced care and treatment of mentally ill.

    2. Superstitions, ignorance, and mysticism influenced past treatment.

        a. Possession by demons as a punishment for sins was widely believed in early times.

        b. Some disorders were regarded as divine.

        c. Affected people were often locked in dungeons or jails.

    3. Movement toward more effective treatment has been slow; attitudes towards mentally ill have changed gradually.

    4. Some misconceptions regarding the mentally ill still exist.

    5. Recent reforms contributed greatly to a growing knowledge of prevention, cause, and treatment of mental illness.

        a. Facilities are expanded and emphasis is placed on treating clients before hospitalization is necessary.

        b. Psychiatric units are located in general hospitals.

        c. Community mental health facilities often provide treatment, outpatient treatment, partial hospitalization, and 24-hour emergency care where crisis intervention is a major focus.

        d. Halfway houses provide help for clients during the transition from a hospital to the community.

        e. Foster family care may be used instead of hospitalization or as a transitional stage back into the community.

        f. Nursing homes are often a potential source of help with the milder psychiatric issues and with the aging person who has mental or emotional problems.

        g. Sheltered workshops provide employment for mentally ill clients.

        h. Areas of focus of mental health care are:

            i. Prevention

            ii. Deinstitutionalization

            iii. Community-based care

            iv. Public mental health

E. Role of the community

    1. Develop programs to enlighten and educate public concerning needs of mental health field.

    2. Establish institutional facilities for mental health.

    3. Establish recreational facilities for all age groups.

    4. Establish day and night care for all age groups - halfway houses, foster homes, and after care (should be included in all community planning).

5. Alcohol and drug-abuse programs should be coordinated for maximum benefit of community.

6. Sex education should be taught in elementary and high schools in order to provide correct and intelligent information for children and to help prepare young people for marriage and parenthood.

F. Mental health treatments and rehabilitation

1. Drugs - tranquillizers, sedatives, etc.

2. **Milieu therapy** - safe, structured environment in which to do mental health work

3. **Occupational therapy** - structured tasks that help enhance self-esteem and improve mental health

4. **Electroconvulsive therapy** (ECT or electroshock therapy) - application of electrical current to the brain; increases circulating levels of neurotransmitters

5. **Psychotherapy** - planned sessions with a trained mental health practitioner to address issues and improve mental health

6. **Psychoanalysis** - in-depth work with a psychiatrist to explore the psyche and resolve subconscious issues

7. **Behavior modification** - a structured approach to altering behaviors and improving interpersonal functioning

II. **Elements of a Therapeutic Relationship**

A. **Therapeutic relationship** - one in which nursing activities are purposeful and goal-directed, and in which the client is helped to become a healthier, more appropriate, and productive participant in the community.

1. It is important for a nurse to understand his/her own behavior.

2. Nurses use their own personalities as a therapeutic tool.

3. Honesty, trust, and empathy are the tools the nurse uses.

4. Observation and knowledge of therapeutic communication are important to client treatment.

5. Nurses help clients make positive changes in behavior.

6. Nurses help create and maintain a therapeutic environment (**milieu**) that is conducive to improvement and recovery.

B. Basic principles of mental health nursing

1. Have self-awareness - an important therapeutic tool.

   a. Nurse should seek to understand self.

   b. Knowledge of one's own needs and motivations is very useful in understanding the needs and motivations of the client.

2. Accept client as he or she is. *Positive Regard*

   a. Display genuine interest.

   b. Show patience and understanding.

   c. Act in a nonjudgmental and nonpunitive manner.

      i. This does not necessarily mean approval of behavior.

      ii. Demonstrate acceptance of client regardless of behavior.

3. Establish trust.

   a. Be honest.

   b. Be consistent.

   c. Don't make any promises you can't keep.

4. Offer reassurance.

   a. Demonstrate nursing competence.

   b. Attempt to see the situation from the client's point of view.

   c. Do not minimize client's fears and anxiety.

   d. Show sincere interest in client.

5. Encourage reality experiences.

   a. Do not support unrealistic ideas.

   b. Encourage healthy and appropriate communication with staff and others.

6. Promote safety and provide consistency in experiences.

   a. Consistency is useful in routine.

   b. Attitudes of staff toward clients are important.

   c. Clients are made to feel more comfortable by knowing what to expect.

7. Avoid promoting unnecessary anxiety.

   a. Limit demands on the client.

   b. Avoid use of unfamiliar, professional jargon.

   c. Concentrate on client's strengths, not weaknesses.

   d. Be sincere.

8. Maintain objectivity.

   a. Do not allow personal needs and feelings to take precedence over those of the client.

   b. Be accurate and free of bias in reporting and recording observations.

9. Maintain a realistic relationship.

   a. Recognize the difference between friendliness and a professional relationship.

   b. Focus on client's needs.

   c. Offer warmth and understanding, but not intimacy, in relationships.

C. Nurse-client relationships

   1. Relationships consist of the interactions between nurses and clients, with focus on the client's needs.

   2. Relationships offer clients opportunities to modify behavior.

   3. Nurses' actions are directed toward meeting client's needs.

   4. Nurses use a healthy personality to promote mental health in others.

   5. Therapeutic relationships provide security for clients and enable them to grow and develop to potential.

PEARSON

6. Effective relationships do not necessarily mean doing what clients want, but they do require providing for client needs.

D. Communication skills

1. Communication involves all modes of behavior by which people influence one another. It is a two-way process in which the purpose is to promote understanding.

2. Modes of communication are

   a. Verbal

      i. Spoken word

      ii. Written language

   b. Nonverbal

      i. Gestures

      ii. Mannerisms

      iii. Voice tone

      iv. Body movements

      v. Facial expressions

      vi. Silence

3. A nonverbal component is always present when verbal communication takes place; for example, inflection of voice carries sentiment when a statement is made.

4. Characteristics of successful communication are:

   a. Feedback - opportunity for listener to respond. It may serve to clarify, extend, or alter the original idea contained in the communication.

   b. Appropriateness - reply is relevant to the communication received; there is neither too much nor too little information.

   c. Efficiency - language used by the parties is understood, and enough time between verbal responses is allowed for the listener to perceive and evaluate them.

5. **Therapeutic techniques** of communication are methods used to facilitate communication.

   a. Listening - an opportunity to understand the message and provide feedback.

   b. Silence - gives the opportunity for meaningful reflection by both participants.

   c. **Exploring** - interjecting appropriate comments during conversation to show interest and attentiveness. ("Go on." "Tell me more.")

   d. **Reflection** (flashback) - repeating all or part of an individual's statement. It assists people in understanding their own thoughts and feelings. (The person states, "I feel worried about my condition." The responder may say, "You feel worried?")

   e. **Open-ended statements** - comments referring back to a topic that has been previously mentioned in order to obtain more information. ("You were telling me about. . . . "). They suggest the desire to hear more than "yes" or "no."

   f. **Clarification** - request for more information; should be used carefully and appropriately. Questions are often helpful when there is need to clarify. (The client refers to "they". It would be appropriate for the nurse to ask, "Who are 'they'?") Questions are also useful in eliciting necessary information.

6. Blocks to effective communication are:

    a. Persistent questioning or **probing** for information. Avoid asking "why" and "how" questions since they place the client on the defensive.

    b. Failure to listen - intended message is not received.

    c. Overloading or underloading the conversation - talking too much or too little.

    d. **Clichés** – common statements that provide pat answers and false reassurances ("Don't worry, you are going to be fine.")

    e. Using value statements, such as "good" or "nice." Although well-intended, it indicates that the nurse is judging the client as good or bad.

    f. Giving advice - this often carries the suggestion that the client is not capable of directing his or her own activities.

    g. Changing the subject - results in avoidance of discussions.

E. Nursing assessment of the psychiatric client

    1. Observation of data, of the person, and of the situation

        a. Involves all the sense organs, not just the eyes

        b. Is important for planning interventions

        c. Has legal ramifications

    2. Important aspects to observe include:

        a. Appearance - includes everything that can be seen:

            i. Hair

            ii. Eyes

            iii. Facial expression

            iv. Skin

            v. Clothing

            vi. Posture

            vii. Movements

        b. Behavior - all of client's actions in such areas as:

            i. Sleep

            ii. Appetite

            iii. Hygiene

            iv. Elimination

            v. Medications

            vi. Treatment

            vii. Social interactions

        c. Conversation

            i. Relevant or irrelevant

            ii. Loose or appropriate thought connections

   iii. Possible hesitancy or silence

   iv. Rapid or extremely slow speech

  3. Aim of assessment is to identify client's strengths, weaknesses, and needs.

  4. Assessment outcomes:

   a. Enable nurse to plan care

   b. Enable nurse to anticipate needs

   c. Afford better understanding of client

  5. Client should still be considered nurse's primary source of information.

III. Personality Development

 A. Human **personality** - somewhat predictable behavior response patterns that are unique to the individual

  1. Behavior is both conscious and unconscious.

   a. Intellectual and physical qualities

   b. Social behavior patterns

   c. Psychological and emotional attributes

   d. Awareness of individual self

 B. Factors in personality development:

  1. Physical makeup

  2. Genetics

  3. Birth order

  4. Family composition

  5. Early childhood experiences

  6. Family attitudes, feelings, and values

  7. Satisfaction of physical and emotional needs

  8. Social environment

 C. Theorists

  1. Sigmund Freud

   a. Founded psychoanalytic movement

   b. Explored the unconscious part of the mind and developed dream theory

   c. Categorized human drives

  2. Other theorists

   a. Alfred Adler

   b. Otto Rank

   c. Carl Jung

   d. Karen Horney

   e. Erich Fromm

   f. Erik Erikson

3. Four basic concepts of personality development on which almost all psychoanalytic groups agree:

   a. All behavior is meaningful.

   b. The role of the unconscious is important in determining behavior.

   c. All behavior is goal directed.

   d. The foundation for later personality development is laid in the early years of life.

4. Personality theory according to Freud

   a. **Id** - pleasure-seeking instincts

      i. Present at birth

      ii. Concerned with biologic drives

      iii. Seeks immediate gratification of needs

   b. **Ego** - the "self" or "I"

      i. Begins to develop toward the end of the first year of life

      ii. Develops from experience

      iii. Guides and controls actions of the individual

      iv. Seeks to postpone immediate satisfactions until appropriate time

   c. **Superego** - conscience or sense of right or wrong

      i. Begins to develop around the second year of life

      ii. Reflects the demands of society

5. Levels of awareness (Freud)

   a. **Unconscious** - repressed memories, thoughts, feelings, or wishes of which the individual is unaware

   b. **Conscious** - memories, thoughts, and feelings of which the individual is aware

   c. Preconscious/ **Subconscious** - that which may be brought into awareness with some effort

6. Freud's developmental stages of the personality

   a. **Oral phase** (birth to 1 year of age)

      i. Focuses on oral satisfaction

      ii. Relationship with mother is of prime importance.

      iii. Love and satisfaction of physical needs help develop security.

      iv. Good experiences set firm basis for future development.

   b. **Anal phase** (1 to 3 years of age)

      i. Child learns pleasurable bodily sensations relating to passage.

      ii. Period of conformity commences as toilet training is begun; child learns to give and take.

      iii. Toilet training should begin only after sphincter control develops, usually around 15 months of age.

      iv. Child needs love and understanding during toilet training, which should be accomplished without punishment.

    v.   Child begins to relate to others and use words to communicate.

    vi. Motor skills and independence increase.

c. Phallic phase or **Oedipal phase** (3 to 6 years of age)

    i.   Child becomes aware of own body and differences between sexes.

    ii.   Curiosity about body results in self-exploration.

    iii. Positive attitude of parents is important in handling masturbation.

    iv. Boy becomes attached to mother and sees father as rival.

    v.   Girl is antagonistic toward mother and desires to take mother's place with father.

    vi. Oedipal conflict is resolved as child takes on characteristics of parent of same sex (identification).

    vii. This phase is the most crucial period of development for social and sexual adjustment; children need stable figures with whom to identify.

d. **Latency phase** (6 to 12 years of age)

    i.   Energy is directed towards intellectual growth and socialization.

    ii.   Child learns to compete with others, and to give, take, and compromise.

    iii. Hero worship and identification with figures outside family

    iv. Groups become important: child has strong group loyalties, wants to be one of the gang, and seeks acceptance of the group.

    v.   Companionship with members of own sex is outstanding characteristic of the phase.

e. Adolescence (12 years of age to maturity)

    i.   A period of many conflicts, it begins with onset of physical maturity and ends with acquisition of patterns with which to handle conflicts.

    ii.   Physiologic changes include glandular changes, growth of pubic hair, voice changes, and changes in body shape.

    iii. Desire for independence often leads to conflict with parents (ambivalence), and rebellion against rules, regulations, and family restrictions.

    iv. Dating begins as adolescent expands socially and seeks sexual companionship.

    v.   Group identification continues

        (a) Adolescent conforms to group standards.

        (b) Group ideas tend to be idealistic.

        (c) Group offers security.

    vi. Outcomes of this phase are:

        (a) Selection of vocation

        (b) Emancipation from parents

        (c) Adjustment to opposite sex

    vii. If experiences have been successful throughout this stage, a mature person emerges.

      f.   Maturity - emotional maturity is an ideal state and includes:

         i.   A realistic view of life

         ii.   Ability to see own strengths and weakness

         iii.   Ability to give and receive pleasure, have friendships and love

         iv.   Ability to learn and profit from mistakes and successes

D. Coping mechanisms

    1. Need for mechanisms:

      a.   All humans experience conflict and tension; life is a constant struggle between desires and obstacles.

      b.   When conflicts arise, individual must learn patterns to cope with them (adjustment).

      c.   One way of handling increased tension is through ego defense mechanisms.

    2. Characteristics of coping mechanisms (defenses):

      a.   Ego **defense mechanisms** are a means of managing emotional conflict and anxiety.

      b.   They usually operate without individuals' conscious awareness.

      c.   They are utilized by all humans in times of stress and anxiety.

    3. Commonly used defenses:

      a.   **Repression** - barring of unacceptable thoughts and feelings from consciousness

         i.   A way of excluding painful, unpleasant material from awareness

         ii.   An example is an upsetting event in childhood that is pushed from awareness and may not be recalled at will.

      b.   **Suppression** (a conscious act) - process of deliberately forgetting unpleasant thoughts and feelings

         i.   Unlike repressed material, suppressed material can be recalled into awareness.

         ii.   An example is a student who chooses not to think about her argument with her spouse until after work.

      c.   **Denial** - refusal to accept reality; avoidance of an unpleasant or threatening truth

      d.   **Reaction formation** - mechanism by which individual expresses attitudes and behavior that are the opposite of his or her true repressed feelings

         i.   An example is an overly friendly, overly polite person who has unconscious feelings of hatred toward others.

      e.   **Projection** - process of attributing undesirable thoughts and feelings to others

         i.   Individual fails to recognize personal faults by finding them in others.

         ii.   An example is a wife who is frequently critical of husband, saying that her husband is always finding fault with her.

    f. **Rationalization** - process by which an attempt is made to explain or excuse oneself for unacceptable behavior

        i. Rationalization serves to hide real motives behind behavior.

        ii. An example is a student who does not study for examination, fails, and then says poor teaching was the cause.

    g. **Displacement** - process whereby an emotion is transferred from the original object onto another object.

        i. Displacement occurs when it is unsafe to express feelings directly.

        ii. An example is an employee who has a misunderstanding with the boss, goes home, and is mean to his or her spouse.

    h. **Sublimation** - mechanism by which energy associated with primitive drives is channeled into acceptable social activities

        i. An example is the aggressive boy who becomes a prize fighter.

    i. **Identification** - process whereby a person adopts characteristics, feelings, or attributes of another.

        i. Identification is a necessary mechanism for a child; it is a method by which the child learns gender roles.

        ii. Examples are a little boy who develops mannerisms like his father and a girl, like her mother.

    j. **Conversion** - unconscious mechanism by which psychological conflicts are expressed through physical symptoms.

        i. An example is a wife who develops deafness upon hearing that her husband wants a divorce.

    k. **Regression** - process whereby an individual utilizes patterns of behavior characteristic of an earlier phase of life

        i. Regression helps a person to escape a painful reality temporarily.

        ii. An example is a hospitalized person who cries easily or shows excessive dependency needs.

    l. **Compensation** - making up for real or imagined deficiencies by excelling in another area

    m. **Undoing** - attempting to right a wrong with another unrelated action

        i. An example is making an embarrassing scene in front of the spouse's peers and then making reservations to treat the spouse to dinner at his or her favorite restaurant

    n. **Fantasy** - use of wishful and imaginative activity to relieve tension

        i. Fantasy is frequently used when no satisfaction can be found in reality.

        ii. An example is daydreaming rather than focusing on the present.

IV. Mental Status Assessment

    A. Areas evaluated

        1. General appearance

          a. Appropriate

          b. Grooming

      c.   Expression

      d.   Stereotypical movements

      e.   Rigidity

      f.   Catatonia

2.   Level of consciousness - sensorium

      a.   Oriented to time, place, and person.

      b.   Alert, awake, somnolent, lethargic, stuporous, comatose

3.   Memory

      a.   Immediate

      b.   Remote

      c.   Recent

4.   Judgment - insight

      a.   Appropriate

      b.   Inappropriate

5.   Intellectual ability

      a.   Concentration - attention

      b.   Knowledge

      c.   Reasoning

      d.   Concrete

      e.   Abstract

6.   Thought processes

      a.   Appropriate

      b.   Delusions

      c.   Hallucinations

      d.   Obsessions

      e.   Phobias

7.   Affect and mood

      a.   Appropriate/inappropriate

      b.   Labile

      c.   Ambivalent

      d.   Hostile

      e.   Depressed

      f.   Flat/blunted

      g.   Euphoric

8. Speech

    a. Relevant or incoherent

    b. Flight of ideas

    c. Neologism

V. Mental Health Care Team

A. The psychiatric team

  1. Psychiatrist

  2. Psychologist

  3. Psychiatric social worker

  4. Psychiatric nurse

  5. Licensed practical/vocational nurse

  6. Psychiatric aids

  7. Occupational therapist

B. The role of the nurse

  1. General principles

    a. Focus care on the client as a person.

    b. Avoid physical and verbal force.

    c. Communicate on level of client's understanding.

    d. Be consistent in attitude for client's security.

    e. Extend yourself to client.

    f. Anticipate client's needs.

    g. Reassure client.

    h. Know client.

    i. Understand client's behavior.

    j. Plan for client's care.

    k. Implement plan.

    l. Evaluate results of care.

    m. Share your observations with members of healthcare team.

  2. Preventive measures

    a. Early detection of symptoms

    b. Establishment of healthful living patterns

    c. Expanded mental health research

    d. Stable home life

  3. Clients requiring constant observation

    a. All new clients

    b. Depressed clients

    c. Drug-addicted clients

      d.   Alcoholic clients

      e.   Suicidal clients

      f.   Clients who talk about suicide

      g.   Clients receiving special treatments

      h.   Clients who lack impulse control

      i.   Clients with persecution complexes

      j.   Hypochondriac clients

VI. Mental Health Disorders and Nursing Care

A. **Anxiety:** a vague, uneasy feeling in response to real or imagined stress

    1. Generalized anxiety disorder

        a.   Motor tension, autonomic hyperactivity

        b.   Nursing care:

           i.   Provide calm, quiet environment.

           ii.   Help client to recognize anxiety-causing situations.

           iii.   Teach relaxation techniques.

    2. Panic disorder

        a.   Apprehension, fearfulness, chest pain, dyspnea, tachycardia, elevated BP, fainting, sense of impending death

        b.   Nursing care

           i.   Provide quiet, nonstressful environment.

           ii.   Administer anti-anxiety medications.

           iii.   Remain with client.

    3. Obsessive compulsive disorder

        a.   **Obsessions:** persistent, unwanted thoughts

        b.   **Compulsions:** persistent urges to perform some action

        c.   Nursing care

           i.   Avoid ridiculing the client.

           ii.   Avoid interrupting rituals.

    4. Phobic disorders

        a.   **Phobia:** an intense, irrational fear of a known object

        b.   Nursing care

           i.   Help client learn relaxation techniques.

           ii.   Help client and family identify primary and secondary gains.

           iii.   Encourage desensitization techniques.

5. **Somatoform disorders:** involuntary physical symptoms without any physiological causes

    a. Nursing care:

        i. Nonjudgmental approach

        ii. Avoid focusing on physical complaints.

        iii. Teach relaxation techniques.

B. Psychotic, neurotic behavior; characteristics:

    1. Agitation

    2. Suspicion

    3. Worry

    4. Guilt

    5. Loneliness

    6. Illusion

    7. Insomnia

    8. Repression

    9. Compulsions/obsessions

    10. Somatic complaints

    11. Delusions of grandeur

    12. Hallucinations

C. Care of clients with personality disorders

    1. Establish therapeutic nurse-client relationship:

        a. Negative behavior will not receive approval.

        b. Positive behavior will receive approval.

    2. Anxiety and frustration

        a. Must be identified

        b. Must be allowed to be expressed

    3. Aggression and hostility

        a. Accepted

        b. Channeled into appropriate outlet

    4. Appropriate praise and encouragement must be given.

D. Care of schizophrenic clients

    1. Establish therapeutic relationship; maintain nonthreatening environment.

    2. Assist client in maintaining good personal hygiene.

    3. Stimulate social behavior.

        a. Assist client in developing feelings of trust.

        b. Assist client with development of sense of self.

4. Help client to reestablish effective contact with reality.

5. Teach client and family about the importance of maintaining medication regimen.

E. Organic behavioral disorders

1. Can be caused by traumatic experiences

2. Can be from nervous system injury

3. Acute form

   a. Cause - presence of toxins in body

   b. Treatment

      i. Removal of toxins

      ii. Prevention of complications

   c. Nursing care

      i. Provide reassurance, security, and consistency in routines.

      ii. Provide well-balanced, easily digested food.

      iii. Assist client in recognition of intellectual and emotional limitations.

      iv. Protect client from emotional upsets.

      v. Protect client from ridicule.

      vi. Assist client in maintaining good personal hygiene (including bowel and bladder hygiene).

      vii. Keep client comfortable.

      viii. Help client to use his or her abilities.

      ix. Extend empathy and kindness to client.

      x. Help maintain client's individuality.

      xi. Follow physician's orders.

      xii. Avoid excessive stimulation of client.

      xiii. Observe client closely.

4. Chronic form

   a. Other designations

      i. Senile dementia

      ii. Alzheimer's disease, Pick's disease

      iii. Multi-infarct dementia

   b. Treatment objective is to help client function to the best of his or her ability.

   c. Nursing care

      i. Help reestablish feelings of worth.

      ii. Provide companionship.

      iii. Provide social acceptance.

    iv. Help develop self-respect.

    v. Provide medications as ordered.

  F. Deviations from normal behavior

    1. Aggressive behavior patterns

     a. Openly expressed hostility

     b. Extreme mood changes

     c. Nursing care

      i. Provide quiet, consistent environment.

      ii. Provide adequate rest.

      iii. Avoid stressful situations; lead away from area in a calm, nonthreatening manner.

      iv. Allow client to express hostility.

      v. Answer questions directly.

      vi. Do not criticize or condone inappropriate actions.

      vii. Avoid challenging client.

      viii. Recognize escalating behavior and ask for help.

      ix. Be alert to nonverbal communication.

      x. Protect persons from injury to self or others.

      xi. Distract person with food or activity.

 G. Affective disorders

    1. Bipolar-manic depressive disorders-marked by mood swings

    2. Manic phase (overactivity)

     a. Traits

      i. Excessive, undirected, frantic physical activity

      ii. Elation, grandiose behavior

      iii. Delusions

      iv. Poor judgment

      v. Rapid speech and thought patterns

      vi. Bizarre behavior

      vii. Little attention to physical needs

     b. Treatment

      i. Lithium carbonate, valproic acid

     c. Nursing care

      i. Handle client calmly.

      ii. Provide quiet, nonstimulating environment.

      iii. Provide physical outlets.

      iv. Provide outdoor recreational activities.

PEARSON

       v. Provide opportunities for client to develop talents.

      vi. Provide opportunities to pursue hobbies.

     vii. Keep client from injuring self.

    viii. Maintain nutrition and fluid needs.

3. Depressive phase (underactivity)

    a. Traits

        i. General state of depression

       ii. Extreme apathy

      iii. Lack of self-esteem

      iv. Sense of unworthiness

       v. Isolation from others

      vi. Decreased appetite

     vii. Altered sleep patterns

    viii. Somatic complaints

    b. Treatment

        i. Antidepressants

       ii. Electroconvulsant therapy (ECT or electric shock therapy)

      iii. Psychotherapy

    c. Nursing care

        i. Provide for regular exercise.

       ii. Give special attention to personal hygiene.

      iii. Administer good skin care.

      iv. Observe for circulatory complications.

       v. Maintain musculoskeletal activity.

      vi. Prevent client from standing or sitting in one position for long periods.

     vii. Show interest in client.

    viii. Provide objective, accepting attitude.

     ix. Provide nutrition.

4. Suicidal client

    a. Traits

        i. Client threatens to take life.

       ii. Cause stems from extreme feelings of unworthiness, depression, and despair.

    b. Warnings

        i. Earlier attempts with drugs, poisons, etc.

        ii. Statements that provide a warning.

            (a) "I want to end my life."

            (b) "Life isn't worth living."

            (c) "I'd be better off dead."

        iii. Giving away possessions

        iv. Moods

            (a) Depression

            (b) Defiance

            (c) Dissatisfaction with dependency on others

            (d) Disorientation

            (e) Sudden, unexplained cheerfulness

    c. Nurse's role

        i. Listen to client.

        ii. Show acceptance of client.

        iii. Show client that he or she is worthy of respect and attention.

        iv. Report any attempt at suicide or early warnings.

        v. Observe client closely.

        vi. Anticipate client's behavior.

        vii. Never leave client alone.

        viii. Remove any articles that could be used for self-destruction.

H. Drug addiction

  1. **Addiction** - condition caused by dependency on substances (drugs, alcohol)

    a. Drugs used in order to adjust to or cope with conflict

    b. Excessive misuse of drugs

  2. Commonly misused drugs

    a. Opiates

    b. Cocaine

    c. Demerol sodium

    d. Methadone

    e. Barbiturates

    f. Hallucinogenic drugs

        i. LSD (lysergic acid diethylamide)

        ii. Mescaline

3. Symptoms upon withdrawal

   a. Irritability and extreme agitation

   b. Muscle cramps

   c. High blood pressure

   d. Diarrhea

   e. Prostration

   f. Nausea

   g. Less severe symptoms - weakness, insomnia, and anorexia

4. Treatment and rehabilitation

   a. Long-term rehabilitation

   b. Counseling

   c. Psychotherapy

   d. Therapeutic communities

   e. Hypnotherapy

   f. Yoga

I. Alcoholism

1. Causes

   a. No one specific cause

   b. Alcohol provides an "escape" from emotional problems.

   c. Psychological dependency.

2. Symptoms

   a. Impaired motor activity

   b. Disturbed motor coordination

   c. Depressant effect on brain and nervous system

   d. Physical effects of toxicity

   e. Delirium tremens in cases of alcoholism for five to ten years

      i. Delusions

      ii. Agitated mind

      iii. Hallucinations

3. Treatment and nursing care

   a. Watch client closely in order to prevent self-injury or injury to others.

   b. Avoid physical strain and/or exhaustion.

   c. Administer medications prescribed by physician (medications often include tranquilizers).

   d. Prevent respiratory infections.

   e. Determine time of last drink; observe for seizures.

f. Treatment for prevention of delirium tremors or DTs (onset 24-48 hours after last drink). Treatment includes vitamin B, anti-anxiety medications (Librium), and supervision.

g. Maintain adequate fluid and electrolytes and nutritional intake.

h. Provide calm, quiet, well-lit atmosphere.

i. Avoid criticism.

j. Prevent additional complications.

k. Use of aversion therapy - disulfiram (Antabuse) - caution clients to avoid taking or eating anything with alcohol.

l. Group therapy in the form of Alcoholics Anonymous

VII. Nursing Responsibilities in Drug Therapy

A. Goals

1. Relieve client's anxiety in regard to administration of medication and its effect on illness.

2. Relieve symptoms and signs of illness.

3. Administer drug correctly- correct client, drug, dose, route, time, and documentation.

4. Assemble proper equipment for administration of ordered medication.

B. Procedures

1. Medications are given only on physician's order.

2. All orders should be complete.

C. Responsibilities

1. Observe client's reaction to drug.

2. Record all signs and symptoms.

3. Immediately report any untoward signs after administration of drug.

4. Make certain client swallows medication during oral administration.

5. Chart medication when given.

6. Chart omission of scheduled dose and report immediately.

7. Question reason for refusal.

8. Educate client about the name of drug, how to take it, and what reactions to expect.

Additional Resources Found on MyNursingLab

- Neurosynapse (animation)
- Drug Chart: Drugs for Mental Health Disorders

MODULE 8.1

Disaster Nursing

Learning Objectives

8.1.1. Describe principles of basic life support.

8.1.2. Describe emergency management for common physical emergencies.

8.1.3. Discuss the nursing role following natural disasters and acts of terrorism.

I. **Basic Life Support**

    A. Airway obstruction - Heimlich maneuver

        1. Assess for signs of distress: clutching of neck; weak, ineffective cough; increased respiratory distress; and inability to speak or cough.

        2. Standing, conscious client

            a. Stand behind; wrap arms around client's waist.

            b. Make a fist; place thumb side of fist against the client's abdomen; grasp fist with other hand.

            c. Press fist into client's abdomen with upward and inward thrust.

        3. Unconscious client

            a. Position client on back.

            b. Kneel astride, facing client's head.

            c. Place heel of one hand against client's abdomen, slightly above umbilicus, below xiphoid process.

            d. With the other hand over the first, press into client's abdomen with quick, upward thrust.

        4. Adult/child 1-rescuer CPR

            a. Check for response.

            b. Activate emergency system/call for AED.

            c. Open airway using head-tilt/chin-lift.

            d. Check breathing (*minimum 5 seconds; maximum 10 seconds*).

            e. Give 2 breaths (1 second each).

            f. Check carotid pulse (*minimum 5 seconds; maximum 10 seconds*).

            g. Locate CPR hand position.

            h. Deliver the first cycle of compressions at a correct rate: less than 23 seconds for 30 compressions.

            i. Give 2 breaths (1 second each).

   j. Deliver the second cycle of compressions at a correct rate: less than 23 seconds for 30 compressions.

   k. Give 2 breaths (1 second each).

   l. Deliver a third cycle of compressions of adequate depth with full chest recoil.

  5. Adult 2-Rescuer CPR with AED

   a. Turn AED on.

   b. Select proper AED and place pads correctly.

   c. Clear away from the client when the AED is analyzing the heart rhythm.

   d. Clear victim to shock; press shock button (*maximum time from AED arrival is less than 90 seconds*).

   e. Resume chest compressions after 1 shock.

   f. Deliver a cycle of compressions at the correct rate: less than 23 seconds for 30 compressions.

   g. Pause to allow the other rescuer to give 2 breaths.

   h. Deliver another cycle of compressions using correct hand position.

   i. Pause to allow other rescuer to give 2 breaths.

  6. Infant 2-rescuer CPR

   a. Check for response.

   b. Activate emergency response system.

   c. Open airway using head-tilt/chin-lift.

   d. Check breathing (*minimum 5 seconds; maximum 10 seconds*).

   e. Give 2 short breaths (1 second each) with visible chest rise.

   f. Check brachial pulse (*minimum 5 seconds; maximum 10 seconds*).

   g. Locate CPR finger position.

   h. Deliver first cycle of compressions at correct rate: less than 23 seconds for 30 compressions.

   i. Give 2 short breaths (1 second each) with visible chest rise.

   j. 1st rescuer pauses to allow 2nd rescuer to give 2 breaths.

   k. 1st rescuer delivers cycle of compressions.

   l. 1st rescuer gives 2 breaths during pauses in compressions using bag mask (2 cycles).

II. Hemorrhage

 A. Control external bleeding: use direct, firm pressure; elevate affected part; use a tourniquet only with traumatic amputations or as a last resort when bleeding cannot be stopped by other means.

 B. Control of internal bleeding with no direct signs of external bleeding

  1. Usually prepare for emergency and pharmacologic therapy.

III. Shock

 A. Loss of adequate circulating blood resulting in inadequate organ and tissue perfusion

PEARSON

    B. Causes:

        1. Hypovolemic - loss of blood - most common

        2. Cardiogenic

        3. Neurogenic

        4. Anaphylactic

        5. Septic

    C. Goals: identify cause, restore and maintain tissue perfusion.

    D. Treatment: maintain airway and circulation.

        1. IV fluids

        2. Blood replacement

        3. Intake and output (I&O)

        4. Vital signs monitored

        5. Pulse oximetry

        6. Electrolytes monitored

        7. Central venous pressure (CVP) monitored

IV. Drowning

    A. Aspiration of fluid with asphyxiation

    B. Causes: accident, injury

    C. Treatment and nursing care

        1. Begin CPR if no pulse or breathing

V. Wounds

    A. Minor to severe

    B. Types: laceration, abrasion, ecchymosis/contusion, hematoma, puncture wound

    C. Cleansing wounds

        1. Cleanse with saline or other agent.

        2. Primary closure: sutures or staples

        3. Delayed primary closure: in tissue with moderate or high potential for infection, wound is splinted, immobilized, and elevated. Tetanus prophylaxis may be given.

    D. Special wounds

        1. Animal bites

            a. Dog bites - concern exists for rabies potential.

                i. Rinse wounds using antiseptic.

                ii. Notify authorities and healthcare provider.

                iii. Tetanus prophylaxis if needed.

                iv. Rabies treatment if needed.

            b. Cat bites or scratches

                i. Rinse wounds using antiseptic.

                ii. Watch for possible infection.

PEARSON

    c. Snake bites

       i. Clean wound and try to remove venom.

       ii. Immobilize area.

       iii. Notify healthcare provider.

       iv. Transport to hospital.

    d. Insect bites

       i. Clean wound.

       ii. Remove stinger if present.

       iii. Apply ice.

       iv. Check for history of allergies.

       v. Transport to hospital if respiratory symptoms present.

    e. Parasite bites: tick

       i. Remove insect.

       ii. Wash with soap and water.

       iii. Seek medical attention.

VI. Trauma

  A. Fractures and dislocations

    1. Types: simple, compound, incomplete, complete, and greenstick

    2. Assess for pallor, pulse, paresthesias, and paralysis.

    3. Immediate pain care; control bleeding, if any; immobilize affected part; splint; apply ice; and observe.

    4. Treatment

      a. X-ray

      b. Cast

      c. Surgery

      d. Traction

  B. Sprains and strains

    1. Assessment for pain, tenderness, dislocation, swelling, and loss of function

    2. Nursing care: elevate affected part, apply ice in first 72 hours, bandage, and immobilize.

  C. Head injury - trauma from blunt or penetrating force

    1. Skull fracture

      a. Assessment

        i. Airway

        ii. Control bleeding.

        iii. Observe for shock.

        iv. Observe for signs of intracranial pressure (ICP).

       v.   Assess level of consciousness (LOC).

       vi. Monitor vital signs.

   b. Treatment

       i.   Surgical intervention

       ii. Antibiotic therapy

2. Brain injury - concussion, contusion

   a. Assessment

       i.   Nausea, vomiting

       ii. Headache

       iii. LOC

       iv. Delirium

       v.   Seizures

   b. Treatment and nursing care

       i.   Close observation; maintain airway.

       ii. Maintain hydration.

       iii. Provide nonstimulating environment.

       iv. Seizure precautions

3. Intracranial hemorrhage

   a. Types

       i.   Epidural

       ii. Subdural

       iii. Subarachnoid

   b. Assessment

       i.   LOC

       ii. Airway

       iii. Vital signs

       iv. Hydration

   c. Treatment and nursing care

       i.   Maintain airway.

       ii. Administer O2.

       iii. Monitor vital signs.

       iv. Monitor motor strength and mobility.

       v.   Monitor ICP.

4. Eye injury

    a. Foreign body

        i. Assessment and treatment

            (a) Invert eyelid and remove foreign body.

            (b) Irrigate with sterile saline.

            (c) Provide rest.

    b. Corneal abrasion

        i. Assessment

            (a) Pain

            (b) Light sensitivity

            (c) Twitching

            (d) Excessive tearing

        ii. Treatment

            (a) Cleansing of eye

            (b) Antibiotic eyedrops or OTC artificial tears or lubricants

            (c) Rest, possible eye patch; cornea usually heals quickly.

D. Spinal cord injury

    1. Assessment

        a. Airway and circulation are first priority

        b. Pain, absence of feeling, numbness, tingling, paralysis

        c. Alteration in motor function

        d. Observe LOC.

        e. Observe for shock.

    2. Treatment and nursing care

        a. Maintain airway.

        b. Treat and prevent shock.

        c. Immobilize to prevent further damage.

        d. Monitor hydration, careful I&O.

E. Chest injuries

    1. **Pneumothorax:** negative pressure loss by air entering pleural cavity

        a. Symptoms

            i. Chest pain

            ii. Tachypnea

            iii. Decreased breath sounds

            iv. Dyspnea

       b.   Treatment and nursing care

           i.   Establish airway.

           ii.   Position in semi-Fowler's.

           iii. Administer O2.

           iv. Prepare client for chest tube insertion.

VII. Injury from Environment

    A. Hyperthermia: heat stroke

       1. Assessment

          a. CNS dysfunction - confusion, delirium, coma

          b. Hot, dry skin

          c. Tachycardia, hypotension, tachypnea

       2. Treatment

          a. Cool sheets, towels

          b. Ice packs to neck, groin, and axillae

          c. Cooling blankets

          d. Iced saline irrigation via NG tube

          e. IV therapy

          f. Monitor vital signs.

          g. Monitor LOC.

          h. Observe I & O.

    B. Hypothermia: cold injury; frostbite

       1. Assessment: numbness, tingling, burning

          a. Edema, numbness

          b. Blister formation

          c. Discoloration

       2. Treatment and nursing care

          a. Remove wet clothes.

          b. Use warm soaks.

          c. Give conscious clients warm drinks.

          d. Immobilize affected part.

VIII. Poisoning: Ingestion of Contaminated Food, Toxin, Pathogen, Drug, or Toxic Chemical

    A. Botulism - caused by improperly canned foods

       1. Symptoms

          a. Headaches

          b. Nausea and vomiting

          c. Changes in vision

          d. Lethargy

        e.   Difficulty breathing or swallowing

        f.   Talking

        g.   Seizures

   2. Treatment

        a.   Maintain airway.

        b.   Give antitoxin.

  B. Food contamination

   1. Causes

        a.   *Staphylococcus aureus*

        b.   *Salmonella*

        c.   *Escherichia coli*

   2. Symptoms

        a.   Nausea, vomiting, and diarrhea

        b.   Abdominal cramps

        c.   Weakness

        d.   Fever, chills

   3. Treatment and nursing care

        a.   Bed rest

        b.   Fluids

IX. Sexual Assault (Rape)

  A. Clients mostly female but can be male.

  B. Assessment

   1. Reassure client that she is safe.

   2. Notify proper authorities.

   3. Have someone remain with person.

   4. Provide privacy.

   5. Obtain history.

   6. Obtain necessary specimens.

   7. Provide emotional support and remind client that it was not her fault.

  C. Treatment

   1. STI prophylaxis given as ordered

   2. Refer to counseling.

X. Natural Disasters and Terrorism

  A. Definition of terms

   1. Disasters: ecological disruptions or emergencies of severity and magnitude resulting in deaths, injuries, illness, and or property damage.

2. Disasters may be internal or external nature. They can be natural or manmade.

 a. Natural disasters include: earthquakes, floods, tornadoes, hurricanes, volcanoes, etc.

 b. Manmade disasters include: biological and biochemical terrorism, chemical spills, nuclear events, fires, explosions, accidents, and acts of war.

B. Nursing and disaster preparedness

 1. ANA noted a need for health professionals to be educated in the response to any disaster.

 2. Nurse's role may include:

  a. Triage

  b. Stabilization

  c. Definitive care

  d. Evacuation

 3. Psychological stress is immediate and persists after stabilization.

 4. How a victim or care provider deals with the stress is influenced by many factors.

C. Nuclear disaster

 1. Nuclear explosion is considered the least likely for a terrorist to use. However, the potential exists for it to happen, and even more potential exists for the use of radioactive materials.

 2. Detection - Radiation cannot be detected by our senses, but each type can be detected and identified with instrumentation.

 3. Health risks

  a. Risk depends upon several factors:

   i. Dose (total amount of radiation received). The larger the dose received, the greater the health risk becomes.

   ii. Dose rate (the length of time over which the dose is received). Dose rate exposures are categorized as follows:

    (a) Acute: a large dose occurring over a short period of time (less than 24 hours). Victims may begin to show symptoms within 24 hours, such as burns of the skin, vomiting, and diarrhea.

    (b) Chronic: small doses occurring over a long period of time (months or years)

D. Chemical weapons

 1. Chemical agents are super-toxic.

 2. Relative toxicity: industrial chemicals < mustard gas < nerve gas

 3. Normal states of chemicals are liquid or gas.

 4. Inhalation hazard is greatest concern.

 5. Characteristics

  a. They do not penetrate unbroken skin.

  b. Nonvolatile

        c.   More toxic than normal chemicals by weight

        d.   Undetectable by senses

        e.   Disseminate as aerosols

E. Biological agents

   1. Bacteria, viruses, and toxins

   2. Bacteria and viruses

        a.   Need portal of entry

        b.   Multiply and overcome immune systems

        c.   Some can cause epidemics.

   3. Toxins

        a.   Poisonous by-products of micro-organisms, plants, and animals

        b.   Not living organisms

        c.   Not contagious

   4. Potential biological agents

        a.   Anthrax (bacteria)

        b.   Plague (bacteria)

        c.   Q fever (Rickettsia)

        d.   Smallpox (virus)

        e.   Ebola (virus)

        f.   Venezuelan equine encephalitis (VEE) virus

        g.   Staphylococcal enterotoxin B

        h.   Botulinum (neurotoxin)

        i.   Ricin (cytotoxin)

   5. Protection against biological agents

        a.   Mask

        b.   Clothing

        c.   Sanitation measures

        d.   Decontamination

        e.   Medical treatment

        f.   Bloodborne pathogen Universal Precautions

Additional Resources Found on MyNursingLab

- Shock (animation)
- Performing a Gastric Lavage (video)

MODULE 9.1

Leadership and Management

Learning Objectives

9.1.1 **Discuss leadership and the different leadership styles.**

9.1.2 **Describe the characteristics of a good leader.**

9.1.3 **Describe managers and the functions of management.**

I. **Leadership and Leadership Styles**

    A. Leadership and management concepts are used by all organizations to run smoothly and achieve organizational goals and objectives.

    B. To face the challenges of the 21st century, the practical nurse needs to develop leadership and management skills.

    C. Practical nurses must have leadership and management skills because they are responsible for managing the care of their clients and for supervising others to meet employer's goals.

    D. In their role as practical nurses, LPNs/LVNs supervise nursing assistants. Many times they are team leaders or charge nurses for evening and night shifts in long-term care.

        1. Accountability

            a. **Accountability** is present in all professions and is the obligation to answer for one's actions. This means that if a mistake occurs, the expectation is that the person will take ownership of the problem, rather than blame others.

            b. Individuals have a responsibility to do only those activities that are within the profession's scope of practice.

            c. To perform these actions, the individual must receive training and attain the level of competence necessary.

        2. Nursing service to clients must be in accordance with the professional standards of practice and code of ethics.

    E. Leadership

        1. **Leadership** is the approach used to provide direction and motivate individuals to implement care standards.

        2. Leadership determines how a person gets along with others to complete a task. The focus is to produce change to meet the goals of the agency.

        3. Leadership can be informal when given to a person by a group of people.

        4. Leadership can be when others follow you.

        5. Leadership can be written directions or developed out of experience.

        6. Leadership skills can be taught through training programs.

F. Types of leadership

1. Autocratic/Authoritarian

a. The autocratic/authoritarian leader tells the employee what must be done, when it should be done, and how it should be done without any regard for the employee's input or feelings.

b. Expectations are clear, as is the division between the leader and employee. Communication is downward, from the leader to the employee.

c. Decisions are made independently by the leader without input from the rest of the group.

d. The leader has power over the group using constant observation to control.

e. The leader may often be bossy, controlling, or abusive, and may use coercion, threats, and punishment to get things done.

f. In this type of leadership, individuals are not motivated and morale is low, resulting in absenteeism and high employee turnover.

g. This leadership style is appropriately used in situations where the leader has the most knowledge and there is little time for group discussion.

2. Democratic/Participative

a. Democratic/participative leadership focuses on staff as well as employers. Communication goes up and down.

b. Democratic leadership is a more effective style. The leader possesses the authority to make the final decision and offers guidance to group members while allowing for their input and participation.

c. This type of leader has the respect of the employees, which is a strength that can be used to motivate the group and to encourage work that is more creative and higher in quality.

d. The democratic/participative leader acts as a facilitator or resource person for the group.

e. The leader allows employees to participate in decision making.

f. The quality of work is high. Job satisfaction is high, but because a consensus is needed for every decision, this type of leadership can slow productivity of a company.

3. Laissez-faire/Delegative/Permissive

a. This style of leadership tries to please everyone and focuses on the employee's feelings while ignoring the task.

b. It leaves the group to make the decisions and offers little or no guidance to the group. Accomplishing tasks may be a problem, but the staff feels good

c. Communication is equal. This style of leadership can be suitable for highly skilled professional workers.

d. Leaders who use this style have a need to be liked.

e. This style works best when the group is highly qualified and when workers are experts in the area.

f. If the leader has confidence in the individuals' skills and level of performance, monitors the group's achievement, and communicates back frequently, its potential improves.

g. Laissez-faire style can lead to a lack of motivation by its members and blame of others for goals not met by leadership.

h. Workers take part in decision making and are given a lot of autonomy to complete the job.

i. This style can lead to lack of focus because staff lacks direction. It can cause the employer's goals to be compromised, ultimately leading to job dissatisfaction.

4. Situational Leadership

a. This is a 21st century leadership style that is highly effective. Leadership styles used are varied and determined by the task or situation at hand.

b. One style does not fit all. Therefore an effective leader can switch between autocratic, democratic, and delegative styles instinctively, based on the employees and the work to be accomplished.

c. Autocratic style is best in an emergency when the instruction is clear (e.g., evacuate the building) or with a new employee just learning a job.

d. Democratic style can be used for day-to-day operations, such as when a team of workers knows the job and the leader knows the problem.

e. Lassez-faire or delegative style is best when all team members are skilled, know their jobs, and can make independent decisions.

5. Transformational leadership

a. Transformational leadership is the dominant style taught today. This style looks at meaning, inspiration, and vision.

b. The leader has a goal and leads by inspiring others to share his/her vision.

c. Leaders spend a lot of time with the employee in free open communication to give a clear sense of the mission.

d. Leaders delegate responsibility among team members, with clear rewards for a job done well.

e. In nursing the goals are clear for the nurse and the leader, and the mission is to help people at the most vulnerable time in their life cycle.

f. This fusion of goals is powerful enough to make the mission a success.

II. Characteristics of a Good Leader

A. Good communication skills

1. Communication occurs between two or more people and involves the exchange of information.

2. Communication uses active listening to be sure a clear message is given.

3. Communication is a major tool the leader uses to accomplish the organization's objectives.

4. Only through communication can the organization's policies, procedures, and rules be developed and delivered.

5. Agreement is not necessary for communication to be successful.

6. Formal channels for communication occur downward as directives from high-level leaders.

7. Upward communication from the subordinates to the top can be informative or reporting.

8. Informal communication is the grapevine; messages are shared from one person to another.

    a. The grapevine is an informal and unsanctioned information network in every organization that helps employees find emotional release for their stress.

    b. The grapevine is unstructured and not under the complete control of management; therefore, information moves through the organization in every direction.

B. Effective personality style

  1. Personality style should be assertive, not aggressive or passive, but flexible in given situations.

  2. Persons with assertive personality styles can express their feelings and ideas and direct others without lowering the other person's self-esteem, placing blame, or being hurtful to others.

  3. Persons with **aggressive personality styles** are demanding and use language that is demeaning and hurtful to others to accomplish things.

  4. Persons with **passive personality styles** cannot express what they are thinking and feeling and avoid unpleasant interactions with others.

C. Personal characteristics of good leaders

  1. Credibility, honesty, knowledge, and clinical expertise are key factors.

  2. The effective leader is able to think critically, be open-minded, and ask questions.

  3. Leaders show initiative and can come up with measures to solve problems.

  4. Leaders are risk takers; they minimize the risks but accept that risks are involved in solving problems.

  5. Leaders are persuasive and can motivate others to achieve goals.

  6. Leaders possess business sense. They are able to be cost effective in delegation and team building, which is very important in the amount of time spent for care.

D. Good leaders are change agents.

  1. A **change agent** is a person who embraces change as a part of life and as a way to continue growth.

  2. Change, however, takes an individual out of his/her comfort zone; as a result, it is natural to resist change.

  3. The individual resists change for a variety of reasons, including threats to his/her position or power.

E. Good leaders are able to resolve conflict.

  1. Conflicts arise from interpersonal or intrapersonal interactions.

  2. Conflicts arise because beliefs, values, goals, or decisions are different.

  3. Stages of conflict

    a. **Disbelief** - first emotional reaction

    b. **Disconnectedness** - confusion and shock at the conflict

    c. **Obsession** - period when conflict consumes the individual, causes disturbed sleep, and enters all conversations.

    d.   Frenzied activity - period of increased energy output to decrease pain, bad feelings, and frustration

    e.   **Balance** or **burnout** - apathy without depression, which places an emotional and physical distance between the individuals.

    f.   **Caution** - the individual reflects on the conflict to gain insight on how to handle future conflicts.

  4. Conflict resolution should be based on principles of integrity and a willingness to negotiate or compromise.

    a.   To **compromise** means working to find a solution to satisfy others as well as oneself.

    b.   To **be accommodating** means setting aside your own goals for the other person's.

    c.   Conflict resolution is achieved by standing up for one's own rights or those of others.

    d.   **Collaboration** is meeting the needs of all involved.

    e.   **Avoidance** is moving away to avoid further conflict.

  5. Anger management

    a.   Anger is an emotion and clue that something is wrong. It can help by stimulating action.

       i.   Anger can be justified.

       ii.   Expressions of anger are found to be aggressive actions.

       iii.   The physiologic response to anger is a rush of adrenalin that causes blood pressure and heart rate to increase.

    b.   Management of anger begins with the acknowledgement of anger. Steps in anger management:

       i.   Remain calm.

       ii.   Avoid confrontation.

       iii.   Manage the feeling through relaxation.

       iv.   Respect the opinions of others.

       v.   Make your own feelings clear.

       vi.   Look to see what happens after the anger.

       vii.   Be patient and listen. Don't take things personally.

III. Managers and the Functions of Management

  A. Management:

    1. Management gets things done through and with people, by directing efforts of individuals towards a common goal.

    2. Healthcare managers organize care to meet client's needs over a period of time. The role is assigned to an individual by the employer.

    3. This begins with an organizational chart indicating how each group relates to the others within the organization.

B. Managers

   1. Managers may not be effective leaders. Both leadership and managerial skills have to be developed to make effective decisions for the entire team. Managerial skills can be learned.

   2. Previously, manager charts were based on a hierarchy.

   3. Today's management charts are horizontal and give more responsibility to middle managers.

C. Functions of management

   1. Management is like a circle or ladder. Objectives are all interdependent and if the objectives are not met, we go back to the beginning. Three important processes in all managerial functions are decision-making, communication, and coordination.

   2. Planning: Determine in advance what should be done and set up the goals, objectives, policies, and procedures of the organization.

   3. Organizing: Determine how the work will be divided in order to complete it by assigning jobs and duties to different groups.

   4. Directing: Influence and motivate individuals to achieve the goals and objectives of the agency. This is accomplished by coaching, teaching, and supervising others to get the job done.

   5. Controlling: Determine whether or not the existing plans are being carried out and how to correct any deviation if things are not proceeding as planned.

   6. Staffing: recruit the number of qualified employees necessary to get the work done.

D. Authority or power

   1. Power or authority is delegated to a position, not a person, and within that authority the manager has a legal or rightful power to act. Without this, the manager cannot carry out his/her function and the organization becomes disorganized and chaotic.

   2. This power/authority allows a manager to ask a subordinate to perform or not to perform a certain task.

   3. Power or authority allows for sanctions if an employee refuses to carry out a manager's direct instructions.

   4. Power or authority includes the right to take disciplinary action by which employment could be terminated.

   5. Power must be used only as a last resort. It is better for the manager to speak about the task or the person's duties and responsibility than simply to exert power.

E. Empowerment

   1. Empowerment allows the individual to feel powerful. Things that advance employee empowerment are having their work valued and being respected, as well as the following:

     a. Right to self-determination, such as how you will do the work that has to be done.

     b. Finding meaning in one's work

     c. Confidence in one's ability to do the work

     d. Having one's ideas listened to and accepted

F. Types of managers

1. Managers have many roles in an organization. Being an effective manager means knowing what style of management to use to handle each situation based on skill and personality.

2. Frontline managers in healthcare

   a. They manage and coordinate the individuals who provide care to the clients. They are the team leaders, charge nurses, and patient unit managers.

   b. The LPN/LVN manager is usually a first-level manager working under the supervision of the professional nurse, physician, or dentist.

3. Middle managers

   a. They supervise the staff, prepare and coordinate the work schedule, and write and implement the agency's policy to maintain quality of care. They are assistant directors of nursing and clinical specialists.

   b. Middle managers rely on the practical nurse to think critically, solve problems, and report.

4. Top level managers

   a. They are nurse executives who supervise a number of teams.

   b. Nursing directors and vice presidents and directors of the nursing services are responsible for all departments and teams.

G. Managing client care

1. Planning

   a. Planning is the first managerial function; it involves deciding in advance what must be done in the future.

   b. Planning sets the objectives to be achieved and how to get them done.

   c. Planning must be cost effective for the efficient use of personnel.

   d. Planning can be short term or long term.

   e. In nursing, the plan is written and set up by the manager. This includes the number of clients assigned, their rooms, the names of the caregivers, break time, and name of relief.

2. Delegation

   a. Delegation is another important part of management and is assigning the individuals able to provide care based on scope of practice.

   b. It means outcomes are achieved by sharing work with others while obeying the rules established by the Nurse Practice Act.

   c. Delegation does not mean loss of accountability. The one who delegates the task retains responsibility for it.

   d. The practical nurse must be careful when delegating tasks to unlicensed personnel and should follow the guidelines developed by the American Nurses Association.

   e   Delegating the task to the right person means knowing the individual's work ability and ensuring the client's safety at all times.

PEARSON

     f.   Delegating the right task means matching the task selected for delegation based on the Nurse Practice Act.

     g.   Delegating under the right situation means ensuring that the setting and the timing promote safety.

     h.   Delegating using the right communication means providing clear, concise, and accurate instructions.

     i.   The delegator listens for feedback to be sure the message is understood.

3. Time management

     a.   Time management is important to all organizations. Poor time management prevents the organization from reaching its full potential.

4. Documentation

     a.   The client chart is a legal document and assists the federal government and insurance companies in determining what care has been given and what should be reimbursed.

     b.   Documentation is also confidential and comes under the Health Insurance Portability and Accountability Act (HIPAA) guidelines.

     c.   Time of documentation is determined by management policies.

     d.   Documentation must be legible, accurate and concise, and signed using the full signature of the healthcare professional.

5. The physician's order

     a.   Physician's order is a type of documentation which can be generated by computer, verbally, over the telephone, or in writing following agency guidelines.

6. Case management

     a.   Case management uses a multidisciplinary approach to plan, document, and deliver cost effective care.

     b.   The emphasis of case management is on predicting outcomes for specific groups of clients using critical pathways, care plans, or concept mapping.

7. Reporting

     a.   Done at change of shift to share pertinent information and client progress. Reporting can be verbal, written, recorded, or by telephone, based on agency policy.

     b.   Fax or e-mail can be used to send large documents, such as laboratory and progress reports.

8. Nursing conference

     a.   A group of nurses meet to work towards reaching a goal or to help to promote a client's ability to cope.

     b.   An incident report records an unexpected event and is documented as defined by the organization. It often involves medical error or injury to employee, child, or visitor.

     c.   An incident report is not part of the medical records. It is filed with the risk manager; it is done to plan corrective measures and prevent recurrence of the event or problem.

9. Evaluation is the follow-up and can be formal or informal.

   a. Informal evaluation is frequently given verbally by simply asking if the task is done.

   b. Formal evaluation is given periodically. It is usually written and gives an analysis of the overall performance of the individual.

Additional Resources Found on MyNursingLab

- Communicating Effectively (video)